HIGH RELIABILITY FOR A HIGHLY UNRELIABLE WORLD

HIGH RELIABILITY FOR A HIGHLY UNRELIABLE WORLD

PREPARING FOR CODE BLUE THROUGH DAILY OPERATIONS IN HEALTHCARE

Daved van Stralen, Spencer L. Byrum, and Bahadir Inozu

ISBN-13: 9781974506378
ISBN-10: 1974506371
Library of Congress Control Number: 2017912712
CreateSpace Independent Publishing Platform
North Charleston, South Carolina

CONTENTS

Praise for High Reliability for a Highly Unreliable World

"The industrial revolution, for over a century and a half, has pushed us hard to reduce, control, regiment, and essentially dehumanize human systems in order to eliminate accidents. But the irritating reality is that we humans are inherently incapable of individual perpetual perfection, no matter how much regimentation we're forced to use. That reality continues to frustrate our best efforts to be completely safe in high risk endeavors such as naval operations, nuclear power generation, and the sector of the building trades that involve highly complex structures – as well as the airline industry. Even when great progress has been made in adapting imperfect human behavior to the broadened reliability of teams, aviation-spawned programs such as "Crew Resource Management" (or CRM training and discipline) are insufficient by themselves to get to zero accidents and near misses.

The greatest promise, however, for guiding the human nature of human systems into accident-free enterprises comes from understanding what happens when collections of humans engaged in the same common goal achieve the status of being very – or highly –reliable. The resultant descriptor, High Reliability, has been increasingly used as a battle cry in medicine in particular as a way of explaining how certain companies and industries (such as the airlines) managed to reduce accident and incidents on a replicable basis. The problem with the concept of a High Reliability Organization is not the need or desire for one, but the widespread lack of understanding of what actually constitutes such a beast. How to conceive of High Reliability, how to understand it, and how to apply it and sustain it as a way of organizational life is the subject of this very comprehensive and very needed work by Spence Byrum, Daved van Stralen, and Bahadir Inozu.

In my view, the highest value and the basic thrust of *High Reliability for a Highly Unreliable World* is that no one can effectively nursemaid an organization to true High Reliability status without a full and detailed understanding of the HRO as a living, breathing, constantly contradictory and constantly challenging framework of principals, tactics, and strategies all designed to get the best out of we imperfect humans. In other words, and somewhat predictably, a Highly Reliable Organization is just as messy and convoluted as normal human interactions. The difference is that HRO's work to create real safety, while the traditional methods don't.

The extent to which an HRO is at odds with tradition and culture and even human nature itself is also a measure of how much this work - and its deep dive into the structural anatomy of HRO's - is needed. Certainly nowhere is that more true than in healthcare, where 440-thousand patients a year lose their lives unnecessarily through medical mistakes.

No, this is not a beach read that will keep you up through the night. It WILL, however, give you a backdoor master's degree into the why and how of successful HRO's, and most importantly - whether for the individual practitioner or an entire organization - this outstanding and comprehensive book allows the readers to build a rock-solid foundations beneath the changes which are the pathway to HRO status.

And in that, you might say, this book in itself is highly reliable, as well as a must-own and must-read for anyone in a position of responsibility who is serious and honest about espousing the transformation from the traditional to the highly reliable."

-**John J. Nance**, JD, Author of: Why Hospitals Should Fly, American College of Healthcare Executives (ACHE) 2008 Book of the Year

"The health care industry has laudably embraced the principles that characterize high reliability organizations in its ongoing efforts to provide better care to every patient and prevent harm in each case. To that end, healthcare high reliability has focused on leadership, processes, and metrics, all vital to build and sustain a highly reliable organization. However, in its quest to transform health organizations to high reliability, the methodology to do so has often not focused on the complex, contextual or concomitant aspects of healthcare delivery. Dr. Van Stralen's book takes the reader on a high reliability journey designed for healthcare delivery environments on the system, team, and personal levels of involvement. His work provides context to high reliability through stories and examples common to high-risk environments but unique to health systems and patient care. Without deviating from established HRO principles, Dr. Van Stralen introduces health care organizations and its workers to theories and tools not generally associated with patient care delivery but that encourage introspective analysis of beliefs, behavior, and work processes and importantly, a simultaneous bottom-up, top-down acceptance and adoption of a sustainable, contextually relevant highly reliable health organization."

-**Patricia E Sokol**, RN, JD,

George W Merck Family Fellow, Institute for Healthcare Improvement 2010-2011

"Much is available about strategy and tactics for avoiding waste, unnecessary variation, defects, hazard, and catastrophe in health care. However, very little demonstrated success or validated outcomes are from within the health care delivery industry, particularly when the relatively controlled environment of inpatient anesthesia is excluded. Healthcare delivery in the community is an extraordinarily complex, uncertain, and high risk environment, and we haven't yet achieved any reasonable degree of safety, value, service or reliability.

High Reliability in a Highly Unreliable World provides a modern-day Rosetta stone for translating other industries' success in quality, safety and reliability to health care. It draws heavily from contributors' expertise in human performance in aviation, defense, law enforcement and maritime industries, to give breadth, depth and practical wisdom not yet available within health care. Much value, concept, context and content rests in the many stories and sidebars they provide.

This work is dense–steeped in theory as much or more as in practice. As such, it is not a stand-alone handbook for implementation. References to complexity science, anthropology, physiology, neuroscience, epistemology, logic and general philosophy will capture the interest of scholars and content experts; beginners and novices will want this book close at hand as a reference to frame future practice."

-Roger W. Bush, MD, MACP, SFHM,

Director, American Board of Internal Medicine Commissioner, The Joint Commission

Director, American Board of Medical Specialties, Multispecialty Portfolio Program

"The book's authors seek to explain what High Reliability Organizing (HRO) is, how it developed, what it does, and how it works. Their thesis, held by many including this reviewer, is that HRO can have a significant positive impact on the safety and reliability of industries overall and specifically healthcare. Building their case on a strong historical theoretical foundation of disciplined research, they share extensive evidence with examples and application from specific industries. Throughout, they are attentive in the translation of that learning across industries and roles. An emphasis is also placed on what doesn't work; what are the mental models and defensive routines that get in the way. Providing illumination throughout the book are narratives and learning from their own wide-ranging personal experiences and learning in environments on an HRO journey.

What emerges from this book's pages is extraordinary rich content, presented with discipline and including illustration, citation, and narratives. Stimulated, in this reader's mind, were lots of questions, some confusion, and an occasional feeling of being overwhelmed. As a student of HRO for over 15 years, I expected my "training wheels" would have prepared me for a relatively smooth read of this text. Instead, I encountered a rush of concepts foreign to me. I was wishing I had an author, co-reader, or even a class, who was also reading this book so that

I could run this new content by them. In the process, the book helped me realize that while I knew "a little bit of this and a little bit of that" related to HRO, this text was systematically taking me far into the depths of understanding and applying HRO. Throughout the reading, and re-reading, the authors' case for the application of HRO in healthcare was built stronger and stronger.

Noteworthy also are the chapters on leadership and culture. While content in these areas is well known to this reviewer, I was struck over and over with the number of new/reinforced concepts and citations. Since reading it, the phrase "the quality of leadership is reflected in their subordinates" stays top of mind with this leader/reviewer.

High Reliability for a Highly Unreliable World is an important content-rich reference publication for those seeking to unleash the power of HRO to their industries and specifically to healthcare. Yes, it is a difficult, time-consuming read of high value optimized for the reader when matched with an appropriate learning community (teacher, leader classroom, study group, book club, leadership academy, or the like) and with effective sustained execution and continuous improvement."

-**Jim Conway**, Trustee Lahey Health, Chair Board Quality of Care Committee Trustee Winchester Hospital
    Adjunct Faculty Harvard TH Chan School of Public Health (retired)

"*High Reliability for a Highly Unreliable World* is the long awaited primer on High Reliability Organizing (HRO) for the medical care professional that presents a definitive set of ideas and tools for managing the complex decision processes in the medical care environment. Interpreting and expanding upon the five HRO Principles from the previous definitive work of Weick/Sutcliffe in the three editions of *Managing the Unexpected*, this book further defines the five Attitudes and six specific Values that can be developed and are found in most HROs to facilitate more efficient and effective daily operations while training the entire medical care organization to anticipate and perform well in uncertain situations.

    As both the Joint Commission and the Department of Defense continue to emphasize and encourage expanded use of HRO principles in health care, this book fills the void with specific recommendations, techniques, and procedures along the journey of higher reliability and enhanced patient safety."

In Memory of
Linda Anne Aldridge
1931-2017
Educator, Storyteller

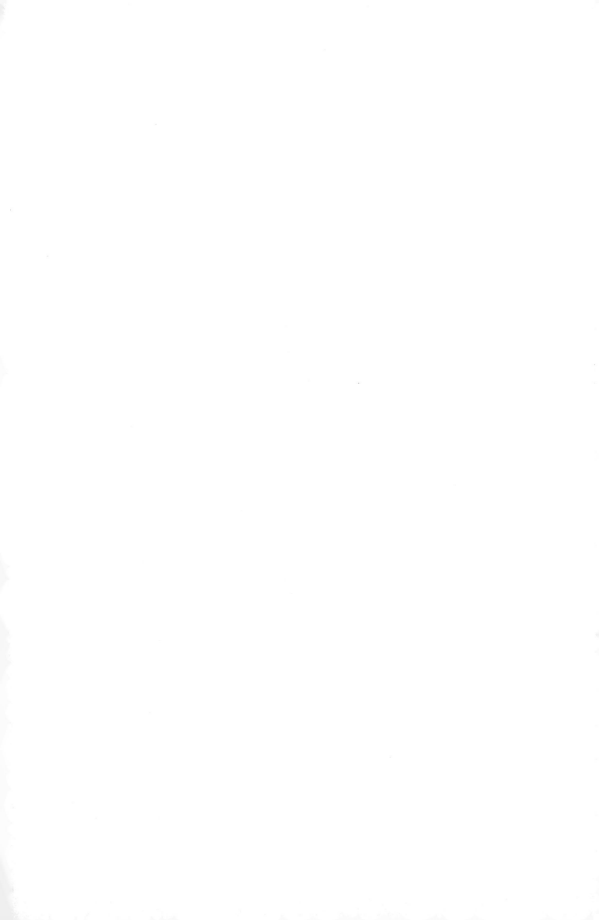

FOREWORD

E ven though the organizational form referred to as a High Reliability Organization has been discussed for a relatively short period of time, the basic idea has already been elaborated with credibility and breadth. Those elaborations are on full display in this encyclopedic volume. That does not mean that this is the 'official' statement of HRO, although it certainly supplants a host of other less thoughtful efforts that basically do little more than market the phrase and the image.

The present authors live by a 72-hour rule: "what I teach today must explain yesterday or be used tomorrow." The density of ideas presented in this book might seem to preclude explaining either yesterday's simplified determinacy or tomorrow's indeterminacy. But that's not necessarily the case. True, the variety of literatures and ideas and concepts and applications that are discussed is stunning. But so are the connections back to a much smaller set of foundations of High Reliability Organizing. Thus, the variety in this volume provides multiple points of entry into a finite set of principles, attitudes, and values that cohere around the management of complex surprises.

What is especially distinctive about this synthesis of High Reliability organizational forms, is that it is the product of deep practical experience in emergency medical services and critical care medicine informed by and infused into deep theoretical experience with research on neuroscience, physics, biology, sociology, social psychology, and organizational studies. There is respectful, informed use of all of these domains. Throughout there is an ongoing sensitivity to the fact that "If it happened once, it can happen again; if it happens again, it can happen worse." And throughout, there is also an insistence that decision makers should keep asking themselves, is this "too soon" or "too late," and "too much" or "too little."

As the argument moves from the general nature of reliable functioning under adverse conditions to a more specific focus on healthcare, the health examples take on a richer meaning. If the reader had started at the end of the book with the examples and then read toward the beginning, seasoned health workers might say "sure: happens all the time. So what?" Read from front to back, however, those "same" examples will be harder to dismiss, more filled with meaning, and now be seen as more powerful moments of leverage to make systems more reliable.

Sustained reliable functioning in an uncertain world is neither as obvious nor as intuitive as people often presume. It is tempting to simplify pathways to reliable functioning, tempting but misleading. The beauty of this volume is that pathways to more reliable functioning are made explicit even if, at times, that explicitness feels daunting. A close reading coupled with sustained, alert implementation, will produce the kind of informed awareness verbalized by a Los Angeles firefighter who said, "I may not know what is happening, but I know what to do."

Karl E. Weick
Rensis Likert Distinguished University Professor of
Organizational Behavior and Psychology, Emeritus
Stephen M. Ross School of Business at the
University of Michigan

Preface

W hen we said we were writing this book, friends, colleagues, and reviewers invariably asked, "Who is your intended audience?" They asked
this because we teach in diverse fields but also from the belief that
authors should write for a specific group. Sean McKay gave us the answer we now
use: "I wrote it for you." Sean is a friend and colleague who also draws on diverse
disciplines to attain better performance in diverse fields. Sean will coauthor an
adaptation of this text for public safety, "high-angle" rescue, and special-opera-
tions forces. High-angle rescue refers to rescue using a rope harness with angle of
terrain greater than 65° requiring the rope to carry the full weight of the rescuer.

While we use healthcare examples throughout the book, we present the concepts independently of medicine or healthcare. Those who are not in the healthcare field can readily access the concepts, and our healthcare examples may help
these readers better understand a discipline they will inevitably encounter.

Our concern in writing to a particular audience is that doing so may influence us to write for what that audience wants (or what we think they want). To be
accepted by that audience, we may limit any evidence that disconfirms that audience's strongly held beliefs. We may categorize information to fit their sincerely
cherished preconceptions. We would write to be successful by being accepted
by our selected audience. We would have written what the Harvard psychology
professor Ellen Langer describes as "mindlessness." Not only would we not serve
our audience, but we also would have reinforced walls between our audience and
"others."

We wrote this particular book based on the principles of the High Reliability
Organization (HRO) and the principles of the approach we have collectively
used for over fifty years. Our guiding rule was to go to the originating science or
discipline for any model, concept, or principle, then build up from there. In that

way, we learned that some popular ideas are quite weak; they are not well supported by the originating science.

The work you are currently reading is for those who want an explanation of HRO—how it developed, what it does, and how it works. You want your knowledge as pure as possible and with a minimum amount of bias from the interpreter or author. You want to know, "How will this help me?"

You are the one we wrote this book for.

Some industries developed High Reliability through their experience from devastating failures, while others are in the process of developing High Reliability by using those lessons they've learned from other industries. Healthcare professionals have several beliefs that often impede the effective adoption of High Reliability methods:

(1) The complexity of disease processes causes most unwanted or unexpected outcomes, thus diminishing the effect of individual initiative.
(2) Sound science (and the use of scientific principles) protects us from errors and mistakes by reserving decisions for those with the proper body of knowledge.
(3) Successful High Reliability processes should be accepted selectively, conditionally, and free of any originating context.
(4) The inherent dangers in healthcare are unique: they depreciate HRO traits that disconfirm strongly held principles.

Reliability, safety, and High Reliability Organizing draw on many disciplines. Bringing concepts from disparate disciplines to a new discipline in a haphazard or incoherent manner risks the creation of "silos." People pick and choose what makes sense to them or what is easiest to incorporate without regard to how others use the same knowledge. The idiosyncratic adaptation of knowledge creates barriers to communication. For example, the well-developed concept of culture in anthropology or sociology becomes, in healthcare, "culture change" after acceptance of a singular, new program. Healthcare seems to routinely adopt the use of new words, phrases, or clichés; use outside stories and "narratives" to teach new concepts but without the original purpose and context; or initiate the context-free adoption of new processes.

Blocked or impeded horizontal communication also creates silos between vertically integrated groups such as disciplines, specialties, departments, hospital units, programs, etc. Silos will also develop when a supervisor requires subordinates to channel all communications to outside groups through the supervisor.

The isolation from silos creates barriers and contributes to patient harm and lowers quality of care.

High Reliability concepts are rich and enriching but can easily be manipulated to reinforce conventional approaches and prevent organizational change. Translations of High Reliability disciplines can become layered and misleading the further they are from the original science or industry. There is also the risk conforming to the purposes or personal views of the authors of such books.

In this book, we started with what worked for those who taught us, those whom we taught, and ourselves. We then searched the published material from the originating sciences, disciplines, and/or individual research scientists or academicians. We followed the principle, building on existing work to make it applicable and practical, and we kept our eye on comprehensibility for the High Reliability novice. In our experience, both novices and veterans can operate in an HRO fashion. If the novice cannot understand something, then it is unlikely an element of HRO.

Healthcare must, as all industries must, search for the best program. Such programs are often developed in industries that share a threat but experience it differently or uniquely. William Harvey, the English physician who first described the systemic circulatory system and the heart as its pump, believed that "the best fertilizer for medicine is the progress of other and quite different sciences" (in Kevles 1992).

This book breaks through the walls of silos.

Those readers who work in healthcare may already be aware that the Joint Commission views High Reliability Organizing as the gold standard in healthcare. For those outside of healthcare, the Joint Commission accredits and certifies healthcare organizations and services at a national level and provides education and similar services internationally. Through the Joint Commission Center for Transforming Healthcare, the commission advocates for HRO use in healthcare facilities. (See http://www.centerfortransforminghealthcare.org/hro_portal_main.aspx.)

The authors of this book are not associated with the Joint Commission. We have written this material from our personal experience, with the point of view of helping like-minded people come to HRO. HRO is a process for better operations when faced with an adverse or hostile environment. In our experience, HRO is not a program that an executive, administrator, or supervisor can implement and then walk away from. All members of the organization change, and it does not take long for them to notice and appreciate the change.

The Science of the Practitioner

Business schools study High Reliability Organizing within the field of organizational behavior; contributing sciences include social psychology and cognitive psychology, among others. In our pursuit to better understand HRO, we have made use of the sciences, disciplines, and research in decision-making, neuroscience, psychology, social psychology, mathematics, physics, physiology, and numerous other fields.

Daved van Stralen's use of this approach in medical school (1980–84) elicited much criticism; he was told that he was clearly wrong and that the people who had taught him were also wrong, whether mountaineers, fire service, or military veterans. This started his search to identify the science that *would* support combat veterans, firefighters, ambulance workers, law enforcement, nurses, and physicians. These are the people who have to be pragmatic to make an effective decision because of the limited time available and their limited knowledge of events. Counterintuitively, all these groups share the same way of thinking. This book brings together the science to support those who naturally work in a High Reliability manner and those who taught us. It contains the information we use to support those who are starting out in this arena.

Each chapter has some redundancy. Developing the science of each topic and chapter led to a longer book than we anticipated. To remedy that, we included in each chapter necessary information from supporting and complementary chapters. Readers can start by reading the particular chapter of their interest and find descriptions of most of the new concepts they encounter in the chapter.

At times, we wrote the same thing from different points of view; some will view this as a useful strength, while others will find it overly redundant. Teaching in this manner comes from years of teaching HRO. People learn HRO within the context of their life or work experiences. Presenting a view that is coherent with a person's life experiences keeps the material from becoming overly complex. Another benefit is that the person who understands it first can soon help others appreciate HRO.

Here are three vignettes in which Daved van Stralen describes this principle.

(1). *Decision-making:* Teaching a particular technique for decision-making to a group of respiratory care practitioners (RCPs) frustrated me. The RCPs kept placing the technique into the approach they use for written standing orders. (These are orders the physician writes for a particular patient and situation; the RCP can then carry out the order when the triggering event occurs.) Frustrated, I looked over at Craig Davenport, a former military police officer and Vietnam veteran. "Craig," I asked, how would you have done this in Vietnam?" He answered, "Well, when we were setting up a .50 caliber machine-gun nest, we would…" The first RCP asked, "You set up a machine-gun nest? That must have been the safest place to be." Craig answered, "No—you were the one the enemy wanted to shoot first." Then Craig explained how the decision-making technique I was teaching would be used in an operational combat situation and how he could use it to manage a child on a ventilator. That opened the whole group of RCPs to using decision-making as we present in this book; Craig became the conduit for teaching.

(2). *Criticism and management*: One manager criticized the "wrong" decisions his team made. He worked with me one morning, and I waited until he started in with his criticisms. I asked him what he did for a hobby "Dirt-bike riding in the desert." He would ride off-road exploring various routes. I asked if he had ever driven up a box canyon, a canyon with an inlet but ends in vertical walls, blocking passage to another area compared to canyons with a sloping terminus that permit continued exploration. The rider would need to return over ground just covered. "Yes," he answered. "Why?" That is, why decide to start up a canyon if it is a "dead-end?" He silently understood we do not know it is a box canyon until you reach the end, that we do not know it is a bad decision until it fails. He never again criticized a decision that made people go back down a path they'd just covered.

(3). *HRO*: I sometimes discuss HRO as being similar to dating. There are rules and guidelines to follow; some parents even develop policies. But in the end, we date and interact and learn about the other person. Then we think about long-term relationships. We may break up. Was the dating a failure? Did we date too long? Had we left sooner, would our lives have been better? Or, had we dated longer, would we have figured out how to overcome the errors and difficulties of two independent beings living within the same event?

We recommend reading the first three chapters before you go shopping for chapters that interest you. Those three lay out our philosophy and some basic thinking rules: our "logic of operations" for HRO. The third chapter appears philosophical, but our experienced colleagues tell us that this is what differentiates HRO from other programs, explains how HRO works, and shows the internal validity of HRO (that is, why HRO makes sense to those who have naturally operated this way). This chapter makes the "HRO mind-set" accessible. Our fourth chapter clarifies how we see the environment in which the HRO operates.

More Books on the Way

"I know this is what Dr. van Stralen taught you, but this is how we really do it." This simple sentence will destroy thousands of dollars of education and training. Jim Holbrook, professor of EMS at Crafton Hills College, told van Stralen, "Simple. Tell your students how it will help them." So, van Stralen would only teach students what would immediately help or what would explain their recent experience. Fairly soon the students would teach themselves to fill the gaps in what van Stralen taught. The pool of *what* information to provide has grown and the style developed into his teaching maxim, "What is learned today must explain yesterday or be used tomorrow."

Students returned to tell van Stralen how this material helped them, being specific to what he taught and when they learned it. This could be twenty-four hours to thirty years later. Once something worked, van Stralen studied it and continued sharing the knowledge.

In this book, when the science is imperfect or lacking, we rely on experience: this is informed experience, validated with scientific principles, and it comes from one of us or the person who has lived it. Just as we cannot use a cliché when lives are at risk, we cannot use second-hand information.

This book grew out of those two rules for teaching: (1) it must help the student and (2) be solidly grounded in experience or science. We originally started out writing two books from those two rules. A "handbook for HRO implementation" was to be a practical guide that would enable you to start performing as a High Reliability Organization immediately. A "primer of HRO" would have explained in straightforward, clear text the underlying principles of HRO.

Laying a solid scientific foundation for the ideas in the two books led to this larger text, now the storehouse of knowledge and reference for the smaller, more accessible books. We have, to the best of our ability, kept the ideas in this text straightforward, coherent, and well developed. After publication of this book, we will immediately start on our original two books.

This book is also the sourcebook for our book series *Practical High Reliability*. Other books include a public safety and special operations version with Sean McKay (www.ElementRescue.com); a personal version for life and work with Thomas A. Mercer, RAdm, USN (retired); a version for educators for kindergarten through twelfth grade with Dale Marsden, superintendent, San Bernardino City Unified School District; and a business enterprise book.

Why This Book?

The search to improve reliability and safety in healthcare, as in other organizations, has turned to industries with better-than-expected safety records and adoption of scientifically developed models. When we take these approaches from their original context, we lose vital information and disrupt reliable routines. We inadvertently create inaccurate models. *Inaccurate models in an adverse environment can kill.*

One approach to improve reliability and safety is HRO, which was codified from US Navy aircraft carriers, naval flight operations, nuclear power plants, and electric power grids. Some observers can readily extract visible characteristics but may easily miss subtle and nuanced interaction between people and with the environment. Some characteristics are not visible, such as the moment of realization that things have just gone terribly wrong. What does the person think? What is the first action to take?

As attractive as HRO is, many of its principles and characteristics are counterintuitive. An accurate description of HRO operations is counterintuitive, since it is full of paradoxes and contradictory propositions or beliefs. We must use initiative but conform, improvise but not freelance, decide with imperfect information, use the cognitive and affective domains, and so on. (We will discuss these domains in later chapters; for now, "affect" describes values and how we experience feelings or emotions, while cognition describes the mental processes we use to acquire knowledge and to understand what is around us.) Using HRO is to accept the decisions of people of lower rank and less experience. Paradoxes and the counterintuitive nature of HRO are a few of the obstructions to its acceptance.

High Reliability Organizing developed as a means to engage confusing, threatening situations with minimal technology, often by teams of less experienced people led by people with greater experience. Various industries have begun adapting HRO in more diverse environments such as chemical processing, petroleum refining, and education for use by a larger array of organizations. Understanding the environment and the limits of cognitive function in these situations will provide a better grasp of what HRO can accomplish.

The elegance of HRO and its principles has expanded its use to numerous and diverse industries. This comes at the risk of simplification, loss of vital characteristics, and shifting to an inaccurate model. Connecting to HRO's roots and creating a foundation from the primary sciences can reinforce accuracy in HRO models, thus facilitating translation to those who have not experienced the live-or-die circumstance from which HRO emerged.

This book explores the environment of HRO and the inevitability of crises. Energy transforms and dissipates, communication corrupts information, uncontrolled behaviors confound our need for control, and threat responses hijack our ability to reason. These factors create the unpredictability of events and our responses. HRO describes various methods to bring control toward a desired end-state.

This book explores the mental processes of HRO and effective responses in adversity. Scientific rationality is bounded by the HRO environment. Planning, leadership, "sensemaking" ("Sensemaking" means to give meaning to the environment), and decision-making models presume the effective use of our cognitive capabilities which is made difficult when the environment appears unstructured, random, and disordered. Yet stress impairs cognitive function, and threats distort reasoning—a critical defect addressed in this book. The crisis that disrupts our rules for operations and thinking requires practical rationality and a different logic of operations, something HRO practitioners have become adept at using. These different methods and rationality to modulate threat responses are new in this book and fundamental to making HRO operational.

High Reliability Is Not a Business Model

Some executives and business leaders want to see a business model before they adopt HRO. HRO must directly and concretely support and benefit the business. They must see clear causality between HRO elements and measurable improvement in their business performance.

Some executives and business leaders want HRO to guarantee safety. But High Reliability Organizations originally developed to operate in environments where harm can come internally from operations or from the business situation itself. HRO in the native state does not distinguish safety from business operations. An injured member reduces the performance of the team; therefore HRO methods embed safety into operations.

Today's leaders want to see quantifiable interventions and results with clear, predictable causality to produce benefits to the organization. It is instructive to look to the actions the US Navy has taken. In 1954 the navy lost 536 people, and 776 aircraft were destroyed in flight accidents. The navy did not isolate safety as a separate entity: safety was an important means to maintain operations that was integral to the function of the navy. Rather than search for a proven intervention, the navy studied itself, identified weaknesses, corrected them, then searched for more weaknesses. One seldom-discussed effect on accident reduction was the change in assignment of aviators and the selection of command leaders, from those with connections to those with the most qualifications. The actions and approach to problem-solving the US Navy took that created safer flying conditions and strengthened operations laid the groundwork for HRO (Heggie 2012; Dunn 2017).

This book does not provide solutions and does not guarantee success. This book describes how to think and operate when the rules around you have changed and the internal logic of the system has been lost. HRO is a way of thinking and a way of organizing.

In some sense, Daved van Stralen's search began when, as a paramedic, he asked an emergency medicine resident physician how to straighten a fractured femur when the victim was trapped in a sports car and extrication equipment was not available. She answered, "That would make it easier for you, not for the patient. Do it without straightening the leg." She closed with: "A little knowledge is a dangerous thing." Then she walked away.

She was right, of course. A little knowledge *is* dangerous. Alexander Pope warned us of that. He wrote, "A little learning is a dangerous thing; drink deep, or taste not the Pierian spring: there shallow draughts intoxicate the brain, and drinking largely sobers us again." The Pierian spring, in Greek mythology, provides knowledge and inspiration. We hope this text gives you knowledge and inspiration.

Daved van Stralen
Spencer L. Byrum
Bahadir Inozu

June 2017
Los Angeles

DEDICATION

From Daved: To my wife, Febra Johnson, for understanding the amount of work and listening that were required as I refined ideas for this book. To my children, Kara and Ryan, for their sacrifice as I worked on these ideas, and to my mother, Linda Aldridge, who challenged me during childhood to discover something no one else knows. To my students and colleagues, who told me how this material helped them. And to Karl Weick, who acted as an ecologist for my wanderings in the environments of VUCA-T.

From Spencer: Many terrific people have contributed significantly to the work that I have incorporated in this book. Captain Tom Morgan, USCG (ret.), was the person who made my flying career possible. My business partner, Lee Flowers, has provided remarkable support and a framework for HRO in a host of different applications for over a decade and a half, and Captain Brian Kelley, USCG (ret.), has been a roommate, best man, friend, and confidant as my passion for HRO has grown over the years. Charles Wurtzburger, John Nance, and Alan Reider became mentors, friends, and role models for me as my interest in applying HRO in other disciplines grew. Finally, my coauthors, Daved and Baha, have created the desire to write a comprehensive synopsis of what we believe to be best practices a reality.

Most importantly, I need to thank my family for all they've done to support my dreams. My career has caused me to be away from home a great deal, yet my sons, Zach and Blake, can tell you more about High Reliability than many far older and more experienced people. My wife, LeAnn, has provided untiring support for me, my career, and my passion to share this information with others. None of this would have been possible without her. High Reliability operations cannot be sustained without a team, and I thank God every day for the team that is my family and my friends.

From Bahadir: To my loving parents, Ayşe Berruh and Mehmet Oğuz İnözü.

To our contributor, Michael "Mike" A. Johns (1951-2017), Assistant US Attorney, former wildland firefighter, for integrity and his dedication to educate wildland firefighters in decision making and critical thinking as a science.

Acknowledgments

*F*rom *Daved van Stralen*: Don Connors, my high school English teacher, taught me to use literature to understand science and to better understand life; Jules Crane, my community college zoology professor, taught me to find the basic principles that drive biology; Bill Corr, my fire captain, taught me to look for the underlying construction of anything, even life, and shared his concept of success: a thirty-year firefighter is successful because he has provided shelter and food for his family; and Ron Stewart, my paramedic instructor, taught me to describe my situation and patient accurately and treat from physiology in our environment. But most of all, Dr. Stewart and Capt. Corr encouraged me to apply to medical school and modeled their view that operators on the line are our most valuable assets, and we must support them.

An approach of this size can only come from shared experiences and mutual learning. These are the people who spent hours in discussion, trial, revision, and, most important, sparring with me to develop an approach to high-risk operations that would be practical for the novice and useful in the worst of situations: Jim Holbrook, Racquel Calderon, Gary Provansal, Dan Kleinman, Susie Moss, Sean McKay, Chris Hart, Jim Denney, Joe Martin, Bert Slagmolen, Marc Flitter, Ron Perkin, and John Mace. Sparring was our most vital interaction; as Joe Martin said, "You don't want your friends to go into a fight without them knowing their weaknesses and without making them stronger." George Williams's comprehensive review and critique of several chapters greatly improved the presentation of our ideas. When I almost joined a private practice pediatric group, Jim Conway kept me engaged with reliability and safety studies for healthcare, which led to this book.

Tom Mercer, skipper of the USS *Carl Vinson*, provided two decades of friendship and counsel for practical HRO, connecting actions and attitudes with goals and objectives. Most significantly, Tom made HRO visible as effective and safe operations and started things moving with his invitation to the "Berkeley academics." Karlene Roberts identified the approach Ron Perkin and I had developed to be a functional HRO. Karl Weick's two decades of friendship and intellectual challenge have enriched both my life and this book. One early description of ecology is that the Indians know where the deer are; the ecologist knows why they are there. Karl Weick, to us, is the ecologist. He studies our work closely enough to be an ecologist but without becoming one of us. And we are the richer for it.

I thank Kara and Ryan van Stralen, my daughter and son, for "growing up HRO" and showing to me that HRO works in life. I thank my wife, Febra Johnson, for living an HRO lifestyle, traveling and recovering, and for tolerating countless digressions as I worked out concepts—how do I know what I think unless I say what I think?

A special thank you to the staff of Children's Subacute Center, Community Hospital of San Bernardino, who took these principles to enhance the lives of profoundly disabled, technology-dependent children. Daily, they reach their goal of a smiling child.

Most of all, I must acknowledge the men and women I have worked with who taught me this approach and those who came to me from twenty-four hours to thirty years later to tell me how they had used this knowledge. They described the specific circumstances in which they learned the knowledge and the specific manner in which they used it. Because they told me how it worked to help them, I better understand this approach called HRO. This book is for them.

From Spence Byrum: My parents, H. S. (Biff) and Muriel Byrum, instilled in me a sense of confidence that there was nothing I could not do. That's the good news. The bad news came when I discovered that many things, particularly flying in the Coast Guard and working in the healthcare environment, involved an element of risk that required an increased level of personal discipline and High Reliability that took years to refine. Now back to the good news: those lessons have already been learned, and this book demonstrates that there is absolutely no reason that healthcare practitioners need to make similar mistakes; nor does the timeframe for incorporating HRO into daily operations need to take nearly as long.

Visionary physicians such as Drs. Ed McCabe, Paul Abson, Jerre Freeman, Steve Clark, Tom Green, and John Crockarell helped me understand the pivotal role of physician leadership in implementing and sustaining meaningful change. Healthcare administrative leaders Diane Ridgeway, Ruth Westcott, Cam Welton, Jan Meyers, Joyce Carver, Ann Latstetter, Kathy Wilson, and many others had the courage and vision to know how important it was to bring these concepts to care providers. Finally, I would like to thank my coauthors for making me want to write a comprehensive synopsis of what we believe to be best practices.

From Bahadir Inozu: I would like to thank Seza Gulec (MD, FACS), professor of surgery and nuclear medicine at Florida International University's Herbert Wertheim College of Medicine, and my business partner, Curtis Doucette, for their support and guidance. I would also like to thank all the people who have helped me to understand the science of reliability and to improve reliability and safety at different platforms, from ships to hospitals, including professors Anastassios N. Perakis and Steve Pollock at the University of Michigan.

We would like to thank our reviewers: Karl Weick, Jim Conway, Roger Bush, George Williams, Pattie Sokol, Dana Lagunas, Tom Mercer, Sean McKay, Racquel Calderon, Jim Holbrook, Jay Shiver, Sanem Ozdural, and Bruce Spurlock.

CHAPTER 1

WHAT IS HIGH RELIABILITY ORGANIZING?

A practical definition of High Reliability Organization (HRO) has been elusive. The name itself is somewhat divisive, as if an organization strives for low reliability. It is well accepted that an HRO operates in an environment of risk factors and complexity where we would expect severe accidents, if not catastrophic failure. After that, the definition becomes less explicit: the HRO does not experience such events, avoids these events, or has no errors. Left unanswered, is "Why would an organization enter such an environment?"

The types of organizations initially described as HRO either entered these environments purposefully, such as the military or wildland fire, or they managed dangerous, large-scale technologies, such as nuclear power, the electric grid for power distribution, and air traffic control. These primal HROs worked in or were proximal to live-or-die situations. Uniquely, these organizations adapted the traits for high-risk situations to use in their routine operations. This resulted in a reduction of the number and severity of these negative events in normal times.

HRO, and its explicit definition, matters because any individual or organization will encounter a situation that does not have clear structure. This may be due to the novelty of the situation to the individual or organization, imperfect information about the situation, or turbulent events surrounding the situation. It does not matter of the degree, only that the individual or organization cannot detect the structure.

We want to understand HRO and to do that we must find a practical definition. It is often easiest to understand the principles and dynamics of HRO when viewed as effective means to operate when the environment has suddenly lost its structure. This loss of structure, unfortunately, occurs suddenly as if we had crossed a threshold into its bleakness. The principles of HRO appear counterintuitive before crossing the threshold but are lifesaving after we have crossed it.

First, let us state that there are no low reliability organizations. That does not mean to say there's no such thing as *lower* reliability, only that *low* reliability is not a target, though it could be a consequence of organizational design, operations, or leadership. Lower reliability stands in contrast to the High Reliability we strive for. HROs have certain characteristics, these are natural characteristics every organization possesses and of which the HRO makes full and effective use. This makes implementation of HRO a little smoother because we are enhancing what we already have, but it makes it more difficult for those who want to measure these attributes. Measuring HRO attributes is to make arbitrary choices to value one attribute over another when they interact and build on each other. It also requires dividing attributes along a spectrum, like measuring the individual heights in the group of people *after* defining what we mean by "tall."

Second, the HRO has shared goals of avoiding serious operational failures and maintaining short-term efficiency (La Porte and Consolini, 1991). The challenge of this, operationally, is (1) to avoid major failures in the management of complex, demanding technologies and (2) maintain the capacity necessary for sudden and unexpected, very high peak demands (La Porte and Consolini, 1991).

Third, let us state our belief that HRO is a response to the local environment rather than adherence to a prescribed set of beliefs. HRO is an interaction between cognitive processes and "affective" processes. HRO is pragmatic and adaptive rather than normative, that is, meeting a standard of correct structure and actions. More of our beliefs will come out as you read this book but the most significant is that HRO is enacted by individuals working together.

Fourth, we do not have an explicit definition of an HRO but we will describe what we have found useful and effective in moving individuals, teams, and organizations toward HRO. We would define HRO as an organization prepared to unexpectedly cross a threshold into an environment without structure. While this occurs to all organizations, the HRO has the five principles identified by Weick and Sutcliffe in 2001 and will therefore more likely achieve a better end-state.

You are the most qualified person in your organization during a crisis. This mantle will fall on you at some time when an unexpected High Reliability situation (HRS) arises. Others may be more experienced, but if they are not available, they are not qualified to act. In a High Reliability Organization (HRO), every member is the most qualified person for the job he or she is currently doing. In an HRO, each person is supported to be the most qualified. What makes an HRO different is the support of scientific processes so that people may work in uncertain and ambiguous situations in which time becomes compressed.

Failure *is* an option.

Something startles us and catches our attention. We see a discrepancy, and maybe our work is disrupted. Whatever the reason, something has aroused our attention, and we take notice.

Arousal describes our sudden increase in alertness. In our aroused state, we may simply observe the situation, studying it to learn more about it. Whatever aroused us, however, may also initiate a fear reaction, which causes us to back away or act to protect ourselves. We may engage the situation by interacting with it to learn more about it or to control it. In the worst case, whether we remove ourselves from the situation or move forward and engage it, we may become disoriented because the system has lost its recognizable structure and a sudden, serious threat now confronts us.

How we respond to this arousal, whether it is from a minor situation or full loss of organizational structure, determines our level of reliability. When we take arousal as a challenge for engagement we learn as we gain control, we and our organization then move toward High Reliability. When we avoid interaction, because we experience it as being aversive, and at best observe the situation, reliability will slip away. We can engage and move forward, or we can seek escape and move away. As Daved van Stralen recalls (we will include numerous firsthand accounts such as this throughout the book),

An aphorism about pediatric emergencies is that "kids look OK, then deteriorate rapidly." It was not uncommon to be called for a cardiac arrest in various units or facilities and find a twelve-to-twenty-four-hour history of a heart rate over two hundred beats per minute. We began requesting staff to record the blood pressure, respiratory rate, urine output, and other physical signs, even if normal or relatively normal values, to identify subtle trajectories. We began to teach the "covert, compensated state," where the child looks OK but is in an unrecognized state of hidden deterioration. In each location, these children were then more likely to receive intravenous fluids, antibiotics, and a full evaluation for severe infection.

One time, a senior pediatric resident physician apologized to me for sending three kids to the pediatric intensive care unit (PICU) in one week. Two had been transferred back to the ward the next morning. I reviewed the records with him: the two had heart rates over two hundred, received fluids and antibiotics, and responded to treatment. The third stayed in the PICU, receiving a drug to help the heart beat stronger and have closer monitoring. This child was in septic shock.

I pointed out that he had saved three lives. In two, sepsis was captured, and the children responded quickly to early treatment. The third child was saved in the same manner but was more seriously ill.

This situation represents recognition of the early signs of system dysfunction (the covert, compensated state), where interventions are more

effective and less costly. But the healthcare professional must recognize the situation and immediately engage.
      —Daved van Stralen

In organizations where these situations are the norm, arousal from the unexpected, detection of a discrepancy, or disruption in a routine is generally considered a challenge to be engaged. Engagement of a challenge is a social response that is learnable and teachable; most importantly, engagement can be modeled.

Modeling Attitudes, Behaviors, and Strategies
Aversion due to arousal, discussed above, inhibits the personal initiative necessary for independent engagement. Engagement of a particular situation or uncommon event requires some level of improvisation, a process that is learned through trial and error and observation of others.

As social creatures, people observe the behaviors of other people, and the consequences of those behaviors, the observational learning process described by Bandura in Social Learning Theory (1986). The more experienced members and leaders in an HRO use this process to teach, or assist the novice in learning, the attitudes, behaviors, and strategies necessary to engage a particular situation or uncommon event. Positive and negative consequences are openly discussed as another method to support the novice and adopting HRO attitudes and behaviors. This is particularly important between members with the same level of experience as they learn better from each other than they do from those with more or less experience.

Authentic leadership theory (Avolio, et al. 2004) describes this as "leading by example," a form of role modeling by setting high moral standards, demonstrating honesty, and maintaining integrity. The goal is to evoke similar attitudes and behaviors in others, shared throughout the organization. The leader also models positive emotions, attitudes, and high levels of performance, elements of both social learning theory (Bandura 1986) and authentic leadership theory (Avolio, et al. 2004).

We differentiate this type of modeling from role modeling because the novice is not learning a role but is learning how to perform an HRO, particularly to support engagement of the unexpected events. Because this is not specific to a particular role, it will permeate environment of an HRO to constitute its "attitude ecology."

The member of an HRO achieves authenticity by personifying, in their behaviors and attitudes, the abstract concepts we discuss for HROs. Personification is more than internalization, it is embodiment by grounding the individual's cognitive and affective processes and bodily interactions with the environment (Meier, et al. 2012).

High Reliability Organizing (HRO) describes a dynamic, interactive style of engagement that is effectively used in these situations and for operations in these environments. In this book, we use this approach to describe HRO, from the mundane with the potential to fail to the extreme, where death is real. High-reliability operations engage the High Reliability situation and enact, shape, and create. This is what happens in High Reliability environments.

HROs interpret arousal as a challenge, not an aversion.

One afternoon, Rebecca Martin, a respiratory care practitioner (RCP), noted thickening secretions in the airway of a child who was on a mechanical ventilator. She evaluated the child and found an increased heart rate, cool extremities, and a temperature margin below the knee. (In this situation, the skin temperature changes from warm to cold in one inch, or two and a half centimeters, and is associated with low blood volume.) She called the charge nurse for further orders, but the charge nurse felt it could wait until morning. The RCP told the nurse that these findings were associated with low blood volume and how she had observed several other children benefit from fluids. The nurse did not want to disturb the physician.

At one a.m., the child had to be transferred for emergency treatment. After receiving a large amount of intravenous fluids, the child returned to the unit. Rebecca and I discussed this situation: how healthcare culture can frighten people from engagement or calling for assistance.

—Daved van Stralen

Culture allows the extension of humanity into austere, adverse, and even hazardous environments.

The High Reliability Organization

We recognize that the term "High Reliability Organization" is more commonly used to describe organizations that avoid catastrophes in environments in which accidents might be expected. A deeper look reveals that HRO is not an approach academic researchers have developed but a model that academics have codified after observing successful organizations purposely operating in unforgiving, hazardous environments.

It is the complexity, dynamics, and threats of High Reliability situations and environments that create the risk factors we face. HRO represents a social response we can learn. It is not something one can design or impose on people. When faced with a sudden or unexpected demand, people typically respond in a way that will make sense to them in the moment. Our response, counterintuitively, is generally proportional to the suddenness and novelty of the situation rather than the magnitude of the threat. That is, a person who interacts with a new situation will interact with any situation in the same manner until that moment when demands exceed the person's ability to perform. While it is beyond the scope of this book to discuss "live-or-die" interactions, we do wish to point out that HRO, as codified by the academics, was originally derived from these very situations.

High Reliability Organizing, in this operational approach, describes the processes and structures organizations use to achieve success when encountering the unexpected or in unstructured environments—something individual people and the larger organization are constantly dealing with. This is an interactive approach. Because the most inexperienced and newest member of the organization often initiates this HRO response, it is crucial for senior leadership and executives to set the tone by modeling these beliefs and behaviors during the challenges in their daily routines. Learning the HRO approach from senior leadership should occur long before these challenges present themselves to the novice.

> Shamel Abd-Allah, my critical care fellow, requested a ride-along with the Los Angeles City Fire Department paramedics. He wanted to meet the type of emergency professionals I had worked with and see the environment I had worked in. After he returned, he said, "Now I know how you resuscitate patients." Confused, I told him that I resuscitate like other physicians do and use the same treatments and protocols. "No," he said, "you resuscitate like the paramedics." He meant my demeanor, decision-making, and leadership were all similar to those of the street medics. That is when I realized I had witnessed very few resuscitations; instead, I always participated whenever possible. I had continued to use my rescue ambulance approach as a medical approach to emergency and critical care. They fit.
> —Daved van Stralen

When we use HRO to simply describe an organization, we can lose the meaning of the mind-set, principles, and processes that emerge from routine operations to form High Reliability Organizing. HRO can then become, and has been, a designed program: a set of plans and processes for the rare, unexpected event.

The organization will then shift operations to "HRO operations." HRO becomes a skill we teach for emergency use rather than a method of performance and operations for daily use.

The methods and structure of HRO emerged within organizations that conduct routine high-risk operations in environments where the cost of a mistake can be severe injury, even death, to some or potentially all the members of the team. Most obvious are military combat operations, law enforcement activity, and firefighting.

HRO, supported by scientific concepts, is practical wisdom.

Knowledge as Science versus Wisdom

Some people, when they encounter uncertainty, search science for guidance. Unfortunately, science does not have the certitude necessary for engagement; even if it did, we are unlikely to match our perceptions, reality, and scientific principles to make the "right" decision. This quandary was well known to the ancient Greeks, as Aristotle described in his book *Nicomachean Ethics*. Aristotle described five virtues of thought: *technê*, *epistêmê*, *phronêsis*, *sophia*, and *nous*. These virtues distinguish knowledge from wisdom and the theoretical from the practical. We find the virtue phronesis, practical wisdom, more enlightening than episteme (theoretical knowledge or science) or techne (practical knowledge or technology). This is discussed in more detail in chapter 12, "Leadership, Authority, Command, and Team Formation."

Two virtues are types of knowledge (Parry 2014):

- *Episteme*—translated into modern English as "knowledge" (epistemology is the study of the nature of knowledge), for Aristotle it was pure theory, but combined with the accuracy and certainty of experimentation: what we today would call scientific knowledge.
- *Techne*—translated as "craft," "craftsmanship art," or "skill," this represents pragmatic, context-dependent knowledge, or what we would call practice. Techne is the application of knowledge for the practical ends we call technology.

Two virtues are types of wisdom (S Ryan 2014):

- *Sophia*—theoretical wisdom, or reasoning concerned with universal truths, is the knowledge of necessity—wise in general but not in one particular field. (The Sophists were teachers in ancient Greece who taught argument. Later in Greek history, the Sophists became known for their skill in reasoning in order to make an ingenuous or specious argument, rather than a sound argument. Hence, sophistry is a tricky, misleading, fallacious form of argument; "sophisticated" is a measure of educated tastes.)
- *Phronesis*—practical wisdom, or the capability of rational thinking that takes into account context (or contingent facts); it accounts for the particular. One places value on information that may change with events. Aristotle considered this the first of the four cardinal virtues, because ethics guides the individual to place the community's good ahead of one's personal good. Phronesis is acquired by both practice and observation: practice creates the experience, while observation of elders who model this virtue leads to phronesis. (Providence of foresight is the source for our word "prudence"; the Romans translated *phronesis* as "prudence." Phronesis is now more commonly translated as "practical wisdom.")

We can also separate these four virtues as being purely theoretical (episteme and sophia) and as purely practical (techne and phronesis).

Nous, the fifth virtue, is the intellect—the basic process of rational thinking, compared to perception or reasoning (*logos*)—which develops naturally through experience.

HROs place priority on practical wisdom rather than universal principles.

Karlene Roberts and her working group of academics from the University of California, Berkeley, initially codified HRO from their direct observations of the performance of the crew of the aircraft carrier USS *Carl Vinson* (La Porte et al. 1988). It is remarkable to find these characteristics across dissimilar industries across the United States (and elsewhere): the civilian air traffic control system and electrical power grid system (Roberts 1989), nuclear power generation (Roberts 1990), nuclear-powered submarines (Bierly and Spender 1995), structural firefighting and wildland firefighting (Bigley and Roberts 2001), and commercial aviation safety (Commercial Aviation Safety Team, or CAST) (Soliday & Erickson, 1999; Shin, 2000).

These industries all function in environments where failure is catastrophic, and they all rely on every individual to prevent catastrophic failure. From this perspective, we can readily see that all members of an HRO maintain vigilance for anything that might cause a failure. When an organizational member observes an early sign of a failure, that member will engage the situation and articulate it as clearly and concisely as possible to the team; the person will subsequently be supported by the entire system and organization.

From this concept emerged the five principles Weick and Sutcliffe (2015) presented in their first edition of *Managing the Unexpected*:

- *preoccupation with failure*—vigilance toward system vulnerability; early engagement of problems
- *reluctance to simplify*—the complexity of multiple interactions at the local level; the organization is *reluctant* to simplify or to keep simple in order to capture this complexity
- *sensitivity to operations*—the priority of local discrepancies, disturbances, and interruptions *while* maintaining strategic operations
- *deference to expertise*—the importance of local knowledge from interacting with the situation
- *commitment to resilience*—support of the open-ended working of a problem until resolution

Because HRO supports the rapid expansion of a system during a crisis, it must accommodate the routine operations immediately before the event. There is no confusion about when to shift operational methods from routine to crisis. Daily activities, in effect, become regular practice exercises for an emergency, and the team, whatever that team may be, will then be better prepared to respond appropriately should the situation escalate.

Preventing Failure versus Responding to Failure

It would make sense that the five HRO principles would differ between two industries such as nuclear power, where you would want to prevent failure, and wildland firefighting, where you are responding to failure. The elegance of the five principles is that they can support these different structures and allow transitions between the different processes that use HRO (Roe and Schulman 2015).

For example, the control operators of a nuclear power plant or electrical grid system have identified various processes to prevent system failure. Any deviation from these accepted processes are these industries' discrepancies signifying early failure. On the other hand, when the system has failed, rigorous adherence to processes limits the fluid responsiveness necessary to bring control to the emergency. For our purposes, we will call this dichotomy *control operator* verses *emergency responder*, yet it is important to note that we operate in both modes simultaneously. We are controlling and responding during all operations and functions.

This is a critical element to understand, as successful practitioners of HRO are able to "toggle" between the discipline necessary for optimal system function and the flexibility to react to emergent situations that are part and parcel of high-risk environments. That is, from the lessons we learn, we develop rules that prevent failure, and we then adhere strictly to these rules. On the other hand, in an emergency we use rules when they apply and interact with the situation based on local knowledge and responses.

HROs developed as effective and successful responses to highly dangerous situations. These processes from different environments converged to the programs we see today. Some, such as the aforementioned CAST (Commercial Aviation Safety Team), did not begin as a program to become HRO, but rather to solve a problem of imminent threat to the health of the commercial air transportation industry. Although the accident rate was low, an increasing volume of air traffic would produce more air crashes. Travelers respond to the *number* of air crashes, not the rate, and an increased number would negatively affect the industry. Another, the human performance improvement process, actually is a modification of US naval nuclear propulsion from Admiral Hyman Rickover. The nuclear power industry's human performance improvement (HPI) program developed from an industry need for public acceptance following the Three Mile Island incident and Perrow's work (1984) on normal accident theory. Nuclear power also had a history of responses following early accidental releases of ionizing radiation that caused acute radiation syndrome (Perrow 2011).

The following sidebars describe High Reliability organizing principles in the period HRO studies were commencing. The first is from RAdm Thomas A. Mercer who invited academicians from the University of California, Berkeley, to evaluate the performance of his crew. This directly led to the HRO studies. Next a sidebar written by Christopher A. Hart, Chairman of the National Transportation Safety Board, describes the efforts of commercial aviation to make flying safer, with the finding that safety reduces costs in a manner other than the absence of air crashes. Cockpit (now Crew) Resource Management emerged from efforts to identify why a well-trained crew in a well-designed and maintained aircraft will crash. We end this set of sidebars with the aviation error reporting system described by Mr. Hart.

The Beginnings of HRO on the USS *Carl Vinson*

Upon reporting aboard USS *Carl Vinson*, July 1983.

Operational record. The *Vinson* deployed less than one year after commissioning as the first new West Coast carrier in twenty years and had a mixed air wing and battle group, with units from both coasts. The *Vinson* was also the first carrier to have what is now called Intranet and Internet, which allowed for command of the ship's crew through an Internet-type system. To prepare for this situation, the crew spent an extended period of precommissioning time in the shipyard with officers who had spent their entire tour at the Carnegie Mellon Institute of Computer Science.

The first cruise was a complicated cruise with limited logistic support. The ship visited the Mediterranean, the Ivory Coast, the Arabian Sea, and Australia. The *Vinson* failed her first operational readiness exam, but it was initially unclear whether this was because of the high-tech development of the ship versus operational emphasis or because of something else. Fortunately, the ship had a good aviation safety record but not nearly as good an operational reputation. The captain sets the tone, climate, and culture of the ship.

After assuming command in Australia during the first voyage, my goal was to bring the *Vinson* to operational excellence by improving the following:

- inter-ship communication of goals and priorities to the crew;
- ship and air wing cooperation, which led to the *Vinson* receiving the Ramage Award (named for Rear Admiral James "Jig Dog" Ramage), in recognition of the top aircraft carrier / air wing team for best performance as an integrated unit and excellence in navy aircraft carrier operations;
- gradual increase in operational demands and expanding the envelope; the "envelope" of a plane or ship marks the boundaries within which performance is safe and effective; to expand the envelope, we worked as a team to improve performance and safety beyond the initial limits;

The indicator of our successful results was receiving the Admiral Flatley Memorial Award based on a comprehensive evaluation of contributions to aviation safety.

The early HRO studies from the Berkeley experience (1983–1986 USS *Carl Vinson*, CVN-70) were instrumental in later HRO development. The USS *Carl Vinson* was the most recently commissioned aircraft carrier (March 1982) and was assigned to the Pacific Fleet. I had invited professors Karlene Roberts, Todd La Porte, and Bob Bea aboard the *Vinson* to study the crew performance, which resulted in a study over a three-year period. They had full access to the ship, except for the nuclear plant. This grew into the HRO project, which had other nodes at the FAA Oakland Center, the Diablo Canyon Nuclear Plant, the Chevron refineries in the San Francisco Bay area (including shipping operations), and the experience of fire on oil platforms (such as the 1988 Piper Alpha disaster on the North Sea). The term "HRO" was coined around 1988.

The results of the initial studies revealed that aircraft carriers were "well organized" for operational oversight; they even showed a greatly improved safety record since the 1950s. Some of this came from major aircraft carrier improvements (for example, the angle deck) as well as from aircraft improvements (for example, jet-engine reliability). The training of aircrews had improved over the years, and the navy centralized pilot assignments and promotions to leadership positions.

The Berkeley group generally focused on the more active flight deck operations and mostly shadowed the air department and air boss. (The "Air Boss" is the air officer who controls the takeoffs, landings, those aircraft in the air near the ship, and the movement of planes on the flight deck.) They did not do a lot of observation of the bridge activity or officer in command.

Important to the true performance in what is now called HRO was the style and philosophy of leadership and management throughout the ship. The chief petty officers, whose authority crosses lines of command, have an important role in creating and maintaining the climate of HRO. There is the belief that you are always training your own relief and moving up. The record is based on many lessons and from previous experience. These lessons were learned in blood in the 1950s and 1960s; the crew must always remember that. There is attention to small detail in the belief that anyone can stop the operation if they observe something they believe is significant.

—Thomas A. Mercer, RAdm, USN (retired)

Commercial Aviation Safety Team

The commercial aviation industry in the United States enjoys an amazing safety record. One of the major reasons for that safety record is a program called the Commercial Aviation Safety Team, or CAST.

The industry created CAST because, in the early 1990s, the fatal accident rate, after decreasing substantially for the previous several decades, had begun to approach a plateau. The substantial decrease had resulted largely from new technologies such as jet engines (much more reliable than piston engines), simulators (thus enabling the training of pilots that would otherwise be dangerous to conduct in real airplanes), and automation (which helps pilots perform more efficiently and effectively), but those technologies were reaching their "asymptotic improvement" limits. The concern was that the volume of commercial flying was projected to double by 2010 or so, and if the volume doubled while the rate remained stuck on a plateau, then the public would see twice as many airplane crashes in the news. At that point, it would not be helpful to inform the public that the *rate* was low; what the public cared about was the *number* of events.

The industry realized that in order to get off the accident rate plateau, it had to do something different. At this point, two key leaders played an important role: the administrator of the Federal Aviation Administration (FAA), which is the regulator, and the vice president for safety at a major airline. Together they recognized that the solution was not the typical response by a regulator to improve safety: more regulations and more enforcement by the regulator. To the contrary, the system was already highly regulated, and the accidents had not generally occurred from lack of compliance with regulations; instead, the solution was a collaborative approach in which the industry and the regulator would work together to figure out how to improve the safety of a complex system.

More specifically, the aviation industry is a complex system that consists of several subsystems that are coupled with one another and must work effectively together in order for the entire system to work. Because the subsystems are coupled together, any change in one subsystem can have effects in one or more of the other subsystems. Hence, one of the challenges in making changes to complex systems is "system think," which refers to understanding what a change to one subsystem might do to the other subsystems. Unless the interactions are well understood, the change will be highly likely to lead to unintended consequences.

The aviation industry accomplished system think by bringing everyone to the table—the airlines, the manufacturers, the pilots, the air traffic controllers, the airports, and the regulator—in order to identify the potential safety concerns and decide how best to address those concerns. That collaborative program, which is entirely voluntary, is called CAST.

The results have been phenomenal. In less than ten years, the flat, stuck rate—which many already believed to be exemplary and not likely to get much lower—decreased by more than 80 percent. And, contrary to the conventional wisdom that improving safety generally hurts productivity (and vice versa), productivity improved at the same time safety improved. This was a key result that helped ensure the sustainability of CAST, because the hard reality is that safety programs that hurt the bottom line are not generally sustainable. Adding to the success story is that the process did not generate any new regulations, which was consistent with the FAA administrator's pronouncement that the solution would not be to have more regulations. Finally, safety was improved with very few unintended consequences.

—Christopher A. Hart, chairman, National Transportation Safety Board

Crew Resource Management

Crew resource management (CRM), originally cockpit resource management, came about because of widespread recognition that flight crews were flying functional aircraft into mountains, oceans, and the like due to the failure of the crew to function as a team. CRM addressed the problem of "how could a well-trained flight crew, in a well-maintained aircraft, crash the plane?" Beginning in the late 1970s, crews were trained that CRM involved bringing the crew together to function as a team; developing clear, timely, and solution-driven communications; maintaining a level of individual and team situational awareness (SA) judged to be critical for safe and efficient flight operations; and developing a process for effective decision-making in which *all* members of the crew would provide as much pertinent information as necessary for the captain to make the best decision possible.

It should be noted that many of the old-school, John Wayne–type pilots, who invoked a highly autocratic leadership style, did not initially look favorably on CRM. But requiring all flight-crew members to actively participate in CRM ultimately led to a marked decrease in crew-related

errors, which in turn resulted in entire years in which no fatal accidents occurred among the major US carriers.
—Daved van Stralen, Spence Byrum

The Fuel for Improving Safety

If an organization seeks to improve a characteristic of its operations—for example, productivity, reliability, throughput, or profit—the most effective fuel for that improvement process is information about what is working well and what is not on the front lines in daily operations. Such information is also useful for determining whether improvements and other changes are having the desired effect without generating unintended consequences. When the characteristic to be improved is safety, two excellent sources of information in the aviation industry are near-miss reporting—reports from pilots about things that almost went wrong but fortunately did not—and digital information from flight data recorders.

More effective use of information from near-miss reporting and digital recorders is especially valuable in commercial aviation, because accidents are so rare in the industry that the obvious safety indicator—the number of accidents—provides little "granularity" about whether safety is improving. The use of more and better data provides a means to spot adverse trends early and address them long before they result in an accident.

These information sources present two challenges: obtaining the information and using the information.

Obtaining the Information

When the National Transportation Safety Board (NTSB) investigates accidents, it frequently discovers that the problems that resulted in the accidents were known before the accidents occurred. Unfortunately, however, the problems were usually known by the front-line workers who experienced them in actual operations but not by anyone who had the authority and the resources to address the problems. The challenge is getting those who know the information about potential problems to provide it to those who are in a position to fix the problems. The nature of this challenge depends on whether the reporting is directly from front-line employees or from other sources.

Reporting by Front-Line Employees

The seminal aviation accident that resulted in the development of near-miss reporting programs for pilots in aviation was the crash of TWA 514 in Virginia in 1974 as it was approaching Dulles airport (IAD). As with most airline crashes, many links in the chain contributed to the crash, one of which involved the "approach chart" that pilots use to determine how to get to the runway from their present location when they are unable to see the runway because they are in the clouds. The approach chart they were using contained ambiguous instructions, and the chart, in conjunction with their instructions over the radio from the air traffic controllers, created confusion about when to descend—enough confusion that the pilots in the cockpit debated the subject. They descended too soon and crashed into a ridge west of the airport, killing everyone on board.

In the accident investigation, the NTSB learned that other pilots had been similarly confused by that approach chart; the pilots of one airline, for example, had reported their concerns up the chain of command, which led that airline to spread the word to all of its pilots who flew into IAD. Thus, that airline's pilots who flew into IAD were aware of the ambiguity on the chart, but these TWA pilots were not, and TWA 514 crashed into the ridge.

As a result of that accident, the aviation industry developed a near-miss reporting program to help ensure that systemic issues such as this approach-chart ambiguity would be known by all pilots who needed to know that information. The ultimate remedy in this situation was to address the ambiguity in the approach chart and to revise the instructions that the controllers who controlled the traffic provided, but meanwhile, the program provided a process for immediately spreading the word of caution to all who needed to know it.

Getting the information from where it was—the pilots—to where it needed to be—those who can address the concerns the pilots raised—brought up several important issues. Two related issues were (1) how to ensure that the near-miss reports would not be used for enforcement or other punitive actions and (2) how to get pilots to file near-miss reports. The two issues are related, because one of the major benefits to pilots for filing near-miss reports was the assurance that, with certain exceptions (for example, situations involving criminal or intentional wrongdoing), information from reports filed in a timely manner would not be used for enforcement.

Clarity about enforcement is crucial, because the line between when to enforce and when not to enforce is not always clear. Regarding the approach chart, for example, pilots would be concerned that, unless they happened to reach the same conclusion from the arguably ambiguous chart as the regulator had, they might face an enforcement action for failure to follow the chart. In response to this concern, the FAA announced that, with certain exceptions (as noted above), information from the reports would not be used for enforcement purposes.

Unfortunately, the pilot community's mistrust of the FAA ran so deep that the nonenforcement policy statement was not enough. In addition, the program offered anonymity to those who filed reports, and it was structured in such a way that the pilots would file their reports with an independent (nonenforcing) third party—NASA was selected for this role—and NASA was only permitted to provide de-identified information from the reports to the FAA.

This anonymity presents at least two challenges. First, if more information was needed about the near-miss report to make it understandable and meaningful, then the insistence on anonymity would prevent NASA from calling the filer of the report for clarification. To address that problem, NASA initially reviews incoming reports to see if clarification is needed before de-identifying the report. Second, too much anonymity can reduce the value of the reports, which has resulted in changes to the de-identification regimen based on experience in an effort to achieve a more effective balance between anonymity and the need for information. For example, de-identification early in the life of the program included the removal of information about the number of engines on the airplane. That, in turn, made it difficult to identify any issues about certain types of aircraft. Similarly, removing the airport identity made it difficult to spot issues related to specific airports.

De-identification helped alleviate the pilots' fear of filing near-miss reports. The developers of the aviation near-miss reporting program were concerned, however, that getting pilots to file reports necessitated more than just removing the fear; it also necessitated providing an incentive. The incentive was that if the FAA found out about a potentially enforceable situation from a source other than a near-miss report, then the timely filing of a near-miss report involving that situation would immunize the filer of the report (with the usual exceptions noted above) from enforcement related to that situation. Thus, immunity goes far beyond an agreement not to use the information in the near-miss report against the filer (commonly referred to as "information immunity") and extends to protection from enforcement in relation to the entire situation (commonly referred to as "transactional immunity").

Other Types of Reporting

In addition to reports filed by pilots, the commercial aviation industry generates large quantities of digital data because all airliners (as well as many other larger airplanes) are required to be equipped with flight data recorders. Early flight data recorders recorded analog information on magnetic tapes and foil strips, listing fewer than ten parameters such as engine exhaust, temperature, fuel flow, aircraft velocity, altitude, control surfaces positions, and rate of descent. Recorders on modern airliners are digital and record thousands of parameters many times a second.

Although the requirement for recorders on airplanes resulted from a desire to provide more information to accident investigators to help them determine why an airplane had crashed, the recorders have also been found to be very useful by providing information that can be used proactively to help prevent accidents. Most US airlines now voluntarily and routinely provide information from their flight data recorders to a program known as the Aviation Safety Information Analysis and Sharing (ASIAS) system in the Center for Advanced Aviation System Development, which is operated by the MITRE Corporation, an American not-for-profit organization. ASIAS now contains digital information from millions of flights.

As with the near-miss reports, the airlines' voluntary submittal of information from flight data recorders to ASIAS necessitated the FAA's assurance that the agency would not use the information for enforcement purposes. Unlike with respect to near-miss reports, however, the incentive to submit data to ASIAS came from the airline industry's desire to prevent accidents rather than from any special protection provided by the FAA.

Using the Information

The combination of removing concerns about enforcement with providing an incentive has resulted in pilots filing as many as forty thousand near-miss reports a year. In addition, as noted above, MITRE is the custodian of the ASIAS database, which contains digital information from millions of commercial airline flights. That large quantity of data presents significant issues about how to use the information productively. For the digital data, the industry is continually developing new tools to help mine the data more effectively and efficiently. Mining the data is far more challenging with near-miss reports, which are free text, ordinary language lacking the constraints of format or coding. Thanks to the need of other industries to develop better ways to mine textual data (for example, in efforts to detect fraud and to prevent terrorism), ever-improving text-mining tools are increasing the industry's capability of using near-miss text reports proactively.

Ideally, this wealth of digital and textual information will be useful not only for identifying potential safety issues but also for generating quick feedback on whether the interventions that were put in place to address the issues—as well as any other changes to procedures or equipment—are accomplishing the intended result and not generating unintended consequences.

A major caveat regarding the aviation industry's data-analysis programs described above is that they are voluntary, so they do not provide a basis for statistically valid conclusions about the frequency of occurrence of a given phenomenon. Experience has shown, for example, that immediately after a runway-incursion scare (i.e., two airliners nearly colliding at an airport), the number of near-miss reports about runway incursions increases. This increase is probably the result of increased awareness rather than an actual increase in the number of events. Similarly, news stories about an airplane that landed with very low fuel reserves will typically lead to an increase in near-miss reports about low fuel.

Conclusion

The aviation industry is demonstrating the power of information about what is happening every day on the front lines to help analysts identify potential safety issues and to reveal whether the remedies that are being implemented to address those issues are accomplishing the desired result without creating any unintended consequences. Other industries can learn from aviation about the steps that were necessary to obtain this information as well as the challenges associated with extracting useful information from large quantities of data.

—Christopher A. Hart, chair, National Transportation Safety Board

---

These vignettes demonstrate that High Reliability Organizing is a set of attitudes, behaviors, and interactions. HRO has a unique but shared mind-set, as we will discuss in the next section.

HRO Is a Mind-Set

HRO is a mind-set of all members of the organization as well as a system within the organization that encourages the identification of early signs of failure or the first signs of the normalization of deviance with appropriate engagement. The danger comes from an overreliance on checklists, one of the methods that control operators (mentioned earlier) use appropriately to *prevent* system failure. When a system failure has occurred, a checklist can provide guidance but is not in itself a process sufficient for emergency responses or managing little surprises.

In addition, total quality management (TQM), continuous quality improvement (CQI), or process improvement (PI), by design, look backward for information that can be helpful in the future. HRO, on the other hand, is real-time interaction; TQI, CQI, and PI do not suffice for reliably *preventing* system failure or as a *response* to system failure. Nor do they prepare the program for *evolving* or novel emergent properties, such as a new and highly complex threat such as SARS or the Ebola virus. Lean, Six Sigma, the Theory of Constraints, and more are excellent at making processes more efficient by eliminating waste and barriers, but they do not address the *dynamisms* in the environments in which HROs necessarily operate. (We discuss these systems further in later chapters.)

HRO engages the problems that we don't want to encounter. It is an adaptive operational approach for environments without structure or in which people can lose structure easily, or they do not readily recognize new, emerging structures. One limiting factor for translation and understanding of HRO in order to make sense of it is the lack of experience most people have across the "liminal threshold" into HRO environments, which makes it difficult to fully translate the salience and meaning of HRO concepts when non-HRO concepts are generally easier to understand and employ. The liminal threshold, a concept borrowed from anthropology, refers to the disorientation experienced during a ritual to mark a change in status within the community. In some societies, this threshold is ritually induced, and the initiate never returns to his or her previous status. Significant in the ritual is the loss of control, threat, and absence of supportive others—an enactment of death.

We use this concept to describe the threshold between the stable, predictable environment and the unstable, unpredictable environment where our known rules no longer apply. A significant and dramatic change occurs in the internal logic of the system. The principles and attitudes of HRO can apply in the routine environment, while those of the routine environment can become unsafe when the liminal threshold is crossed.

The HRO mind-set prepares, or conditions, the individual to perform *during* these events. Encountering time compression or a threat changes how the brain performs. This is similar to crossing a threshold, where familiar processes and rules no longer apply and may become counterproductive and cause harm. To identify what will work, one must engage the problem and environments in order to learn what works through action, thus creating knowledge as the situation evolves. This takes mental preparation, good socialization skills, and strong support from one's superiors.

A child with a complex medical condition who was dependent on a mechanical ventilator was a resident in the nursing home and rapidly developed signs of sepsis and low blood volume (hypovolemia), as identified by the respiratory care practitioner (RCP). The team called 911 for an emergency response by the fire department and ambulance. Gaining vascular access for fluids (i.e., to provide intravenous fluid, or IV, therapy) would be impossible in this setting, but the child's condition indicated the need for immediate fluids.

I asked Gwen Conley, the RCP noted above, to draw small amounts of normal saline, a type of IV fluid, into a syringe. Under my orders, she then administered these small amounts repeatedly into the child's tracheostomy tube, hand ventilated, and then suctioned the airway. It was as I thought: the fluids were not suctioned because they had been absorbed into the bloodstream. We continued this therapy until the fire paramedics arrived.

The situation confused the paramedics when they arrived; they did not have a protocol for combined sepsis and hypovolemia, and the history was of very poor vital signs that had, since the 9-1-1 call, improved from the fluid administration, yet no IV had been placed.

Gwen calmly attempted to explain this situation to the paramedic, but it was not a part of his experience or mind-set. Gwen had learned this mind-set as part of her HRO education.

—Daved van Stralen

One would not expect a long-term care specialist to resuscitate a child as effectively as Gwen. She provides respiratory care in a pediatric subacute facility to children dependent on a mechanical ventilator. Other vignettes in this book describe the use of HRO processes in a subacute facility, some for emergency responses like Gwen's. The mind-set used in the facility is vigilance for early heralds of trouble, communication that is objective and presents the action taken and result, modulate fear and threat responses, and characterization of the duties required by the various disciplines and allied healthcare givers. James P. Denney, EMS Captain, Los Angeles Fire Department, observed, "We do in an emergency what we do every day." The nursing home had adapted emergency operations for use in routine long-term care.

The Five HRO Principles

Weick and Sutcliffe (2015) identified five principles necessary and sufficient for High Reliability Organizing. Though these have reached an almost iconic status, which we agree with, we have found organization leaders have difficulty establishing them in practice. This book will assist you. Individuals will find one or two of these principles more logical and easier to incorporate into their operations than others. The other principles will then naturally flow; therefore, we do not believe in incorporating all five principles at once or in a specific order.

Below we have provided operational descriptions of the Weick and Sutcliffe (2015) principles.

1: Preoccupation with Failure

"Preoccupation with failure does not mean failure of the individual but the system failing."
—KARL WEICK, PERSONAL COMMUNICATION

High Reliability developed in organizations as a necessary response to the vulnerability of operating in hazardous environments. What distinguishes an HRO is how the organization considers any lapse in performance a serious consequence; there are no small failures. People watch for, and respond to, the weakest signals of failure. Rather than viewing outliers as random, independent events that one can ignore because of their rarity or disregard because of their disconnection to the system, the HRO will view the outlier as an early sign or representation of what is possible. Ignoring small failures leads to larger cascading failures and possibly catastrophic events.

Failure has context, industry, and time specificity. We create several objectives when engaging uncertainty; we act to increase our chances of success and to decrease the chances of failure. As the situation evolves, we adjust our objective, because a portion may become out of reach while an alternative becomes more achievable.

> "Failure in community policing is missing a criminal;
> failure in school policing is a student not graduating."
> —JOE PAULINO, POLICE CHIEF, SAN BERNARDINO
> CITY UNIFIED SCHOOL DISTRICT

2: Reluctance to Simplify

HROs are *reluctant* to accept simplifications; this does not mean they do not simplify. Reluctance is an ongoing suspicion of simplicity, we ask what we are missing, we feel something is amiss in this routine (Weick, personal communication). People take deliberate steps to create more comprehensive and nuanced pictures of what they face.

The outlier incident serves as both a sign of vulnerability (Preoccupation with Failure) and an indicator of the complexity beneath the visible surface (Reluctance to Simplify). Taken as a value far outside an expected range, the outlier can readily be discarded, the view of the outlier as statistical random, independent data. The more ominous prospect regards the outlier as an early herald of a disruptive process.

To members of an HRO, the outlier doesn't represent randomness, rather, it is a local, *emergent* structure from within a self-organizing system. These are systems where novel properties "emerge" from internal, simple but non-linear processes within the incident. From this simple start can emerge novel, unexpected properties that create unexpected problems. An HRO will simplify but knows that simplification interferes with evaluating the evidence foreshadowing these unexpected problems.

A characteristic of nonlinear systems is the input does not create a proportional output. The output can be significantly less, taking greater effort to achieve smaller gain; significantly more, small actions produce large results; or vary when taken at different times. Another characteristic of nonlinearity is the inability to reduce nonlinear systems to components with separate solutions for each component. Nonlinear systems trouble planners.

The reducibility and predictability inherent to linearity creates the simplicity necessary for protocols, algorithms, and rapid solutions. For these reasons, planners use linearity rather than nonlinearity for categorization, models, and education.

When we label or categorize, we lose information. Diversity and discussion enable people to see different things when viewing the same event, which brings out hidden information. Complexity contains more information than simplicity.

Self-organizing systems can appear simple or complex. Though complexity is, generally, a global property of self-organizing systems, simple order emerges from local interactions. The continuous dynamic activity of the system creates stability. The system, however, may appear simple when we evaluate only the lower levels of self-organizing processes. Finally, a novel event will appear complex because of our lack of familiarity with the system.

Suspicion of simplicity, a second take on reluctance to simplify, is reluctance to *keep* simple. Big things start simply. If we continue to view these events as simple, we risk missing the point when a crisis starts. We want to respond during the covert, compensated phase, when the failure is hidden because the system works; it is compensating.

It is this simplification, in which we keep to simple explanations, where we miss the developing failure. We ask, "What am I missing?" We know something is askew with the process or our routine. We search for that potential fracture point or hidden vulnerability.

> "Most naval aviators would recognize this feeling: A
> 'leemer' is an uneasy feeling in the pit of your stomach:
> just a sense that something is not going right. Perhaps
> it came from 'leery': 'wary, suspicious of.'"
> —THOMAS A. MERCER, RADM, USN (RETIRED)

When change happens in this covert, compensated state, we must also change and adapt; we do not continue with simple approaches for simple events. Failure to intervene here allows the failure to develop until it becomes overt, decompensated failure. This is the fallacy of overreaction or "crying wolf."

An infant in the PICU had not improved for a week and was receiving mechanical ventilation and drugs for heart function. The pulmonary consultant advised us that the child's lungs had an illness, but it was not so severe as to require mechanical ventilation. The cardiology consultant advised us that the child's heart had a minor problem, but again, it wasn't severe enough to require drugs or mechanical ventilation. Though our consultants had simplified their involvement, we were unable to wean the child off either the drug or the ventilator.

Mark Rogers, the RCP who had been assigned to this infant for several days, administered varying levels of oxygen to the infant and recorded the effect of the supplemental oxygen and ventilator pressures on the oxygen saturation of the blood. His graph demonstrated an increase of oxygen saturation until a specific amount of oxygen was supplied and specific ventilator settings were reached—a "respiratory shunt" had occurred, in which blood was shunted to damaged lung areas and was not picking up oxygen. Then there was no increase in oxygen in the blood, which is called a "cardiac shunt" because the blood shunts across in the heart and is never exposed to the lung.

This infant had combined respiratory and cardiac disease. Either one, taken alone, would not have caused the problem. The infant soon went to the operating room.

—Daved van Stralen

An HRO should be suspicious of simplicity, reluctant to simplify, and reluctant to keep simple.

3: Sensitivity to Operations

Karl Weick added this principle because organizations would disrupt, if not stop, their strategic operations due to the distraction of a tactical situation; he also noticed that organizations that failed did not adjust their plans in real time for changes at the operational level (Weick, personal communication). Operations are where the real work gets done. Sensitivity to Operations is situational and less strategic, thus allowing for continuous adjustment to the operation. Organizations notice and respond to anomalies and outliers rather than disregarding them as random events. Supervisors must know what is going on and adjust their operations accordingly. People may not speak up because of fear they will undermine operations.

> "Operations also include enactment. Sensitivity also means being aware of your *own* impact in displacing, shaping, and creating what you think is merely external and out there: 'I need to be sensitive to *my* impact.'"
> —KARL WEICK, PERSONAL COMMUNICATION

"Fire Rescue Ambulance Responses in an Active Gang Environment" (Chapter 4 HRO and the Environment) describes the inclusion of enactment with Sensitivity to Operations.

4: Commitment to Resilience

Commitment to resilience is the intrinsic ability of the organization to maintain or regain a stable state in a dynamic situation. The organization supports people to report errors, act to keep errors small, and to improvise quick solutions to keep the system functioning. Members of the organization engage the problem to work toward resolution. There is recognition that the system and people are fallible and that errors can be corrected; therefore, there is no blame. Unexpected, unpredictable trouble *will* occur, so we learn from error. The organization teaches "early error recognition and management" rather than "error avoidance," which can lead to ignoring or hiding mistakes and errors. Because it minimizes or eliminates unwanted variability, resilience is a form of control.

5: Deference to Expertise

Deference to expertise is deferring to local knowledge; those who are closest to the problem or who have specialized knowledge can extract meaning from the problem's context. For example, the physician has expertise in diagnosis and prescribing therapies, the nurse has expertise in the patient's immediate condition and events at bedside, and the paramedic has expertise in providing care in adverse environments. Decisions and authority migrate up and down to achieve the agility necessary to manage dynamic situations. While knowledge is important, how the knowledge relates to the situation is of special significance. That is what we mean by expertise.

"Deference" here means respectful regard or concern rather than submission or yielding. This differentiation can be found in the etymology for the word "defer." Defer as respectful regard, "to put off action," derives from *deferren*, a late 14th century word for "to delay" or "put off." Defer as submission or yielding, "to yield respectfully in judgment" or "to refer for decision," derives from *déférer*, a mid-15th Century word for "to yield or comply" or "to carry away." This articulation is important, as some have interpreted "deference to expertise" to mean that the one with expertise makes the decisions even without responsibility for the decision. We *defer* to expertise, not obey it. As we stated above, HRO is judgment for the particular situation: practical wisdom versus universal knowledge.

> RAdm Thomas A. Mercer and I were discussing with senior executives of a national patient safety organization the resistance doctors had toward HRO. We were told that physicians had difficulty with deference to expertise. I asked Tom to define command in the US Navy, and he replied: "Those

duties you cannot legally delegate." (He noted that you can never delegate accountability.) I asked the senior patient safety physician what duties a physician cannot legally delegate. We both quickly identified "diagnosis" and "prescriptive authority." This led us into a deeper discussion of deference and expertise as local knowledge, such as the patient's immediate condition.
—Daved van Stralen

Deferring to the non-physician is where physicians may have difficulty. We have had success with two good approaches:

- "deference to expertise" refers to local knowledge, such as what is happening at that moment with the specific patient;
- "command" consists of the duties you cannot legally delegate: a physician cannot legally delegate diagnosis, prescriptive authority, or surgical procedures except selectively and only with specific procedures in place.

While we separate these principles for discussion, it is important to understand that High Reliability emerges when the five principles interact with one another. For example, when a discrepancy or disruption occurs, the closest person, regardless of his or her position in the hierarchy, will engage it and communicate with (and receive support from) the surrounding team. This action may have to take priority over the current operations, or current operations must continue while also engaging the evolving situation. This situation describes preoccupation with failure, deference to expertise, and sensitivity operations.

Various people may understand one principle more easily than another. There is no first principle to learn, as learning and using even one of them will make another principle more understandable and accessible. In this manner, a program may appear to start slowly, but it will soon begin to grow quickly.

HRO as Attitudes

The High Reliability principles as described by Weick and Sutcliffe (2015) may more effectively be thought of as attitudes, the five necessary and sufficient attitudes for High Reliability: one's attitude toward failure, acceptance of the complexity of even simple events, awareness of how one fits into the scheme of life (situation-centric versus person-centric), perseverance, and respect for the knowledge and experience of others. These items correspond to preoccupation with failure, reluctance to simplify, sensitivity to operations, commitment to resilience, and deference to expertise respectively.

We have found that framing the five principles as derivations from attitudes increases understanding of their purpose and acceptance by members of the organization, from the senior-most official to the most recently hired on the line. For example, senior executives have difficulty with the concept of preoccupation and failure. Many executives have said that they don't see the purpose of always thinking of failure, and they don't want their employees preoccupied, or focused, on any one thing, let alone failure. We can ask these executives about their attitude toward failure. They don't want it? Then what are they doing to identify it early and engage early signs of failure? Do they have a plan to rapidly bring events to a resolution?

Positioned as attitudes, we see how the five principles develop from experience and then frame the processes necessary to reach High Reliability Organizing. The five principles describe natural, effective, adaptive responses to adversity and hostile environments. If we assume that attitudes drive behaviors, careful to distinguish this from creating behaviors, then the five attitudes are reasonably close to behaviors. Our beliefs do not change environments; our attitudes do.

HRO as Specific Values

Values are more strongly held and more permanent beliefs compared to attitudes. We use our values to judge information and actions. Values are personal, but some specific values also bind us to a culture. From their operational experience, Daved van Stralen and Thomas A. Mercer have identified five values that enable an HRO to perform and that are shared with its members through acculturation. Weick has subsequently added the sixth HRO value of resilience (Weick, personal communication).

Dignity. This means acknowledging the value of everybody's contribution. When you discipline a subordinate, discipline that person without taking away his or her dignity. We do not use the term "respect" here, because respect is generally earned and can easily be lost. Some people will search for justification to disrespect a specific person or other people. We may not respect our patient or the activities of the patient, but we give them the dignity of a human being.

Honesty. What someone says represents the circumstances. This is not honesty, as in telling or not telling white lies or when someone intrudes on your boundaries. We differentiate honesty from trust, which is a transaction based on bias and experience. Our descriptions represent what we see, without making efforts to persuade or hide disconfirming evidence; we freely accept evidence that disconfirms our conclusions.

Humility. The unexpected can happen to any of us; we can all fail. This is in contradistinction to hubris and cognitive dissonance: "I am a good person with good intentions; therefore I would not act that way or cause such a failure." Humility can be learned, and it is the team's responsibility to actively discourage arrogance, because no one is impervious to error. When an error or complication occurs, we immediately help: there is no reason to find someone to blame.

Empathy. HROs work in tough situations where people are going to fail, and it could be any of us doing the failing—there but for the grace of God go I. We do not use compassion, which focuses on the other person and is a response *toward* that person. Empathy refers to our internal belief system toward the plight of others. People make the best decisions they can at the time; when things don't work out, we can support the person even if we disagree.

Duty. We will not let others down; we have a duty to our larger community. This does not refer to duty as described by tasks and job descriptions but to duty as an obligation to others. We do not use the terms "responsibility" or "accountability," which can be limiting. Duty has a larger, more deeply held spiritual component that is internalized and comes from within. We engage to help others do their jobs; often, little things we can do will make someone else's work either harder or easier.

Resilience or perseverance. We will get through this together. We will become smarter, stronger, and more cohesive. The future can seem bleak, but we will remain as one, respectful to one another afterward, and we will perform better next time (added by Weick; personal communication).

Resilience as a value or attitude. We work on the problem together until it gets resolved.

Value Shifting

Some values found in HRO seem to oppose each other, such as initiative and obedience. Others appear to be situational: what helps us one minute may have to be quickly discarded when circumstances change. This ability to shift values is integral to the performance of an HRO.

Schwartz (1992) found that some values are in opposition to each other. We do not expect to find opposing values in the same culture. Examples include obedience versus initiative and conformity versus creativity. HROs, however, work in two environments: the structured environments of routine operations, where preventing system failure is the priority, and the unstructured environments of a crisis, where an emergency response is the priority. This explains why opposing values exist within an HRO. Obedience and authority are part of preventing system failure, but during an emergency, creative problem-solving and the initiative to engage become necessary. Having the ability to smoothly shift between values is one of the hallmarks of HRO.

It is this ability to rapidly develop initiative and creativity in an unstructured situation that creates the "leader-leader" construct we desire for HROs. A "leader-follower" construct too easily creates a docile member who awaits instructions.

Values are also situational. Our evaluation of what will help us and ensure safety will change as circumstances change. We must rely on people who have a sense of duty toward the larger organization, a virtue, and their judgment during the event.

Healthcare Environments

The High Reliability Situation (HRS) emerges unexpectedly in the internal and external environments of the HRO. When it occurs within the internal HRO environment it, in effect, creates an external environmental "bubble" within the HRO. Because the internal HRS has internal logic different from that of the HRO we can consider it external to the HRO. In this section, we will introduce some components of the healthcare environment.

Environment describes the sum of the surroundings and conditions that influence healthcare operations. This includes social, cultural, and physical influences, all of which form the basis of High Reliability Organizing and the causes of the High Reliability Situation.

The environmental influence of healthcare on patients follows a full spectrum from their home and work environment to hospital care. Healthcare, itself, follows the spectrum from public health and preventative medicine in the patient's environment to surgical operations and critical care in the hospital environment.

Healthcare environments occur in various structures for delivering care to a single patient at home or clinic to larger groups of patients in hospitals. The scale of this care encompasses the single patient to whole populations.

Healthcare environments operate as both open and closed systems. Walk-in clinics and emergency departments represent examples of open systems. Intensive care units and labor and delivery represent close systems. The most extreme closed system is a surgical suite.

The breadth and depth of the healthcare environment means that a catastrophic incident can occur to a single patient or entire population. Yet High Reliability operations follow the same principles.

In this section, we discuss uncontrolled physiology as the keystone determinant of the structure of a healthcare HRO. Also included are some of the structures and principles unique to healthcare including the medical hierarchy and the duty to do no harm.

Uncontrolled Physiology

This is the basic problem we encounter: we prescribe treatment for a disease process, but we cannot control how the patient's physiology will respond to the disease, how the disease will respond to treatment, or how the patient's physiology will respond to the treatment.

Even if we know the exact diagnosis, we must deal with uncontrolled physiology. Modern research on the molecular and genetic level shows that each patient can be unique in his or her different responses to diseases and treatments. Our decision-making processes must account for this.

The Medical Hierarchy

The healthcare field remains highly hierarchical despite volumes of evidence that collegial, interactive teams make consistently better decisions. Decisions for patient care come from the physician or surgeon and decisions for nursing care come from nurses while organizational decisions come from executives and administrators influenced by insurers (payers) and regulators. HRO accepts that those with the big picture are best situated to develop strategies but HROs emerged from effective engagement of the HRS. Conflicts arise when the problem is local but the authority is central—something that's not in the best interest of the patient.

The merging of sensitivity to operations with preoccupation with failure occurs when a system becomes unstable, most easily understood with a physiologically unstable patient but can also occur in mental health or a home with external disruptive influences. In this small system, the local situation rapidly changes and effective actions often depend on local information and consideration of new, emergent properties. Deference to expertise describes the importance of the local agent such as nurse, social worker, or allied health professional. Here, deference to expertise describes the "bottom up" forces that drive self-organization for effective response to the HRS.

In a larger system, individuals cannot perform complex tasks on their own, making self-organization inefficient. The leader, though, can observe more of the system with better utilization of resources. Distance from the event allows the use of higher cognitive capabilities necessary for complex tasks. Outside directions increase efficiency through top-down control.

> The greatest barrier to adopting HRO principles and practices is a cultural hierarchy where autonomy is the core value. The very people we need desperately to champion a cultural change frequently complain that the applicability of HRO principles is "cookbook medicine." Many claim that tools such as checklists and standardized practices detract from their autonomy and lack a personal touch. Knowing what we know today about human error, these objections are both dangerous and absurd. Very simply put, if you had the opportunity to choose between a facility that could statistically ensure greater safety by using HRO principles and one that did not, which one would you choose? From an ethical perspective, the healthcare field demands that we "get it right" the first time. It is our moral obligation to significantly decrease the chance for harm.
> —Spence Byrum

This is not to say hierarchy is wrong. Originating from the original physician-patient dyad, healthcare has grown in layers directed toward support of this relationship. We must be mindful of the drift away from support directed toward physician-patient and nurse-patient care by interjections of other professions into these relations.

Hierarchical structures are stable (Simon 1962) but this does not imply strict top-down relations of authority.

Medical Practice
The physician is licensed to practice medicine, which we will consider to be the ability to (1) diagnose, (2) have prescriptive authority, and (3) perform surgical procedures. Some of this responsibility can be delegated through specific means and channels, while some of it cannot. It is important to differentiate what can and cannot be delegated.

Duties of Healthcare Professionals
Other healthcare and allied healthcare professionals have duties derived from their specialties. For example, a respiratory care practitioner has a duty to intervene and treat a patient who is struggling to breathe and does not need a physician's order to do so. A nurse has a duty to respond to the signs of pain or discomfort in a patient. Decision-making conflicts can develop between a

physician's legal duty to practice medicine and a healthcare professional's duty to act. We will address this conflict in later chapters.

Scientific rationality, classical logic (also called scientific logic), and deductive reasoning form the basis of decision-making models in healthcare. We see the advantages of this in evidence-based medicine, standardization of protocols, the use of checklists, and critical thinking. The inability of the structure of science to explain and predict individual situations, though, creates a gap between scientific theory and bedside practice. These individual situations occur across a broad spectrum and from the interaction of diverse scientific concepts to create nuanced and subtle complexities. Our patient situations do not easily align with discrete concepts, particularly in dynamic events, in part because concepts are discrete elements while our situations and perceptions are continuous (Weick 2011).

The Reason for HRO

The uncertain, time-compressed, threatening situation has a different internal logic than the routine or normal situations we work with. In addition, emerging circumstances simultaneously disrupt our normal and personal logic of operations. The elements of normal internal logic and our scientific logic of operations include rationality, deductive reasoning, classical scientific logic, statistics and the normal distribution, linear deterministic decision-making, and reductive problem-solving. With uncertainty, time-compression, and threat these elements do not adequately describe how we operate or contribute to individual or organizational effectiveness.

Unrecognized stress or fear impairs objective sensemaking and cognition. For Karl Weick, "sensemaking" is one word because we construct, or create, our sense of a situation, it is an action we actively take (personal communication). (Sensemaking is developed more fully in chapter 10, "The Sensemaking of Noise.") The HRO principles, possibly intuitive as objective principles, become counterintuitive in application or operation. In this book we describe the limits of logic and rationality in these environments, then describe a different logic of operations developed from combined affective-cognitive thought to create a flexible and agile individual and organizational response and an adaptive program for growth and resilience.

This is more than the idea that medical care has become more complex. We can now perform earlier identification of serious diseases, we have the technology and infrastructure to care for complex patients outside acute care hospitals, and we can provide more complex treatments to match the therapy with the disease, the physiology, and even the patient. When serious changes happen, they are initially subtle and ambiguous, yet they must have a strong, educated response. This is what HRO is.

Organizational Change

In the quest for reliability and safety, we look to effective and successful high-risk organizations. We describe safety as a culture, and we focus on error. This removes the desired qualities of high-risk organizations from the contexts and their environments in which they operate. This contributes to the misunderstanding and misinterpretation of the application of HRO principles that prevent failure or contribute to effective failure response. It also creates the oppressive belief that error can occur in a completely novel situation that no one has ever encountered. We reduce actions to decision-making and problem-solving. At their most reductive, reliability and safety become belief-driven factors, independent of the situation and designed as a normative system with an inherent standard of correctness. When we approach things in this reductive manner, we retain strongly held (though maladaptive) beliefs in a futile attempt to design a program for safety and reliability.

High Reliability is contextual, in that these environments give meaning to information while independently carrying information. As a culture, High Reliability is social knowledge developed through the use of technology and effective response to the environment. High Reliability is problem-driven and self-correcting through early error identification and correction. The purpose of High Reliability is to solve interdependent problems to achieve a preferable end-state rather than decompose a situation into independent problems. HRO creates responsiveness in order to change the environment even as the environment changes the organization. To succeed, people must change and be willing to change.

Change occurs not only through response to environments but through leadership. Some leaders are unwilling to change, or they adapt the principles of High Reliability and safety culture to their beliefs in a manner that will allow them to continue their belief systems without change. Because the High Reliability Organization operates in uncertain environments, when the system loses its internal logic, the leaders cannot know which beliefs and behaviors will be necessary for the next situation. For this reason, HROs rely heavily on specific embodied attitudes and decision processes. Though difficult to effectively teach, leaders can readily model these attitudes and decision processes. That is the crux of the problem and the change toward HRO: the leader must openly embody these attitudes and decision processes and model them for other members of the organization to learn.

Conclusions

(1). High Reliability Organizing (HRO) originated as an operational approach for dangerous environments but is readily adaptable to business or healthcare environments.

(2). High Reliability emerges within an organization when an individual person, supported by the organization, engages a discrepancy or system disruption.

(3). High Reliability amalgamates two distinct processes: preventing system failure and responding to system failure.

(4). High Reliability is a mind-set, a way of thinking at all times, that captures the crisis in its early, more responsive stage.

(5). The five principles of HRO, as described by Weick and Sutcliffe, are derived directly from attitudes and normal operations that are adaptive to the unexpected.

(6). HRO is a behavior of individual people, teams, and the organization as a whole.

CHAPTER 2

What Problem Does HRO Solve?

HRO solves the problem of operations and performance in a volatile, uncertain, complex, ambiguous (VUCA) environment.

The Environment

High Reliability Organizing developed as a means to engage confusing, threatening situations with minimal technology, often by teams of less experienced people led by those with greater experience. It is now being adapted to more diverse environments and situations for use by a larger array of organizations. Understanding these environments and the limits of cognitive function in these situations will provide a better grasp of what HRO can accomplish.

VUCA—Volatile, Uncertain, Complex, Ambiguous

In 1995, US Army researchers working in the Carlisle (Pennsylvania) Barracks described the global environment that had developed at the end of the Cold War as VUCA: *volatile, uncertain, complex,* and *ambiguous*. We may find ourselves in similar situations in which we must act before we fully know the situation or before we know what treatment will assuredly work.

Volatility comes from the compression of time in which the leader must act (R. R. Magee 1998). We see this in the healthcare field when a disease process initiates events that rapidly cascade toward a final common pathway of cardiac and respiratory failure, followed by death. Interventions will be the most effective, and will cause the least complication, if they are performed as early as possible in the course of the disease. We want to block the development of unrecoverable failure, whether the failure comes from our actions or from the disease process.

It is the propensity for rapid change that causes time compression, which is a different entity than time-dependence (see below).

Uncertainty describes our lack of precise knowledge about the situation, our need to obtain more information, and the possibility that the information we need may not be available. Many of our protocols, in order to be used, rely on us knowing what the situation is (or at the minimum, defining the situation). But we often find ourselves in a position where we must act before we know the situation (and therefore before we know which protocol to use).

Complexity refers to the large number of interconnected and changing parts that come together to create the situation. Complexity arises from our choices of treatments and the complications that can arise in the process. Much of our planning, and all protocols, rely on predictability. As complexity increases, however, predictability decreases. Complexity also interferes with our choice of protocols when the situation may indicate several protocols competing or conflicting with one another.

Ambiguity describes how multiple interpretations, causes, or outcomes may be possible for one situation. Ambiguity describes how we can fail even though we did everything right or how two people can come to different conclusions when they have the same information. Because of ambiguity, the wrong course of action may look correct until a dramatic failure occurs. Ambiguity also explains how people can differ strongly in their interpretation of a situation. To a great degree, *doubt* is a good accompaniment to ambiguity, as it can prevent premature conclusions or premature diagnoses. Doubt and ambiguity are drivers to preoccupy us with failure (van Stralen 2015).

To operate in the VUCA environment, the US military recognizes that people must have operational flexibility and be provided with a broad range of options (Schmidt 1995). In this chapter, we will discuss how authority to decide can be safely and reliably migrated to the point of the problem.

A perfect example of VUCA in action is the military flight training associated with a low-altitude power loss (LAPL) in single-engine aircraft. All military pilots, from their first day on the flight line, remember the "turn, climb, check, determine, deliver" protocol. This is ingrained from day one because of the criticality of returning to the departure airfield (if practical); gaining altitude (note that to gain altitude, the plane will lose airspeed, which is a worthy exchange for additional time); checking vital instruments; and radioing in a Mayday call to alert the field of a potential impending disaster. This situation ties closely to another ingrained maxim in aviation emergency management: "aviate, navigate, and communicate." This maxim charges the pilot with proper, logical prioritization of actions in order to maintain safe flight despite facing a potentially life-threatening emergency. Get this wrong, and it's invariably fatal. It is the ultimate example of having "skin in the game."

A pilot's maxim for an unexpected crisis is to:

- *aviate*: first, always fly the plane;
- *navigate*: ascertain the desired direction, then fly toward it;
- *communicate*: let others know your situation.

Time compression in the High Reliability situation (HRS) differs from time dependence as used in the decision-making or cognitive literature and time pressure in the psychological literature. An HRS is that situation where the elements of HRO come into operation for prevention, capture, or resolution.

Time is the measure of sequential relations in irreversible succession. Temporal logic (see chapter 3: "Logic of Operations") describes the logic of time sequences. We more commonly discuss time within emergency situations as "time pressure" or "time dependence."

Time pressure, which represents actions that cannot be postponed, is a psychological stress in which people perceive (whether their perception is correct or not) that they have less time available to perform tasks or achieve results than they require. This results in a narrowing of focus and the use of intuition and heuristics. Heuristics are rules-of-thumb we use as shortcuts to reach an answer more quickly. Decision-making distorts from objective processes and the use of the executive functions in the brain to subjective intuition, biases, and heuristics. (The executive functions describe how the brain synthesizes information for the control of behavior.) The psychological stress alone impairs cognitive function (Arnsten 2009). Organizations become overloaded when information exceeds the ability to be processed (Weick and Sutcliffe 2008). The processes of HRO increase the capacity to process information at the level of the organization (Weick and Sutcliffe 2008) and individual (this book). Therefore, we will not directly discuss time pressure as a subject.

Time-dependence has several uses. We discuss time with duration and time intervals, but time dependence generally does not allow an overlap of events. Time-dependence can indicate that an event will occur at a specific time or after a specific time interval, or that it will occur in a time window after certain other events have taken place. Time-dependence can also describe an event that is contingent on the occurrence of another event as a logical sequence. Time-dependence also includes the concept of "rate-limiting," a method that controls the rate of the process. This can be intentional, or it can be beyond the influence of the operator.

Note that time-dependence describes time as a continuously flowing ribbon, river, or road, which is consistent with "monochronic time" as a cultural factor in "low-context" cultures (Hall 1966). Monochronic time is sequential, therefore planning and scheduling are important. In monochronic time ("chrono," Greek for time) people do one thing at a time. Compare to "monochromic," an art term describing a range of tones of a single color. Events, because they tend to be discrete and sequential, do not distract, thus facilitating the ability to concentrate and utilize time management. The focus is on *when* results must be achieved, which is a form of time-dependence.

"High-context" cultures use "polychronic time," doing multiple things at the same time and becoming easily distracted while readily accepting disruptions. Edward T. Hall described these concepts differentiating high and low context cultures. Whether the environment, or context, contains necessary information distinguishes the two cultures. It is fairly easy to see that HRO aligns more closely with a high-context culture. This may contribute to resistance accepting HRO, those who believe organizing is "portable," that is, it can fit any organization independent of the environment, may have a hard time accepting methods of organizing that depend on local information or information in the environment.

Time-variance describes a system with output characteristics that are explicitly dependent on time. In time-variant systems, certain parameters or influences change with time; the system responds differently to the same input, depending on when it occurs. Linear time-variant systems are linear because they follow an equation and time-variant because variability over time (time is a variable) creates a wave form in the shape of a repeated horizontal "S" described as sinusoid. The time variable gives this "sinusoidal cycling" an associated uncertainty principle, what we are measuring will change with time. The more famous is Heisenberg's uncertainty principle when a wave equation is used to determine a particle's momentum, then we do know where it is along the wave form. To know its position, we must stop the particle but then it has no velocity. In a time-invariant system, output is not a direct function of time.

Time compression suggests the objective reduction of time of events pressing together compared to the subjective reduction of time perceived with time pressure. In temporal logic (see chapter 3, "Logic of Operations"), density is the measure of an instant between two instants or events. Time density is a measure of continuous time rather than discrete time (such as with integers). Events can overlap, interact, converge, or branch. Events can also have different time scales (time densities), even when they occur in parallel, which leads to the confusion and complexity of the HRS; unless we recognize this nature of time compression it can impair plans and organizing,

This is similar to the cultural concept of time in "high-context" cultures (Hall 1966). Tasks will be completed, but this will occur in their own time rather than due to the efforts of the operator. Because events can occur in parallel, distraction is easier. The focus becomes *what* will be achieved. (See chapter 14, "Culture.") This topic is discussed more fully in that chapter.

Daily VUCA

We encounter VUCA daily. Though our lives do not have the degree of VUCA found in military or public-safety operations, we can expect to encounter disruptive VUCA situations regularly and can use the same HRO principles to combat them.

Volatility brings to mind explosive violence, where we expect our military to operate. Volatility also describes something that is easily changeable, transient, or unstable. Unfortunately, some people are disruptive, and some people use instrumental anger or fear for secondary gain. In addition to these people's contributions to volatility, we also experience volatility whenever we are in rapidly changing situations such as experiencing abrupt weather changes, driving a car, or caring for a toddler. In fact, a toddler's volatility in behavior, the natural tendency to rapidly change, contributes to the accidental death rate of toddlers: they can overdose on drugs, ingest poison, drown, or run behind a car before the driver becomes aware that the child is missing.

Uncertainty is the norm in life. To know things with certainty, we must observe, interact, and evaluate—actions that are not possible due to time and physical constraints as well as the limitations of our cognitive abilities. The prevalence of uncertainty may be what drives some people to adopt a level of certitude that makes them comfortable, though that comfort is not necessarily based on context or reality. Certitude is possible because limited environmental adversity causes few severe consequences.

Complexity arises whenever interactions occur in a disproportionate manner. For example, providing seating for two people with two chairs is simple. But if you change the age of the people and the size of the chairs and then add a person and mix the ages and genders, then predicting seating arrangements now becomes impossible without having more information.

Complexity cannot be wished away; someone will always find a complicating factor. Because complexity is difficult to work with, it provides an impetus to simplify. With simplification, we lose information and relationships. On the other hand, complexity intrigues many people, since we can connect what is visible and detectable into patterns with explanations that are pleasing to the mind. What we actually sense is the topography of the situation—that is, the surface that is visible or made visible. Beneath this surface are nonlinear interactions, undetectable causations, and emerging properties we find only with time or interaction. This results in simplification of the complex and complexification of the simple.

Ambiguity can represent two equally acceptable meanings for the same thing or two equally acceptable responses for the same stimulus. This can cause arguments. Ask for a spatula in the kitchen, and you can either get a broad flat blade for flipping pancakes or a broad flat flexible blade for removing liquids from a container. This can also start conversations. When meeting new people, ask "soda or pop?" People will spontaneously state their preferred term for a carbonated soft drink. Where this becomes critical is when people converge to work together without realizing how common ambiguity is.

Threat and VUCA: VUCA-T

People outside of the military are increasingly using the concept of a VUCA environment. It is important to remember, though, that this concept is a *military* concept, and military professionals have the implicit assumption that they work in a dangerous and lethal environment of "going in harm's way" (per John Paul Jones). To that end, we must address how threats can cause fear as well as the effect that fear has on thinking, decision-making, and action.

We often disregard threats in the environment.

Fight, flight, and freeze constitute the "fear response" in humans. The brain responds to fear or stress in the stereotypical fashion commonly referred to as "fight or flight." We include the freeze response, common to prey species, and the choke response found during acts of physical performance. Stress and fear impair cognitive function, which is something not well recognized or described in the decision-making or problem-solving literature but well described in the neurophysiology literature. Stress-impaired cognition is vital for us to appreciate, because people lose their ability to carry out plans and rely on cognitive processes when they act in response to fear.

It is simplest to think of the fear responses as fighting or running away from the threat. When we think this way, however, we fail to recognize the variety of fear responses and how commonly they occur. It also becomes easy to dismiss the presence of stress responses in our own thinking and behaviors or the degree to which they interfere with our daily routines.

Fear responses drive actions toward self-preservation and impair the prefrontal cortex (Arnsten 2009), which is the location of executive functions and planning. Less appreciated and unrecognized in the heat of the moment, fear responses distort the higher cognitive functions of working memory, mental imagery, and willed action. We have even come to think that some of these functions, such as anger, are normal or justified, but we fail to recognize the impairment they have on an angry person. Yet, not only do they impair the person, but they also impair the performance of the target person and those who witness the behavior (Flin 2010).

Fear, in the form of "fight," manifests itself by anger and frustration, while as "flight" it takes the form of avoidance and distraction. "Freeze" is confusion, and "mental freeze" is the inability to recall knowledge or use working memory. Not only do these responses come from extrinsic sources; they can also come from intrinsic sources such as a supervisor pressuring somebody mentally until he or she cannot recall information (the freeze response). This creates a cycle of increased pressure from the supervisor forcing the person deeper into the freeze response, thus causing the supervisor to apply more pressure, thinking it will motivate the person to respond. The only result is the loss of an important asset (the person). Because these distortions are driven by the situation, we call them "situational-cognitive distortions."

> "I saw adrenaline and cortisol wash over the team and create fear." The physician was describing an airway emergency with his team, where they had worked diligently and smoothly to acquire and protect the patient's airway. Then an anesthesiologist ran into the room, shouting and making demands. The team looked up and, as a unit, froze. This fed into the anesthesiologist's emotional state and resulted in a more vociferous response, as if a louder voice and more rapid speech would bring the team back to life.
>
> The child was saved, but the team made fewer calls for anesthesiology assistance after that.
>
> Personal Communication to Daved van Stralen

We can quite easily observe these threat responses in others, like the anesthesiologist and the medical team mentioned above, but we may not have recognized the responses as being a consequence of fear or a threat. And we certainly have not accepted them as a result of poor leadership or teamwork. These behaviors we call "unrecognized fear responses." These responses, as mentioned above, impair the performance of others around the person and the team itself. Unrecognized fear responses contribute to the atmosphere one feels when entering a program with poor leadership and teamwork.

Some people can operate in the face of threats or when in danger. It is perhaps from their life experience, specific training they have undergone, or mental and psychological conditioning, but they are able to modulate the fear response to achieve effective performance in threat environments. Fear motivates and drives their actions, as it does others who are unable to modulate their physical and psychological reactions. It is possibly through metacognition that they are able to continue thinking clearly. We call this the "threat response" to differentiate this response from the distorting or incapacitating effects that arise from the fear response.

We will use the term "VUCA-T" to acknowledge the effect of situational threats in the VUCA environment.

Just as the US Army has made VUCA part of its operational environment, we in healthcare also use VUCA-T in our operational environments. Decision-making programs must (1) allow for time compression in volatile medical situations, (2) accept the uncertainty and ambiguity of limited or unavailable information, (3) support the demand to act, and (4) realize the complexity of the patient's physiology complicates the response to disease *and* treatments. Above all, decision-making programs must account for *situational cognitive distortions* and *unrecognized fear responses*.

> Ron Perkin, MD, FAAP, FCCM, explained to me how he taught airway intubation for a child, which is a stressful procedure in most systems. After sedating the child, he had the nurse administer a muscle relaxant, which paralyzed the muscles. The team urgently began the procedure of placing the airway tube, but Ron stopped them. He told each person to hand-ventilate the child in turn. With his presence and with real-time blood-gas monitoring, this was safe to do. Once the team became calm, he proceeded with the intubation. He wanted the team to understand that the mask ventilation was the true emergency therapy and that each person on the team was capable of successfully performing that critical task. When mask ventilation is done well, placing the airway tube is no longer an emergency.
>
> —Daved van Stralen

Threat and fear responses disrupt normal human thought processes.

Internal Logic of the System

We all have an internal logic for how we view and understand the world. Private and public internal logics also exist; private logic is how people intimately explain events only to themselves and a few trusted others, while public logic is how people openly tell their stories and what they openly expect in a situation. This is not a trivial distinction; private logic is quite visible in the first few minutes or hours after a tragedy as events expose the raw beliefs of each person. Because we otherwise have no access to people's intimate internal logic, some behaviors and beliefs may not make sense to us unless we appreciate their private internal logic.

This is the world of storytelling: how people describe and understand situations and events and how they make sense of their actions. When someone talks about events, a consistent set of rules governs and defines that person's universe. These rules of their narrative affect their understanding of the event as it unfolds, how they interpret the results, and how they tell their story. This is how they explain but also how they understand.

We will hear this internal logic, and the shift from private to public, when we listen to their descriptions or we interview them after events have occurred. First, they make sense to themselves, then the story seems to change as they begin to make sense to others. This is not falsity; listen for their internal logic, as it will help explain their actions and how they will act next time.

In a logical or mathematical system, *internal logic* is (1) concrete, (2) empirical in that it is known from experience, (3) particular to the situation rather than a generalization, and (4) contextual or context dependent, in that the local environment influences the system (Smirnov 1988; Vasyukov 1999). Internal validity is "local" truth. Internal logic is the logic of experience; the internal validity for empirical *experience.*

On the other hand, *external logic* is (1) abstract (symbolic, conceptual, or theoretical) and independent of the real world, (2) forms a "topological space" (a mathematical term for a conceptual space that can be mathematically deformed), (3) unites forces and actions in a continuous way, and (4) is structured with categories of objects. External logic describes the functions *between* categories and objects and expected transformations between the objects ("coherence") (Smirnov 1988; Vasyukov 1999). External logic is the logic of science, the external validity for empirical *experimentation.*

This is also not a trivial digression. In the sciences (*episteme*), we are objective and we obtain our evidence-based conclusions independent of the environment. In High Reliability Situations (HRS), events are context dependent, and the operator or agent performs in a pragmatic, practical scale. Practical wisdom (*phronesis*) combines the internal logic of the local system and local truths with the community values necessary to act for the common good rather than self-interest.

Appreciating the presence of the internal logic of systems and processes allows us to make inferences, predictions, plans, and designs for systems and organizations *from* the situation. The VUCA-T environment disrupts the expected internal logic of the environment with a different internal system logic. Minor disruptions—and how to understand the new internal logic—are more commonly learned through reflective experience and practice. During extreme situations, people experience a loss of the internal logic of the system as well as within themselves. The person must then engage a situation having only imperfect information with threat impairing the ability to think clearly. The person now has limited ability for sensemaking and inference.

What this means is that we can no longer logically predict what will happen or what other structures and elements exist in the system. Even though the elements may look familiar, how they are constructed and derived is not familiar.

> "I may not know what's happening, but I know what to do."
> —Firefighter, Los Angeles City Fire Department

Rationality and Reason

Healthcare consists of numerous sciences-medical, surgical, nursing, laboratory, social sciences and so on. We take this basis of science to mean we are rational and objective, and use the methods of critical. This belief works well for slower, deliberate processes but the turbulence and uncertainty of the HRS confuses any information we can collect. The threat inherent to demands for action in this turbulence is compounded when the threat is directed at us.

This describes the limits of rationality and reason. The methods used to reach HRO are effective in these situations. This section introduces these limits and introduces methods to maintain cognitive performance.

Unpredictability—Stochastic and Indeterminate Processes

What makes the High Reliability situation difficult for thinking and operations is the loss of predictability. Of course, this comes from the loss of the internal logic of the system, and the elements of VUCA-T prevent any ability to effectively predict, except over short time periods. What VUCA-T and the loss of logic contribute is based on the loss of predictable or stable probability and from nonlinear interactions from which new properties emerge to influence the system.

Probability values can act as parameters with different values for different functions or distributions. That is, the probability at one state is not the probability for the same system in another state. For example, the probability of brain damage occurring from lack of oxygen changes with the patient's body temperature. If we do not know the parameter (in this case, it is temperature), then we can experience changing probabilities, even though all reactions remain the same. This situation describes the stochastic state. (The term "stochastic" is derived from the Greek word for conjecture.)

Indeterminate processes are the result of the nonlinear or undetectable interactions in the VUCA-T environment. In a determinate system, the state variables and known interactions determine the outcome; for indeterminate processes, this does not happen.

In healthcare, the sciences provide predictability and explanations. The scientific method is the bedrock on which modern medical care is founded and is our method of thinking and problem-solving. This mind-set makes it difficult to understand or accept other ways of thinking and problem-solving during medical emergencies. It makes it easier, instead, to adopt approaches that appear logical and rational in low-tempo periods. Problematically, these comfortable non-emergent strategies tend to fail during unexpected crises. We have a false certainty that predictability brings our future into our present. Unpredictability forces us to enact, or create, our future. The solid, linear methods used for predictability will certainly fail in the unpredictable state.

Hospitals have committees that create and validate plans, protocols, and clinical pathways, among other things. These are best efforts to effectively apply medical science and good judgment to what can be expected and the skill and knowledge set of the bedside caregiver. This is work as planned or work as imagined.

In some cases, the disease does not progress as predicted, treatments do not work as advertised, necessary information is lost or unavailable, and we encounter limits of human perception. This is work as performed.

The difference between "work as planned" and "work as performed" is the gap where HRO operates.

The processes an HRO uses often appear counterintuitive, which makes acceptance difficult. This is because our education and practice are based on scientific rationality. We must remember that experimental scientific studies control the environment and as many elements as possible in order to explain the results and predict later outcomes. In the VUCA-T environment, we have lost predictability, and explanations become only temporary grounding points that help us move toward our next step.

Unpredictability is associated with complexity or chaos theory, but not all situations are completely unpredictable or without probability calculations. Stochastic states develop when the variable(s) have varying probabilities. That is, the situation is similar to solving an equation where the probability value of the variable frequently changes with time, or a series of equations with different probabilities are used in each equation. This produces a rational system that is solvable by equation, except for the fact that the *probability value keeps changing.*

Most of our situations in medicine will be stochastic—that is, rational and even predictable when we know the probability at a particular moment, but the probability value will change. This explains why we can predict things over very short time periods but not over longer time sequences.

Probabilistic thinking limits the imagination of what can happen. To a negative person, imagination of what can happen can also lead to overprotection. The idea of what is possible, and how to prepare using only what the organization has at the time, can create effective and appropriately constrained improvisation in the HRS.

> "It is conceivable that healthcare deals as much with possibilities as with probabilities. Possibilities would suggest that sensemaking is more crucial."
> —KARL WEICK, PERSONAL COMMUNICATION

Probabilities can, and will, change during a process, thus interfering with our ability to predict. To act effectively we must use sensemaking strongly interactive with the situation in real-time as it evolves. This is one reason for "interactive, real-time sensemaking," a slight alteration of Bob Bea's aphorism, "interactive, real-time risk assessment and management," (personal communication).

The ability to plan assumes predictability, or at least some degree of predictability. It was the inability of an organization to adjust plans for discrepancies and disruptions that led Weick to identify the importance of *sensitivity to operations* (Weick, personal communication). He found that organizations typically continue their processes without change or become tightly focused on the unpredictable problem, at the expense of strategic operations.

This is not to diminish the importance of plans or planning, which is the foundation for the control-operator structure of HRO and a principal means of *preventing* system failure in a high-risk program. The control-operator structure requires predictability for reliable rules and safe, functional processes. But even the control operator must shift operations when a discrepancy or disruption occurs. This is the importance of responsiveness at the site of discrepancy or at the time of interruption, the foundation for the emergency-responder structure of HRO. The ability to easily and rapidly shift between stable and unpredictable environments is the hallmark of a true HRO. To summarize:

- the control operator relies on predictability to prevent system failure;
- the emergency responder operates with limited predictability;
- the ability to shift between the two approaches creates High Reliability.

The operational distinction between control operator and emergency responder demonstrates the boundary between the environment where safety culture and lean Six Sigma can operate with predictability and control (the control operator) and the disruptive environment of the emergency responder. Lean Six Sigma without HRO becomes simply orthodoxy and becomes independent of particulars and context. The principles of HRO can adapt lean Six Sigma to the unexpected and to crises.

The control-operator approach may be seen in the design of HRO's policies and procedures to *prevent* failure. It is not uncommon for people to believe they will not make an error; they, themselves, can be trusted. Control operations is not a matter of error-free operations; it is about the system and demands on the system over time. Specialists are not always present during a disruption in operations. For Jens Rasmussen (1983), this is the rule-based structure in his "skill-rule-knowledge" format. For James Reason (1990), the vulnerability in control operations is rule-based errors such as the strong-but-wrong rule, where the operator adheres to the rule, or any rule, regardless of circumstances.

The emergency-responder approach may be seen in the design of standing orders or protocols, which are written in an effort to migrate discretion to the operator at the point of contact. The fullest manifestation of the emergency response is the temporary cessation of rules in a crisis, since the rules, at that time, do not apply.

HRO is the duality of these two approaches; they are not sequential or parallel. While in emergency response, the HRO also prevents system failure, and while it is preventing system failure, people realize they are on the verge of failure. Anything unrecognized or unintended can initiate an unexpected, disruptive event.

By convention, we solve problems stepwise from problem definition to a solution: define the problem, identify the objective, collect information, then generate and evaluate alternatives. Scientific rationality and classical logic move us to the ideal solution.

Thinking: Vertical, Horizontal (Lateral), and Critical
Vertical thinking and critical thinking, by convention, are the more commonly taught and accepted cognitive processes. Vertical thinking is linear, selective, analytical, and sequential; one works within a frame of reference and discards what is not relevant (De Bono 2010). Vertical thinking "drills down" into the problem,

which is a better approach for deterministic processes (i.e., the situation determines our actions, and our actions determine our results).

Vertical thinking is so embedded in most people's problem-solving approach that it becomes their default selection under stress or fear. It is in extreme situations where drilling down into the problem causes people to "cone" their attention and have single-minded focus, disregarding the surrounding environment. In fear conditions, people become severely reductionist and overly concrete in their thinking. We lose the richness of complexity and abstract thought.

For some types of processes, we are better served with nonlinear *lateral thinking*, where we utilize multiple disciplines to find a practical solution. For example, in stochastic or indeterminate processes, probabilities are not known, or the probability constantly changes. In this process, we must use care, as it is possible to lose information when we horizontally or laterally cross into a new discipline or science. This is particularly true when others on the team are not familiar with the new discipline. We more fully develop this idea in chapter 3, "The Logic of Practice and the Logic of Operations."

Critical thinking requires the formulation of clear questions and problems, the collection and assessment of relevant information, and the use of scientific rationality in classical logic to reach a conclusion or solution. With critical thinking, an error can be evaluated and corrected, but in the VUCA-T environment, an error can become deadly in the time required to fully identify the problem or formulate a clear question. Sufficient relevant information may be unavailable or changing. Scientific rationality becomes bounded by our perception, and information that comes in a form for use in classical logic is far too restrictive and slowly obtained for practical operations.

The problem of unpredictability is that minor issues can become highly dangerous, while apparently major issues might resolve themselves. We may ignore our vulnerabilities until too late or take credit for actions that, in reality, had no effect on a positive outcome.

The Legal Significance of Formal Training in Critical Thinking

Mike Johns, an assistant US attorney and senior litigation counsel, defended many physicians and wildland firefighters in the federal courts. HRO lost a strong advocate when he passed away early in 2017. For decision-making queries, both sides in the courts often bring in experts in decision-making cases. It was his firm belief that formal training in critical thinking (CT) and decision-making would obviate much of the need for these experts and shorten testimony on the decision-making methods that are commonly used.

The red card reflects that the person is qualified by training, experience, and certification by a qualified instructor to perform a specific position, such as incident commander or firing boss. I do contend that wildland firefighters become red-carded in decision-making to (1) reduce normal human decision errors and (2) provide evidence in after-accident reviews or litigation that the people who are making the decisions are not just subject-matter experts in their field but are experts in decision-making. If we could also produce evidence that their organizations were in fact implementing critical thinking as dialogue and similar HRO principles, I think it would reduce the tendency to misjudge during hindsight situations and litigation.

A great deal of information is available about hindsight bias. I once even retained an expert attorney-psychologist in that field in a medical malpractice case I defended to testify about the subject; in that case, I retained two medical experts and gave them the same medical file to review, but I withheld the bad outcome from one. As expected, the expert with outcome knowledge was critical of the care, while the expert who lacked outcome knowledge had a few irrelevant concerns but did not see any violation of the standard of care. The results in studies on visual-hindsight bias when reading medical films with outcome knowledge are startling. In litigation, having evidence of expertise in decision-making can open the door to the broader opportunity to educate the court and avoid making biased decisions, rather than just paying lip service to not judging in hindsight.

Critical-thinking skills could be taught. If sufficient staff time is available, for example, using CT as dialogue with another staff member could reduce decision errors. If staff remain shorthanded, it may be difficult to implement CT as dialogue among investigators if the staff have no time to discuss their own cases. Supervisors could possibly perform this function with the investigators.

—Michael A. Johns, assistant US attorney, senior litigation counsel

---

The Limits of Scientific Rationality and Logic

The VUCA-T environment and its necessary processes place a practical limit on scientific rationality and logic. Unpredictability, nonlinear sequences and reactions, stochastic probabilities, and imperfect information all confound the reliable use of scientific rationality. Overlapping categories and ambiguity both interfere with the ability to infer new information from unreliable sources, which prevents the use of classical logic to evaluate events in real time. Threat and subsequent fear responses involving situational cognitive distortions interfere with the perception necessary to evaluate and identify relevant information.

Scientific rationality is generally concerned more with theory than practice and utilizes discrete concepts and categories. Scientific logic—the ability to infer new information from existing information—is also linear and discrete, meaning that categories do not overlap. It is clear, then, that complete reliance on scientific rationality and classical logic is a misguided approach that can quickly become dangerous.

Diseases are discrete entities that physicians diagnose; medical conditions are discrete entities that other healthcare providers treat. For recording information and discussion, we keep diseases and medical conditions as discrete entities. But the complexities of healthcare include the confounding variables involved, any complicating diseases and conditions, unique physiological responses, and, most critically, the patient. This all limits our ability to rigorously apply scientific rationality.

When an emergency occurs and we encounter the stochastic or indeterminate process, it quickly becomes clear that the logic of the situation or system is lost and that we must, somehow, infer reliable information from the unreliable situation. Our categories overlap and are no longer discrete and separate, our discrete scientific concepts may not easily align with the continuous spectrum of our perceptions (Weick 2011; Wolfberg 2006), and time may branch out in unexpected directions.

Logic is the process of inferring new information from current information. We must develop a new *logic of practice* and a new *practical rationality*. In an HRO, we are concerned with both theory *and* practice and how they are dynamically balanced between each other (Sandberg and Tsoukas 2011). That is, theory comes from science that is empirically developed in a well-controlled environment and/or deduced from known facts and accepted theories. Practice occurs in different environments, with limited and imperfect information bounded by our personal cognitive abilities. When we encounter a situation that is not explained by scientific theory, our responses can range from rejecting our science to rejecting our observations. To summarize:

- science is measured, independent of context, and objective;
- practice is variable, dependent on context, and subjective;

- HRO works between the two, bridging if not combining science and practice.

The Indeterminate Problem

The problems encountered in the VUCA-T environment are not precisely fixed or not easily established, a problem compounded by the undefined boundaries of the problem that can reach into the local environment. This is the *indeterminate problem*, which consists of the three independent elements of *uncertainty*, *time compression*, and *threat*.

Uncertainty means more than not having information. Counterintuitively, uncertainty *contains* information, or rather information is a measure of uncertainty. Claude Shannon measured the entropy of information as the *increase* in uncertainty, or randomness, during communication. The change in certainty is measured as entropy. Shannon founded the field of information theory, and his work forms the basis of today's digital information systems. (Shannon also coined the computer term "bit," short for binary digit.)

Shannon considered information somewhat equivalent to energy. We lose some energy by using it and transmitting energy over powerlines is one way we use energy. In a similar manner, we transmit information through communication, one way we use information. He discovered through mathematical means that some information is lost through its use just as some energy is lost when we use energy. The same equation in calculus is shared by thermodynamic entropy and information entropy. We may be familiar with the loss of electrical energy from resistance through transmission in power lines, as this dissipated energy is energy that is unavailable for work. The same concept applies to losing information from noise through the transmission of information (i.e., communication).

He described the most basic information as a digital system—such as heads or tails, converted to 1 or 0—to denote certainty and uncertainty. Shannon considered uncertainty to be information, reasoning that if someone tells you something you already know, you have not gained any information. If someone tells you something you do not know, then you have gained information. This is important for us to consider because, by converting uncertainty to certainty, we have created information. In Shannon's information theory, information is the measure of uncertainty; greater uncertainty means a greater gain of information.

Uncertainty Drives Us to Create Information

Shannon is also a major figure in communication theory. Communication consists of a chain of encoding, transmission, and decoding of information, as shown in figure 1 below. Loss of certainty occurs due to noise (think of distractions or false alarms) and can occur at any point along the chain of communication. In this model, information is a static value, though its degree of certainty is not static but can change during communication.

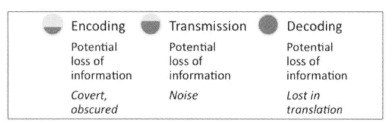

Figure 1—Communication chain

The encoding of information occurs when we collect information about an event and prepare it for transmission. We would like the information to be salient and helpful. These are elements of the affective domain of knowledge and are easily overlooked when focusing on cognitive information.

Information that is *objective, articulate,* and stated in a *succinct* manner is less likely to become corrupted. Though redundancy and the use of a sharp, clear, honest signal both reduce signal corruption, in the "noisy," time-compressed environment, directness of language and behavior may better replace signal redundancy. This directness may come across as harsh in the absence of healthy relationships created before the crisis; if that was not possible, the directness can be softened with humor (see chapter 9, "Threat Responses and Unrecognized Fear"). In healthcare, a team-development program called TeamSTEPPS (Team Strategies and Tools to Enhance Performance and Patient Safety) acts as a toolkit for structured, organized communication that reduces signal loss and noise.

While it may be easy to assume people know that "objective" means without prejudice or bias, they are still likely to insert their opinions and interpretations at some point. Interpretation that is representational of the message for informa-tion flow changes the objective to subjective, while interpretation of the salience of information is a legitimate part of sensemaking.

Many people find it difficult to present objective information without some persuasive effort. In the individual, it may mark inexperience, while in a group of people it may reflect distrust in others or in the system. Complete objectivity is impossible to achieve, because we give the greatest importance to the first thing we hear.

We want the information to be articulate so that it makes sense—that is, the following item is expected and flows from the previous item. Giving information to the receiver out of order the receiver expects is disruptive to reception and risks corrupting communication. The order of information alone will bias the receiver. We can think of articulate (the adjective form of the word) as being fluid, with clarity and effectiveness, but in teaching this concept, we find the verb form (as used in zoology) to be more useful, for example in describing the organization of bones in a skeleton through specific joints. For example, the radius and ulna articulate to humerus which articulates to the scapula and clavicle connecting the lower arm to the arm to the shoulder.

This is a source of miscommunication between different healthcare professions. For example, nurses commonly present the patient by systems, with the problem and treatment provided when each system is presented. The physician presents all the information first, followed by his or her impressions, and ends with the plan and treatments. A nurse may present one problem to the physician and then wait for a reply, while the physician is waiting for the rest of the presentation.

Succinct communication is a separate problem. We do not want extraneous information, or information that is noncontributory. But this goes back to the problem of salience—what is salient to the transmitter and the receiver can differ significantly. This is different from redundancy, where, by design, additional information reduces confusion but can also inadvertently increase the significance of specific parts of the message. This is the source of humor when we see a slide presentation showing how words can be removed from a sentence or paragraph without changing the meaning. What is lost in these presentations is that many of those removed words had the purpose of focusing meaning or bringing out importance.

Information for encoding should be objective, articulate, and succinct. We *identify* what is salient and categorize the information. We then *interpret* the information by placing it in context and giving it meaning. Depending on who we are giving the information to, we may *translate* it into a form the person can better understand.

Information can become corrupted at this point from the use of words and phrases that are trite, ambiguous, clichéd; words that are unique to a specialty (jargon); or words that are developed to separate one group from others (slang).

The act of communication itself can corrupt information. Our methods and purpose in communication is to *identify, interpret,* and *translate.* Communication can corrupt information.

> The medical center assigned me, as a hospital dietitian, to a committee on malnutrition. The purpose was to develop a program for nurses and various physician specialists to understand the threats, causes, prevalence, and incidence of malnutrition in the hospital. To help them understand how we concluded a patient had malnutrition, and to what degree, I described the scientific information and methods plus factors included in the judgment dietitians used to *identify* malnutrition. The overlapping categories and ambiguity of some of the data required registered dietitians to *interpret* this information to find the degree or severity of malnutrition. I then *translated* this information to each group: malnutrition contributes to decubitus ulcers (i.e., bedsores), important for nursing; it reduces the body's ability to make antibodies and perform immune functions, important to internists; and it impedes wound healing, which contributes to dehiscence (the opening of a surgically closed wound), important to surgeons.
>
> —FEBRA JOHNSON

In High Reliability situations, some of our actions are meant to create information and to change uncertain information toward certainty. This is an interactive approach to identifying what we can know and what we cannot know in the moment. This approach is not really one of error or mistake, as any response—desired, undesired, or unchanged—creates information and adds to our knowledge of the system and what is likely to work. While the value of desired and undesired responses is clear, the value of unchanged responses is not. We do not know the reason for no change: Was it the wrong dose, wrong drug, wrong disease, or some other cause? No response to therapy is a common marker or herald of hidden vulnerability.

Ambiguity is the form of uncertainty we can characterize as being more like "dynamic uncertainty" (van Stralen 2015). Ambiguity is far more difficult, though, because for uncertainty we need only gather or create information to develop knowledge. In ambiguity, we must also give *meaning* to the information. This meaning commonly comes from the context in which it lies, as well as our experience.

We give meaning to ambiguous information, most often by interacting with it. Time, as segmented and scheduled in today's culture, easily becomes reduced to a constant and continuous flow of single-point events. This is the model we use today:

scheduling events and measuring time in increments. Today, five minutes is the smallest increment for planning, with days or weeks reserved for more logistic work. As an example, being late in the 1950s was generally considered in fifteen-minute increments; today it is closer to five minutes (Hall 1959, 140). This creates problems when we create protocols based on time segments of five minutes when the actual emergency, being continuous, may demand turnaround responses of minutes, if not the seconds necessary in public-safety or military operations. Time as a path we follow fits well with the concept of time-dependence: that events will occur or responses must be made at certain points amenable to scheduling.

The HRO event compresses time, which makes it difficult to sort out cause-and-effect and discrete events. Time also overlaps, as multiple sequences have their own time flow. The "non-HRO" concept of time as a ribbon or road interferes with the ability to act with effectiveness, whereas "HRO time" better reflects the flux, discontinuities, and parallel interacting events of the VUCA-T environment.

Rather than thinking of time as sequential, single-point events, during which we can schedule actions, an HRO works with time as units of varying lengths; events are allowed to set their own rhythm, and actions take on their own schedule.

Time during an HRO event has a subjective nature related to perception, sensing, cognitive processing, and threat responses. We experience time differently, depending on if we are present *when* the event initiates or accelerates or if we arrive *after* the event started. If the event is in progress, then it is in effect ahistorical, in that we do not have any history of antecedent events. Time compression occurs when the time necessary to process pertinent information interferes with the time available to rectify the situation. By imposing our own rhythm and our own time schedule, we lose information and release our control to the event itself.

Emergencies are *ahistorical* events: we cannot reliably know all that led up to that moment.

Threat is too readily discounted, and stress is depreciated as affecting only less experienced or weaker people. The impact of stress on decision-making is psychologically and physiologically based, thereby having the potential to render a skilled practitioner less than effective when the effects of stress on the person are not recognized and acted on in a timely manner.

Cognitive Function

Decision-making, problem-solving, planning, and leadership presume not only intact cognitive function but a normative component of how people *ought* to act. This leads to the commonly held conclusion that we can prescribe how to make decisions through training, advice, decision aids, and awareness of biases. What these approaches leave out is (1) the effect of subjective valuation of information at a specific time in a specific place, (2) the effects of stress or fear impairing the executive functions and rationality in the prefrontal cortex, and (3) the situational cognitive distortions that result from unrecognized fear.

This is the element of *relativity*: what may appear rational and logical in one frame during a rapidly evolving event that has both time pressure and great demands may easily appear unreasonable from the more distant reference frame, in which we have full information and without threat or time compression. HRO recognizes and accounts for the effects of stress and perception on cognition and performance.

> In US policing, the concept of relativity is embedded in case law governing the police-force response to suspect resistance or threats. In the US Supreme Court case *Graham v. Connor* (1989), the evaluation of force was based solely on the facts known to the officer at the time, without the benefit of twenty-twenty hindsight. For example, an officer can act on the reasonable belief that a suspect is armed; later, the suspect could be discovered to have, in fact, been unarmed. At the same time, any information that is learned later, such as the suspect having a felony warrant for armed robbery, cannot be used to justify the officer's force choices. It is the *context* of the officer's perception that determines the reasonableness of his or her response, not the actual facts that were unknown to the officer at the time.
> —George Williams, international police force and tactics trainer

A system maintains constancy, or homeostasis, using survival or adaptive responses to threats and stress. This situation can become a problem, because the only responses humans are able to draw upon, for even minor disturbances, evolved for survival in primitive live-or-die situations. These responses can ensure safety during exploration of new situations or in response to adversity. On the other hand, when not adequately modulated or recognized, these responses can combine with environmental adversity to become overreaction, thus creating a downward spiral of failure.

Cognitive dissonance and failure from *not* acting can easily prevent leaders from recognizing the benefit of HRO decision-making. The reduction of cognitive dissonance leads people to use *confirmation bias* (i.e., the acceptance of new information that confirms strongly held beliefs) to justify their decisions and almost any outcome (i.e., underscrutiny), thereby preventing error identification and correction. Confirmation bias also inhibits institutional learning. Another manifestation of cognitive dissonance is *motivated reasoning* (i.e., rejecting new information that *disconfirms* strongly held beliefs, or overscrutiny), which leads to the rejection of early heralds of failure.

The dissonance between beliefs and unaccepted reality is the source of many biases and heuristics. Other causes include the limits of thinking and perception from bounded rationality. Bounded rationality, biases, and heuristics are discussed further in chapter 3, "The Logic of Practice and the Logic of Operations," and are also discussed in chapter 7, "Decision-Making in Healthcare."

In people's misplaced sense of safety and to prevent failure—or more accurately to avoid it—people (particularly leaders) often support *not* acting or engaging a situation, but this creates what Weick (1979. 148) describes as failure from *not* acting. Not acting becomes a failure that is not visible and therefore is not correctable. The suppression of engagement of discrepancies or disruptions then readily becomes a part of organizational knowledge. As a result, the group does not gain experience from engaging particular situations. Moral, academic, or scientific opprobrium is directed at any active person to prevent engagement, as doing so goes against the organizational bias of *not* acting. Any negative outcome is accepted as inevitable or being due to extrinsic, uncontrollable influences.

> "Failure from acting can be identified and
> corrected, creating knowledge;
> Failure from not acting cannot be identified, therefore
> not corrected, becoming organizational knowledge."
> —KARL WEICK

Adversity and the response to adversity depend on a person's perceptions, socialization, physiological state, skills, and numerous other factors. We will discuss this more completely in chapter 9, "Unrecognized Fear." To standardize the concept in our text, we will use "adversity" for all unfavorable conditions to which the individual person or system *must* respond across the broader spectrum from undesirable situations to grave crises and along an "orthogonal" spectrum from subjective (interpreted solely by the individual person) to overtly objective, which is seen by all as a grave danger. Orthogonal, 16th Century French for right angle, refers to statistically independent systems but can be pictured as different spectra that are independent yet intersect.

We will use the term "threat response" for real-time decisions and actions that are directed at the effective engagement of adversity and to maintain homeostasis of the system or organization. In the neurosciences, fear is considered an emotion, specifically emotion as a physiological response that may be objectively measured. Fear, on the other hand, is also the term most often used by the public for the subjective sensation. Thus, while the general public considers fear an emotion, neuroscientists consider this type of emotion a "feeling" rather than the physiological sense of emotion. Fear, in the general public's sense, is commonly considered a weakness, while those in dangerous occupations consider it normal and expected. Not feeling fear is a sign the person does not recognize the threat. How one responds to the fear is more critical for our purposes in an HRO.

These objective threat *responses* are the commonly known fight, flight, and freeze. The subjective fear *feelings* are fear and anxiety. The mechanism for the unconscious response to threat is not the same as the mechanism for the subjective feelings of fear or anxiety (LeDoux 2014). We find useful Joseph LeDoux and Daniel Pine's (2016) distinction between the objective threat response, the subjective feeling of fear, and the subjective experience of anxiety.

- The threat response is unconscious, objectively observable, a suite of reflexive responses, primarily subcortical and amygdala, and primarily occurs when the source of harm is imminent.
- The mental state of fear, as a feeling, is conscious, subjective, primarily cortical, and develops when the source of harm is near.
- The mental state of anxiety, as a feeling, is conscious, subjective, primarily cortical, and develops when the source of harm is uncertain or distant in space or time.

The behaviors we identify with *unrecognized fear* have become incorporated into today's culture as acceptable behaviors, if not norms to be emulated. They arise from the well-known fear responses of fight, flight, and freeze but are redirected to more modulated behaviors than the "wild type" we would expect outside the workplace. Unrecognized fear behaviors include anger (including instrumental anger), avoidance, mistaken deference to authority, overscrutiny of disconfirming information, and cognitive dissonance. We label them "unrecognized" because people all too commonly consider them accepted, if not normal, responses.

Stress Impairs Cognitive Function
Unrecognized fear engenders gratuitous stress. While much attention on decision-making focuses on various schemata, the fact becomes lost that threats or stress, at best, affect our ability to reason and access our cognitive abilities; this loss of ability then too easily distorts our thinking and causes irrational actions.

This describes effects from the threat responses of the amygdala (an almond-shaped organ in the brain that is the brain's emotion center) impairing the executive functions of the prefrontal cortex. Through conditioning, however, we can strengthen the influence of the cingulate cortex, a region of the brain that can effectively modulate the amygdala. The cingulate cortex is the cortical area of adaptive decision-making and error recognition.

HRO events are processes that constantly change and evolve. Planning and problem-solving, by their nature, presume a static state. As a process, the event can, at one extreme, self-resolve; at the other extreme, it can cascade toward unrecoverable failure. Processes make it difficult to utilize a protocol or follow a list.

Ambiguity is best clarified through engagement and interaction (van Stralen 2015). To use practical rationality for problem-solving, one must become entwined with the situation and even the problem (Sandberg and Tsoukas 2011). Also, processes cannot be redirected or restrained from outside. HRO describes the methods and structure for these approaches so that we may enter the problem state to engage from within. HROs engage the problem from within the problem space.

Accuracy versus Precision

"Ready, fire, aim!" Army artillery, firing at targets that are out of sight, cannot aim with precision; they do have accuracy, however. That is, they will fire their weapons, take a measure, re-aim, and fire again. In this manner, their rounds hit increasingly closer to the target.

We achieve accuracy through feedback with the environment, changing our actions as we observe how close we are to our target, objective, or goal. Precision initially seems more desirable, but it is an internal measure that is independent of the environment. The action in precision is made independent of the environment, yet it will be affected by environmental influences. Repeated actions will not reliably reach the target point, even though they consistently achieve the same effect. In precision, we hit the same point repeatedly, even if we miss our target. Accuracy allows us to change with the situation, coming closer to the target each time.

A dartboard bull's-eye illustrates this point. We can have precise aim, hitting the same point, but this means little if the hits land at the edge of the target. Digital information such as laboratory values tend to be reproducible and precise. On the other hand, accuracy describes our closeness to the target. Not a bull's eye, but close. Visual evaluations are an example of accuracy, not exactly reality but close. The advantage of accuracy over precision is that we can change our approach in response when we miss and also adapt our effort due to environmental influences.

> "The environment has a vote."
> —James P. Denney, Los Angeles Fire Department captain
> to his fellow fire captains during planning sessions

We achieve accuracy through rapid response to feedback, as our artillery vignette describes. Short feedback loops are more specific to our action and more easily accepted, rightly or wrongly, as being causative. The time compression inherent to the flux of rapid, dynamic events confounds the real-time use of long or indirect feedback loops. To obtain short feedback loops, we must closely approach the environment, even entwining with the environment. Entering the situation shortens feedback loops, thus improving accuracy.

> We in healthcare have developed a bias for precise data at the expense of accuracy in physical examination. For example, we may find repeated laboratory values obtained to track a disease rather than relying on physical examination. Some will obtain an arterial blood-gas value to evaluate respiratory failure rather than conduct an accurate physical examination to determine therapy.
> —Daved van Stralen

In complex, dynamic environments, we are better served if we direct our actions toward error identification and correction and the real-time assimilation of new information. This is a feedback, or cycling, type of decision-making that, when used effectively, becomes self-correcting. We have found John Boyd's loop-decision cycles to be easy to learn and helpful for novices and experts alike. This system consists of four functions, with a loop returning to the beginning function—observe, orient, decide, and act—with observation of the results of action closing the loop. This is commonly called the OODA loop, the name we will also use in chapter 6, "The Boyd OODA Loop."

In healthcare, the treating physician defines both the diagnosis and the outcome; this, to a great extent, defines whether complications and a poor outcome will be inevitable because of interactions between the disease and the underlying patient physiology. The uncertainty and ambiguity inherent in human disease complicate differentiating what can be influenced by systemic interventions and what cannot. This confounds our abilities to identify errors and prescribe interventions to improve the system.

The Loss of Structure

We can now see how easily we can lose the structure of the system in VUCA-T environments, how the logic of processes can be lost during an emergency (Roe and Schulman 2015), and how threats impair our perceptions and rationality. These factors form the basis of the gap that stands between scientific rationality and the practical rationality of HRO.

Any system or program that purports to incorporate or support HRO must (1) include practical rationality, (2) use a logic of practice that allows one to infer reliable information from unreliable environments, and (3) modulate the effects of stress and fear on cognition and behavior.

The greatest difficulty is what is called liminality (liminal = threshold), an anthropology term we used earlier when referring to the crossing of a threshold in life. In anthropology, "liminal" refers to rites that signify changes in status, such as from childhood to adulthood. In HRO, the term refers to the threshold between structured environments and unstructured environments.

The concepts and methods that work between structured and unstructured environments are asymmetric. That is, those methods developed for structured environments are unreliable and are very likely to fail in unstructured environments. The concepts and methods that emerged from, and evolved for, effective operations in unstructured environments can, with modest modifications, prove effective in structured environments.

For this reason, when an organization continues to function well and relies on structured and designed methodology, we can observe complacency develop across members of the organization, although leaders may come to believe they have achieved High Reliability. But this purported success only exists because fear remains unrecognized, and a demanding, unexpected event has not tested the system. The organization has continued to operate within environments with unrecognized structures.

This systemic complacency is in contrast to the complacency of the person who responds to organizational or systemic pathology. Leaders will often characterize this type of complacency as lack of discipline rather than the absence of emergencies or organizational or systemic pathology.

The loss of structure when unexpected events occur is profoundly disorienting, sufficient to create aversive feelings and refusal to engage a situation (or even to make the necessary plans for such situations). The loss of structure creates an unwillingness to discuss our own personal limitations and our need to rely on one another. Some people respond to the loss of structure by finding or creating some form of structure to act as a safe harbor. They do not realize that this new and/or conjured structure simply supports inaction.

The loss of structure is one of the most unsettling experiences one can have. This may cause one to see or conjure nonexistent structures or to apply strong-but-wrong structures—all of which are maladaptive and counterproductive.

The threshold we are discussing is the border between environments we know and feel comfortable operating within and a different environment of disorientation and threat. In more minimal degrees of severity, one can enter somewhat disorienting environments and continue to use the organization's standard operations, rules, and procedures. This may or may not yield success. Danger arises when we use our conventional logic of operations in this liminality—dangers Tempest, Starkey, and Ennew (2007) described in the Mt. Everest liminality, where the climbers who died, the liminal sojourners, did not embody the attitudes and behaviors of seasoned mountaineers. Also of note is that the US Army described the environment of the multilateral world at the end of the Cold War as VUCA. In its early work with VUCA, the army did not develop any new approaches for engagement specific to VUCA or singular elements.

Liminality forms a boundary where the system and operators must toggle between control operators to prevent further failure and the emergency responders who engage system failure. It is at this boundary where we see the limits of lean and Six Sigma; their continued use can result in disaster, as in the Mt. Everest event. One approach for this problem of error management during the loss structure is James Reason's "swiss cheese model," which is an organizational or system-failure model, whereas liminality is experienced by the individual person.

This approach assumes an intact system, an environment that may be described by control operations. Across the emergency-response threshold, such as the liminal state, the environment has lost structure, and the swiss cheese model may not apply. Further, the swiss cheese model is structural, created by the organization, while the liminal state is experienced by the individual person. This conundrum is described further in the next section.

Error Management: Swiss Cheese, Systems, and Enacting

High Reliability situations (HRSs) present disrupted structure and logic to the individual. In the midst of events, we act and observe the responses to our actions. We cannot know if an error is occurring, if we have identified an unidentified discrepancy, or if we are experiencing a new disruption to our operations. We cannot know if our hesitation to engage is not an error. "Look before you leap" may cause serious error during cascading events.

There is structure in our defense against error (defense in depth, described below), but this does not help the operator during the HRS in a VUCA-T environment. James Reason (1998) described the organization's "defense in depth" to protect people and the organization's assets from local operational hazards. These are the various defenses, barriers, and safeguards the organization puts in place to prevent an error. The swiss cheese metaphor allows for visualization of the causes of error and subsequent system failure and the alignment of gaps (the holes in the cheese) in the various defenses (the slices of cheese).

Active, but transient, failures at the human-system interface constantly create new gaps as older holes close. Latent system failures, which typically live longer, arise from the difficulty of anticipating all possible scenarios.

In this model, Reason identified proximal and ultimate causes of error, whether it is an active failure committed by people during an activity (proximal causation) or a latent failure caused by defects in system design and structure (ultimate causation). What is missing is flux in the situation and environment, something more than "dynamic," more like the VUCA-T environment (volatile, uncertain, complex, and ambiguous, combined with threatening).

In the VUCA-T environment, the slices of swiss cheese act more like spinning slices where alignments commonly occur, not just when there is activity. When aligned at the moment of a critical activity, consequential error leads to system failure. Christopher Hart, chair of the National Transportation Safety Board, developed this concept during his career in transportation-safety regulation and accident investigation (Hart, personal communication). Hart discussed this adjustment with Reason, who believed it to be a reasonable assessment.

The holes in the swiss cheese only become apparent at the level of the individual. To identify and then discuss these events, we must have a culture that supports the free flow of information about these failures. Reason identified that a safe culture must have honest information. Punitive or disciplinary measures intended to prevent the supposed aberrant mental processes that led to the error will prevent the reporting of this necessary information. A "just culture," one without blame, will lead to a reporting culture (Reason 2000). We discuss the just culture model further in chapter 11, "Other Systems."

A reporting culture requires that we free the individual from retribution for error; otherwise, there would be no reports of near misses and insufficient information about the circumstances surrounding a failure. This approach will bring attention to the system and enable systemic improvements. After all, the person who "caused" the error will one day leave, and others will arrive who will also "cause" errors. System approaches are independent of the individual.

According to Reason (2000, 770), "High Reliability Organizations are the prime examples of the system approach. For these organizations, the pursuit of safety is not so much about preventing isolated failures, either human or technical, as about making the system as robust as is practicable in the face of its human and operational hazards."

The systems approach uses layers for defense against errors (Reason 2000): engineering, people, and control through procedures and administration. Each type of layer, however, has weaknesses, but it is this layering that makes the defenses effective.

The swiss cheese model presumes errors and mistakes. Actions become mistakes (Paget 1988) at some point late in their development or even after the action. The focus of the operator is on the situation and its responsiveness, where mistakes may not be as visible as they would be to someone farther away in space or time.

Identifying the immediate precursors of errors and mistakes as actions or behaviors presents the same difficulties as animal behaviors do for behavioral ecologists. We do not look until the act or behavior—the transient, antecedent event—has passed.

This discussion presumes that errors come from action. As noted earlier, Weick described the idea of "failure from not acting," which is an invisible form of failure. When encountering a situation, people will often not act, which is an action that provides a sense of security while avoiding failure. But when failure does occur, it is attributed to underlying events: "it was expected."

Failure from acting becomes visible to others, which shows the benefit of just culture and the swiss cheese model. The visibility of failure from acting is what makes learning what works in novel or unexpected HRSs possible and valuable. HRO and just culture support engagement of the HRS toward the enactment of an end-state.

But the visibility of failure is delayed, which interferes with early correction. This is the problem of error: we can discuss the structure of error and prevention, but we cannot identify or capture error "in the act." If we cannot do this, then we cannot teach early error identification and mitigation.

Yet, it remains intuitive to many authorities that an engineering model, no matter how well crafted, designed, and structured (and incorporating signal versus noise and rulemaking), will prepare us for emergencies. The only support for this approach is a hindsight-based approach. We advocate what Robert Bea, professor of civil engineering at UC Berkeley, describes as "interactive, real-time risk assessment and management" (Bea, personal communication). This creates sensemaking in real-time performance toward enactment, as described by Weick (1995) in his description of sensemaking as an iterative process of sensemaking and enactment in which one improvises when encountering the unexpected (Weick 1998).

This is distinct from enactment failure from not acting, which may be a response to social knowledge that action is dangerous. By not acting, we do not learn what caused the failure (or even if a failure will occur). For example, it was once taught that administering adrenaline via aerosol to an infant with croup would lead to "rebound croup." From this idea developed a belief that administering adrenaline via aerosol can actually make the infant's condition worse. In reality, if the child deteriorated later, it was due to the progression of the disease, not the treatment. This situation is similar to ibuprofen's effects wearing off followed by a return of the headache pain. We do not call this "rebound headache."

The systems approach is useful for design and evaluation but is less useful for an operator in the moment when an error has just been identified, is immediately possible, or has already happened.

The famed airline pilot Chesley "Sully" Sullenberger found the swiss cheese model less useful for real-time error management (personal communication), but he recalled once hearing of error described as a ball rolling down a ramp, where speed bumps captured the error. The steeper the ramp, the taller the speed bumps need to be. "Another part of the idea is that it often requires more than one speed bump to finally trap the error. The ball may miss some bumps altogether or may roll over them if it is going fast enough. (So the taller the bump, the more likely it will trap the ball.) Having many speed bumps represents 'defense in depth,' a military concept that we also talked about that day. A multilayered defense system is less likely to be penetrated than a single layer" (Sullenberger, personal communication).

While the swiss cheese model better describes structures' organizational design for defense in depth, the model does not fully accommodate the dynamic nature of the HRS. Christopher Hart identified this limitation with the idea of "rotating slices of cheese." Decision-makers, immersed in the HRS, act to increase the chance of success and concomitantly act to decrease the chance of failure. The "error ball and ramp" model that Sullenberger describes is a dynamic organizational design to reduce system failure that also recognizes the operator's real-time efforts to decrease the chance of failure.

Conclusions

(1). High Reliability solves the problem of operations and performance in the VUCA environment but must be adjusted to the civilian world by including the concept of threat or threatening: the T in VUCA-T.

(2). The VUCA-T environment limits and disrupts scientific rationality, which is addressed by HRO.

(3). Unpredictability is expected in stochastic situations and from nonlinear, indeterminate processes; in these situations, HRO utilizes both vertical and horizontal thinking.

(4). The indeterminate problem the HRO encounters is described by uncertainty, time compression, and threat.

(5). In these events, the system loses known or recognizable structure, which is a challenge for conventional methods of organizing but is effectively addressed in an HRO.

CHAPTER 3

THE LOGIC OF PRACTICE AND THE LOGIC OF OPERATIONS

4 X 6 + 3 ÷ 2 – 5 = ?

This math equation has a correct answer. But it is only "correct" if one has accepted the conventions of mathematics. Answers develop differently when reading the equation from left to right versus right to left, performing addition and subtraction first or multiplication and division first, or using the integers and combinations of operations that are uniquely easier for the individual to perform mentally. This is the logic of operations.

PEMDAS describes the "order of operations" we use in mathematics, a standard to ensure consistency in our solutions. The order is to first perform the operations in *P*arentheses followed by *E*xponents, both powers and roots. Next is *M*ultiplication which takes precedence over *D*ivision, followed by *A*ddition then *S*ubtraction. Following the PEMDAS protocol, the answer to the equation is 20.5, but a set of parentheses around any two numbers would change the answer.

Circumstances in healthcare may cause us to change our direction of operations, contingencies will alter the logic we use, and crises will severely impinge on our logic as they disrupt our operations. Failure to recognize, accept, and adapt to changes in the logic of operations will lead to unrecognized catastrophic failure as people hold tightly to cherished beliefs and continue their strongly internalized routines.

This change in logic is built within the structure of an HRO; the ability to appropriately draw on the correct or adaptive logic of operations is the hallmark of HRO operations. Rather than viewing this change as something new, almost alien, we can see it within our daily lives. The change is basically a formalization of what we have experienced during the act of living.

Introduction

The logic, rational thought, and empirical knowledge we use to create and operate our programs, operations, and organizations readily fail us when we unexpectedly encounter severe contingencies such as the High Reliability situation (HRS). Events severely challenge our system and organization. We often cannot identify the internal logic of the situation or unfolding events (see chapter 2, "What Problem Does HRO Solve?"). Changes occur within changes. The greatest danger to any system occurs when we hold too strongly to beliefs that typically work in normal times but fail in time-compressed, uncertain situations like the HRS. Subjective and adaptive ways of thinking we dismiss as irrational. This is the deadly nature of the gap between work as imagined and, in the HRS, work as demanded.

When the internal logic of the system changes, we may misidentify the failure due to our logic of operations. Science, however, supports the use of subjectivity and does describe the rationality of other ways of thinking, which an HRO uses to its advantage.

In this discussion, we will use various levels of analysis to describe the limits of cognition, rationality, scientific logic, deductive reason, and statistics from the normal distribution curve. We will present the utility of "affect," other logics, inductive reasoning, and the power law (i.e., Pareto) distribution curve. The way in which you respond to uncertainty or threat determines whether you or your organization will attain resilience and adaptability or whether the situation will decompose into disorder.

A structured approach, drawn from principles, rules, or authority, tends to value obedience and conformity while looking to the past for strength. While it is exceptionally effective in what we previously described in the "control operator" mode (see chapter 1, "What is High Reliability Organizing?"), total reliance on structure can inhibit immediate engagement of the problem, thus impairing creativity and innovative thinking. As the circumstances override the ability of the person or organization to respond, this structural inflexibility will lead to potentially preventable failure.

When you engage the situation with the values of initiative and creativity, you look toward the future in order to match the complexity of the response to the complexity of the situation. This creates the risk of failing *while* acting. Errors *while* acting are visible, which makes them open to criticism as well as opening them to revision. An HRO maintains vigilance for early error identification and correction. Acting creates visibility, and in this conspicuity, error becomes correctable in real time by creating safety margins and learning. Successful field operators "are flexible, can learn and do adapt to the peculiarities of the system, and thus they are expected to plug the holes in the designer's imagination," (Rasmussen 1980, 97). This is the result of engagement: failure *while* acting, thus permitting the real-time correction of failures.

On the other hand, "failure *to* act" creates a different type of error that is not observable and therefore not correctable. It is the invisibility of these errors that obscures the actual problem and leads to institutionalized, yet unsupported, knowledge. In this situation, members of the organization cannot learn. Some members of the organization may unintentionally collude to avoid action and will offer elaborate explanations about some presumed danger of why they and others should not act. Failure to act, and the organizational knowledge this type of failure creates, makes change to effective approaches like HRO appear counterintuitive and protects the organization from the need to adapt to the environment.

> In the 1990s, our pediatric intensive care unit routinely ordered epinephrine (adrenaline) in an aerosolized form for severe croup. This would constrict blood vessels that had swollen in the airway. We would give this every forty-five minutes if there was symptomatic swelling and commonly found that the child could be discharged home the next morning.
>
> Invariably, a referring physician would hesitate or refuse to give epinephrine, or one of the resident physicians assigned to the PICU would become alarmed at our relaxed use of the drug. It seems that the emergency medicine and pediatric textbooks warned that the drug can cause "rebound croup," a condition where use of epinephrine makes the croup worse and leads to a hospital stay. No one seemed to want to use it for fear of going against accepted belief. (One resident once personally carried four heavy emergency medicine textbooks into the PICU, opened them to the proper page, and demanded that I read each section on croup.)
>
> Despite repeated demonstrations and reviews of patients who had been admitted with this therapy, we continued with the occasional resident being afraid to "fail by acting." The failure by not acting—that is, by not treating—was invisible and accepted by many. Any problem could easily be explained.
>
> This only began to subside when I asked how to differentiate rebound croup from the epinephrine effect wearing away. That is, do we get "rebound headache" four to six hours after taking pain medication, or did the medication simply stop working?
>
> —Daved van Stralen

HRO is counterintuitive. The farther away from the problem, the less HRO makes sense and the more likely leaders will attempt to force structure onto the situation in an attempt to control the outcome. *HRO is not a structure* but describes a dynamic process, effective in environments incapable of being structured. HRO is the sum of emergent properties coming together from local people who are interacting with a local problem in real time, a form of "self-organizing improvisation."

The greatest problem we have encountered for this change in operations is at the level of the individual. There is often the need to "de-orient" people: that is, demonstrate in some manner that the approach and way of thinking they have used does not work or, at the least, will not work in emergency environments. (Some of this is discussed in the "Motivational Leadership and the Use of Discrepancy for Individual Change" section of chapter 13, "Models of Leadership.")

Learning a new logic of operations is the most difficult problem of implementing HRO and the source of greatest obstruction—it also creates a strong, negative emotional response. For managers and those at even higher levels in the organization, we must recognize that people are successful and that their current approaches and methods of thinking were responsible for their career success and their rise in the organization and promotion. For some, it is even responsible for the respect they receive. *To bring in HRO as a new model is threatening.*

What we have found to be the central problem in adopting HRO was that people did not want to engage unless they were comfortable with the information they had at hand. Therefore, we had to demonstrate, in real time, how one can *create* information through engagement. We also had to demonstrate how to sort through vast amounts of information, some of it redundant and others of varying reliability. In these situations, they must individually place their own value on information.

Most critical for training, however, is the importance of identifying what information and data are salient, knowing that this salience can change, and understanding the critical role of the *early herald* as a trigger to be engaged. The salience of information brings people's attention to the situation, while the early herald explains why they must engage or act and why, in review, they may have appeared to others to have overreacted.

We were working with the risk management department of a large hospital to determine why the neurosurgery department was experiencing a disproportionate number of complaints, reported incidents, and attrition. Our inquiries found that the department head, a very aggressive personality, squashed every input by the staff with the same type of condescension that he displayed to us. He would actually stand three to four inches away from people and loudly demand, "What are *you* going to tell *me* about being a neurosurgeon?"

The salient point is that neither we, nor his staff, were trying to tell this physician how to be a neurosurgeon; rather, we were trying to say that the total stifling of staff inputs and extremely confrontational communications would ensure that concerns about patients, their progress, and their safety would not be communicated to this surgeon. As long as he continued to discount the situational assessment of all others and try to make the facts comport to his version of reality, the early heralds would not only be marginalized; they would be crushed like a grape. Any future efforts by the staff to advocate for the patient would be disregarded and ridiculed, thus setting up a situation where the neurosurgeon would be making critical patient decisions with incomplete information, thereby jeopardizing the patient's safety and limiting, if not precluding, the possibility of an optimal outcome.
—Spence Byrum

Levels of Analysis

Complexity is more than interactions and reactions, as if we can observe complexity from outside the event, teasing apart its elements from afar. Complexity is more than the structure of a problem. Complexity is held by the community using the operation and processes and it is resolved by the community. Complexity occurs across various levels of analysis. Faced with a complex situation, we must enter it, entwine ourselves with complexity, and change our points of view.

> "Make sure you change when things change."
> —Daved van Stralen

We can analyze a problem at various levels, from a line worker who first engages a discrepancy and operates at a tactical level to the CEO who sees the larger picture and operates strategically. Other, less obvious, levels would include the level of reductionism from the psychological to the more complex social and organizational levels. We can also analyze systems based on the degree of predictability for events or outcomes of the problem. We must identify the level of analysis we use in our discussion, because "discussion across levels of analysis can create false debates" (MacDougall-Shackleton 2011, 2076).

Levels of analysis provide a scaffold, or support structure, for understanding decision-making, problem-solving, and the logic of operations for the routine problem as well as emergencies and crises. They can reconcile observed conflicts in explanations that are generated at different levels. While they are less important for defined problems, such analyses become critical when problems or situations are not clearly defined or are manifested in different environments. Time compression, uncertain or ambiguous information, and proximity of threat all create a distinct logic of operations that is incongruous with the logic of operations employed in more stable, deterministic, and linear environments.

Proximate versus Ultimate Cause

The proximate level of analysis is tactical and looks at the immediate cause. While this level plays a greater role in homeostasis and exploration, it also fine-tunes and corrects problems that occur in more routine operations. The ultimate level of analysis is strategic, moving toward long-term strategic improvement and preparation for crises. As described in Weick's *sensitivity to operations* factor, while tactical and strategic operations are at different levels of analysis, we do not sacrifice one for the other. That is, we maintain strategic operations while giving necessary priority and support to the new tactical challenge.

Level of Reductionism

Keeping in mind that behavior and social interactions are emergent properties, we can use reductionism to better understand how people make sense of the situation, bring together the team, and align the workforce with the organization's goals. We find this in the neurosciences and neuro-economics; psychology, social psychology, and sociology; and organizational behavior and culture.

Immediate actions that are made in response to the event—the proximate cause of behavior—differ in sensemaking from those that are taken at a distance—the ultimate cause—where the "big picture" drives strategy.

System Failure—Prevention versus Response

The methods used to prevent failure, such as well-accepted processes and more rigid vertical hierarchy, can be harmful when used as a response to an unexpected and rapidly evolving emergency. Emergency responders must use initiative and creativity to rapidly engage a crisis. What is correct for one system, the control operator who prevents failure by adhering to processes, is counterproductive in the other, where the emergency responder engages the crisis by adapting to the situation. "Deviation from process" is an early herald in the control-operator state, while "rigid adherence to process" prevents agile responsiveness in stochastic environments or impairs safety in a dynamically evolving emergency (Roe and Schulman 2015).

Processes to *prevent* failure *can* conflict with processes that respond to failure.

Vertical Hierarchy

An organization's structure stands vertically from the executive level, administration, and management to the line worker. It is clear that the executive level is strategic, with greater freedom to act, while the line worker is tactical, with greater constraint. We must not forget that managers interpret strategy to the line worker for better performance and transmit the needs of the line worker toward the executive level. Doing so requires expertise in understanding both extremes of the organization and how to translate information in a useful way. Administrators must break the organization's overarching strategy into bite-size operational pieces for managers. Likewise, administrators must translate performance indicators from managers to the executive level. Each level in the vertical hierarchy has a different level of analysis: executive, administrative, management, and line.

Managers are in place to know were problems arise from the line and why the problem is important to administration; managers can then negotiate a solution with the environment.

Each level in the vertical hierarchy operates in a different environment:

- *Executive*—regulatory agencies, finance, competitors, suppliers, public relations, etc.
- *Administrative*—strategic plans, tactical operations, human resources, finance, regulations, the organizational structure, etc.
- *Management*—employee organizations, work and employee productivity, directives from administration and executives, other units in the organization, etc.
- *Line staff*—coworkers, supervisors, work tasks, customers (service industries), etc.

Horizontal Analysis

In this discussion, "horizontal analysis" describes the different level of analysis used between a situation occurring as expected compared to a similar situation where the unexpected happens. At the extreme, there is time-compression, uncertainty, and threat. Because this loss of structure causes threat responses and impairs cognition, we describe change in level as crossing the liminal threshold. (See chapter 1, "What Is High Reliability Organizing?")

Analysis across the liminal threshold of threat is horizontal analysis because, though the physical environments and resources may not change, the presence of threat changes the analysis. Threat impairs cognitive function, and people are at risk to act in self-interest and, in worst-case scenarios, self-preservation. The paradox here is that we can better protect ourselves through collaboration and helping others than we would through personal defensive or offensive actions.

It is difficult, but important, to learn and understand the effectiveness of the logic of operations across the liminal threshold; embodiment of this logic will drive greater performance in adversity.

Exploitation and Exploration

Organizations must grow, which is something they do by exploiting their environment. The environments can change, becoming adverse and impeding growth. On the other hand, organizations must expand, which is something they do by exploring for new markets and products. Exploration exposes the organization to adversity or threat. Hazards also exist in the competitive world of business in the financial climate of the time. These threats can disrupt homeostasis. Exploitation and exploration are two distinct levels of analysis: as March put it, "the exploration of new possibilities and the exploitation of old certainties" (1991, 71).

Causation

Causation differs by level of analysis. In the immediate engagement, we may only be able to consider a single cause—that is, a single stimulus causing the problem. A more tactical view may reveal the convergence of several distinct causes, with each needing consideration and, possibly, separate engagements. At a greater distance from the situation, the leader may recognize causes that combine to make the event. Several causes could stem from a larger group of causes, with one or more from each grouping necessary to come together and set events in motion. The greater the distance the leader is from a situation, the more *unlikely* it is that the leader will notice subtle but important causations. The leader thus may take proactive actions and begin to strategically plan for new events that may develop, with the intent of limiting the entrainment of more problems into the current process (Hilborn and Stearns 1982).

Multiple causes lead to the complex problem. Within a complex problem, some causational factors are not visible in the midst of events, though some become visible only at a distance, and some are parallel while others are interactive. It is fallacious to identify a single root cause when any one cause, at any one time and at any one level, may have the influence to stop the cascade.

From Node to Network

In network theory, the scale-free network is created through linkages with various nodes based on the use of each node. More linkages to a node indicate more use of that node. That is, linkages preferentially connect to the more frequently used nodes. In an HRO, the nodes develop at the incident, and connections are based on the need for resources or information. "Linkages" here represent authority migration and information flow. For analysis, we would evaluate whether nodes can, or do, develop and connect freely and spontaneously as necessary, and whether nodes grow in size due to necessary activity and not as an artifice of the organization's structure. These structural, behavioral, or temporal nodes and linkages may not exist during routine operations (Stadler et al. 2014). HRO, then, can describe the extemporaneous emergence of a scale-free network around the HRS.

Response to Adversity

Behaviors allow animals to survive in hostile environments. The Nobel laureate Niko Tinbergen identified four levels of analysis for these behaviors (1963): causation, development, evolution, and function, as discussed below. We can modify this concept for an analysis of human behavior necessary to operate in adverse environments.

The advantage of this analysis is the differentiation between behaviors general for high-risk environments and behaviors specific to a particular industry. This brings out behaviors common to us as human beings when we are faced with adversity or danger and how we collaborate as social creatures. Such analysis also identifies behaviors for a specific industry we may choose not to emulate.

> *Causation*—this describes the mechanism of the actual behavior, including perceptions, sensemaking, physiology, and threat-reward responses. These are the behaviors that come out in response to an emergency or that conform a person to the organization's ideal. This behavior operates at the level of the individual.
>
> *Development*—these behaviors develop in the individual through education, training, experience, and modeling from others. How events are interpreted and processed has a greater influence on the development of adaptive behaviors than pure didactic pedagogy or instruction. Of even

greater influence is the modeling of behaviors by respected peers and superiors. The use of lessons learned and case reports are methods of development for desired behaviors. This is also the process from competence to proficiency and expert performance in the "Dreyfus" model of expert skill acquisition from beginner to expert (Dreyfus and Dreyfus, 1980). The study of the particular case, the developmental level of analysis, lifts the organization toward expert performance. It is through the modeling of desired behaviors that the novice develops expertise and comes to embody HRO culture.

The Dreyfus brothers studied pilot emergency response behavior for the US Air Force (Dreyfus and Dreyfus, 1979) and the mental activities to acquire skills (Dreyfus and Dreyfus, 1980). From their studies came the levels of skill commonly used today in numerous fields: novice, competence, proficiency, expertise, and mastery.

Evolution—these are behaviors that evolve within an industry. This is the history of those behaviors, and why people in the specific industry care about these behaviors. These behaviors are then passed on as a part of the culture of a specific industry. When we do not understand their purpose, we are in danger of losing effective behaviors that have evolved in healthcare over generations—particularly those behaviors from a "simpler" time when physicians and nurses had more intimate, long-term relationships with patients and families and between one another. We may find it difficult to connect a purpose to these behaviors that we adopted by modeling our respected elders. Any attempts to defend these behaviors to others, in the absence of evidence-based research, cast an idiosyncratic light on them. Others, coming after us, may reject these behaviors and beliefs if they lack the evidence that they work. The evidence that these behaviors work is in the particular, their purpose known only to the person who carries these behaviors. Just as these behaviors evolved in healthcare, a new environment may lead to the evolution of less intimate behaviors.

Function—these behaviors have an adaptive value, or they would be extinguished from the behavioral repertoire. These are the behaviors that are shared across industries that operate in similar situations, such as an HRO versus an organization with a stable operation in predictable environments. These behaviors make the HRO organization more fit for the exploitation of opportunities in adverse or stochastic environments and for exploration into risky situations or the conducting of risky operations. These behaviors contribute to the fitness of individuals and the organization toward cooperation and success within the adverse environments.

The study of behaviors in other and quite different organizations can advance HRO in healthcare, as it can for all organizations. We can identify industry-specific behaviors from other industries and study how they can benefit healthcare. In the final analysis, we must monitor our environment and the members of our organization to refine HRO and make it unique to our organization.

> "The best fertilizer for medicine is the progress
> of other and quite different sciences."
> —WILLIAM HARVEY, FIRST PHYSICIAN WHO DESCRIBED
> THE COMPLETE CIRCULATORY SYSTEM

De-Orientation and Orientation

HRO principles seem to activate a somewhat unusual form of resistance in people. Some believe their mental processes will work well in the High Reliability Situation (HRS). Others view HRO processes as a danger to themselves or their organization. Some will co-opt the principles of HRO into their existing belief system and will agree with HRO principles in public. Not all of these people will continue resistance, they will de-orient from their previous models of thinking to orient toward HRO. The anger expressed later is not from the way HRO was presented but from the de-orientation.

This is a discussion one of us (DvS) has continued with Karl Weick for several years, how to reduce or overcome resistance to HRO and, more critically, the source of the resistance. In that sense, we could have placed this in a section about change. It is likely people perceive the implication that they have not been organizing reliably. That is not the case at all, there are methods that will enhance the processes they have in place. HRO augments what the organization is, what appears to be replacement of the organization's structure is actually the transformation to a new form.

Academia, education, business, and research all build on categorization, linearity, and direct causation. At some point, the sophistication of shared or overlapping categories, nonlinearity, and indirect causation become the focus of education and interpreting experience. Even that, however, may not prepare people to effectively operate in dynamic, complex environments in the presence of immediate threats. "Low-tempo" situations can support the belief that we can rely on scientific logic and empirically proven, independent, and noninteracting principles. (We have borrowed the musical term "tempo," the rapidity of movement, to describe low-tempo slow action and high-tempo rapid action.) The moment when we learn the inadequacy of these strongly held beliefs may be at the edge of chaotic events and the beginning of irreversible failure.

De-orientation from nonadaptive or maladaptive beliefs and behaviors may help implement HRO methods into the organization. Some people readily comprehend the principles of High Reliability Operations. Other people hold strongly to beliefs that have supported them well in routine times. Rather than using catastrophic failure as a method to disabuse people of these beliefs, we can de-orient them from their nonadaptive or maladaptive beliefs and behaviors.

The identification of discrepancies from the use of their approach when faced with VUCA-T environments (see "The Environment" in chapter 2, "What Problem Does HRO Solve?") and the indeterminate problems of uncertainty, time-compression, and threat can begin the discussion. Following their logic and premises to an ultimate conclusion can identify unintended consequences and failures. The inability of their approach to identify or effectively manage "high-tempo" events can also be identified as thought problems. This is discussed in the motivational interviewing approach to leadership in chapter 13, "Models of Leadership."

HRO environments, whether control operator or emergency response, has developed a different logic of practice. Learning this logic before a crisis occurs may prevent the crisis or bring it to a quicker resolution and more desirable end-state. These are two distinct, though interacting, levels of analysis, and the de-orientation to reach each of them is a distinct level of analysis from routine job orientation.

The Expert versus the Initiate

The reason someone continues an activity differs from why that person started it. This is true for professions, vocations, avocations, sports, and hobbies, whether one is a participant or an avid observer. We must remember this during the implementation processes for HRO. Telling novices that these principles will help them manage the unexpected will not go far when their concern is to not respond in fear. Rather than using a standard teaching approach, we must fit our level of analysis and teaching to the experience and interest of the individual.

HRO-implementation programs often encounter resistance and co-optation into current beliefs. Part of this arises when a program is presented by an experienced expert consultant with a graduate degree to an experienced expert business executive or administrator who also has a graduate education. This program is then given to line staff and novices. Several levels of analysis separate these groups. Someone who is not familiar with effective performance in adverse or hostile environments will also use a different level of analysis than someone who is new to HRO and each differ from a veteran of such environments or someone experienced in HRO.

This is not a trivial problem. These levels of analysis are similar to those in the Dreyfus system of expert skill acquisition from beginner to expert. HRO is a fulcrum dividing competence and proficiency. Competence is the skill level for general, context-independent principles used by organizations in stable environments. Proficiency is the skill level for the particular, context-dependent principles where the HRO starts.

> "To change someone's beliefs, you must change their perceptions."
> —DAVED VAN STRALEN

The Limits of Rationality

Rational thought arises from facts and sound reasoning. Though this is a formal process, it is a process all of us believe we routinely use. Facts may come from observation, information provided to us, or knowledge already known to us. Our reasoning strives to consciously make sense of the world and our situation. When necessary, we infer new information from our existing information and create interpretations from our circumstances through the processes of scientific logic. Formally, these are the elements of scientific rationality with its emphasis on deductive reasoning that guarantees the hypothesis with facts and the predictive power of probability.

In VUCA-T environments, however, we cannot meet the standards of facts and sound reasoning for scientific rationality and logic. We know that reality exists, because we experience it. We continue to believe in truth, because we can see the actual state of affairs. What confounds us is rapid change (volatility), unavailable or imperfect information (uncertainty), unidentifiable causations (complexity), multiple interpretations (ambiguity), and impairment of our cognitive function (threat). Probabilities, predictions, the inference of new information from existing information (logic); the evaluation of information and the judgment of consequences (critical thinking); and, most significant, objective thinking (the basis of rationality), have become impossible.

We must become practical and pragmatic when in the VUCA-T situation. We infer new information from unreliable information with the use of inductive reasoning: (evidence supports our conclusion; as we strengthen or discard evidence, we must also adjust our conclusion). We have greater concern for the serious *possible* threat (the ease with which an event can happen), even if it has a low probability of occurrence. That is, an HRO is more concerned about a serious event if it is highly possible, even though it has a low probability of occurrence. These are some of the limits of rationality for an HRO.

Scientific Rationality

Scientific rationality assumes *perfect knowledge* and the ability to process this information deductively. That is, we have access to facts, and these facts guarantee our hypothesis. We must also have a reason for our beliefs and must not act without a reason for the actions.

We are able to infer a truth from facts because we categorize things into discrete, non-overlapping entities having distinct properties. This precludes a thing from having elements shared across diverse categories. For example, scientific rationality has a verge or threshold that defines "failure" and "not failure." We might categorize respiratory failure by separating failure from not failure at the level of CO_2 or O_2 in the blood. In reality, patients form a spectrum from distress to failure and may move between groups based on momentary physiological demands, emotional responses, or medical treatment.

Definitions and categories are necessary to identify what makes things alike or different, to statistically analyze data, and to apply specific and precise conclusions we have deduced using scientific rationality. Definitions and categories, both useful for discussion and research, can impair our ability to combine categories or elements of different categories. For example, an increased heart rate in a patient with respiratory findings may be caused by sepsis, increased respiratory effort, dehydration from inability to drink during respiratory distress, or concomitant heart pathophysiology. Our patient may have elements of various medical conditions extending to various degrees, or he or she may be at a different point in the progression from wellness to illness to being critically ill. This ambiguity confounds practical application of scientifically developed knowledge.

Experimental design, a product of scientific rationality, requires falsifiability—that is, we must state the hypothesis in a manner in which it can be proven false. If we cannot prove it is false, then it must be true. This follows from the idea that we cannot prove truth. The complexity and threat inherent to VUCA-T environments preclude making a hypothesis that is falsifiable or conducting research that purposely endangers the subject or a member of the organization.

Steve Clark, Jan Meyers, and many others (including myself) collaborated to bring HRO to the Perinatal Safety Initiative of the largest for-profit hospital system, the Hospital Corporation of America (HCA). Dr. Clark, a highly respected high-risk OB/GYN physician, offered the following sage advice to a conference of his HCA colleagues on the "science" of medical decision-making: "Evidence-based medicine does not mean: unless you can prove it with multiple prospective, randomized, double-blind, placebo-controlled cross-over trials, it's OK to do anything we feel like. Evidence-based medicine does mean: where there is clear evidence of superiority of one method over another, use it."

Dr. Clark was far ahead of his time back in 2000 by exhorting his colleagues not to wait for the perfect scientific solution when HRO contained the framework for raising the bar on the level of care while simultaneously seeking to validate best practice with science.

—Spence Byrum

Bounded Rationality

Rationality, by necessity and definition, is binary, reductive, and assumes omniscience, thus making it impractical except for the simplest of our problems. The world and human capacity further limit our perceptions, knowledge, and ability to reason. Cognitive limitations and the finite amount of time available for decisions create boundaries to reason and rationality. The Nobel laureate Herbert Simon (1957) called this "bounded rationality."

Decision theories describe the biases and heuristics we use within this boundedness. Generally, academics see these as weaknesses that cripple rationality, but some of these heuristics actually contribute to better decision-making. Simon recognized that, because people have limited time and knowledge, they must make inferences from the information they have available. These heuristics, then, would be specific to a situation and would derive their rationality from the structure of the environment (Gigerenzer 2008; Gigerenzer and Goldstein 1996).

Practical Rationality

A gap exists between modern scientific rationality and the practical rationality of daily work. Scientific rationality consists of three interconnected core assumptions: (1) reality contains discrete entities with distinct properties; (2) we, as observers, are separated from the world; and (3) a representational logic underlies practice. This rationality underestimates the degree to which practitioners are immersed in the environment, ignores unique situations, and detracts from time as experienced by practitioners (Sandberg and Tsoukas 2011).

Though there is no well-developed "practical rationality" as a science, the idea does represent the manner in which practitioners engage and solve problems. Practitioners immerse themselves in the situation, looking for disruptions and breakdowns that will allow an intervention. Entities and events are continuous and constantly changing (Sandberg and Tsoukas 2011). As this working frame changes, as in frame analysis (see chapter 4, "HRO and the Environment"), some rules change, while others do not. The practical part is to identify which rules continue to apply and when they apply.

The complexity and dynamics of the threat environment in which the HRO operates confound the use of scientific rationality. Uncertainty and ambiguity confound perception and cognition, both necessary attributes for bounded rationality. This impairs the use of bounded rationality for HRO operations. An HRO will adopt best practices as soon as practicable while continuously validating new practices and current beliefs. Practical rationality (i.e., the rationality of practice) best describes this type of rationality used by HROs.

"Practical rationality" describes the rationality of routine operations in our everyday environments. Though derived from science and philosophy, the idea differs significantly from the scientific rationality we learned in science and liberal arts education and that is used in academic publications.

Disrupted Rationality

Van Stralen has observed in professionals unconditioned to the threat environment that direct or imminent threat seizes people's cognitive functions in a manner they do not recognize. Without conditioning, threats can redirect our thoughts toward self-preservation and escape. Even mildly acute, uncontrollable stress dramatically decreases prefrontal cortex cognitive abilities (Arnsten 2009) such as the executive functions and rationality. In these most intimate moments, the rationality of survival and escape disrupt cognitive rationality.

Emotion and cognition interact in ways that are starting to become clearer. Emotional responses when we experience threat include emotional memory and learning, influence on attention and perception, processing of social stimuli, and regulation of emotional responses (Phelps 2006). This "affective" side of decision-making, necessary for survival but taxing of cognitive performance, is little recognized in the fields of decision-making and problem-solving, yet it is a synthesis commonly used by experienced HRO operators.

Disrupted rationality is a form of instrumental rationality that coherently identifies the means for achieving the desired ends within the existing conditions. Adaptive and undesirable ends may have to be accepted along the way to reaching an effective, accepted conclusion.

Knowledge in the threatening, unstructured state takes a different form than what we are accustomed to. Knowledge acts as a degree or level of belief that must be updated from information generated during the event. Mistaken beliefs must be identified and corrected, no matter how dearly held. A mistaken belief, compared to an updated belief, may only depend on the mistaken belief's presence at its initiation or the length of time it is held. Events happen continuously, thus creating the need for dynamic reasoning processes and easier acceptance of new, disconfirming evidence. Long-held entrusted beliefs must be freely questioned, which is not an easy thing to do for most people, regardless of their level of skill or logic they use.

Discrete concepts and categories allow for science and the planning necessary to prepare for events; they also contribute to a mind-set that problems are like puzzles: we collect the information and puzzle pieces necessary, put them in place, and we have an answer. In environments without boundaries that are dynamic and in flux, we are better served by mystery-solving rather than puzzle-solving. There are many possibilities, and what helps us on one level can hurt us on another. While we were taught to use categories and discrete concepts, we use continuous perceptions, which creates a gap between what we know and our experience. This is the gap where we use a different logic of practice and a different logic of operations (Wolfberg 2006; Weick 2011).

Those who have the necessary cognitive, affective, and behavioral repertoire may have some protection from symptomatic cognitive dissonance. When we learn to freely relinquish our cherished beliefs in the face of new experiences, we are less likely to hold on tightly to those cognitions that create dissonance with other cognitions. On the other hand, those who hold on tightly to certain cognitions in the face of disconfirming evidence must deal with the discomfort of cognitive dissonance and its concomitant state of arousal. This can lead to unrecognized fear responses, the denial of uncertainty, the failure to recognize error, or the inability to accept the ongoing flux of events.

To summarize, disrupted rationality is (1) loss of the internal logic of the system from turmoil and threat and (2) a state in which the maladaptive fear responses, avoidance, withdrawal, and panic all make sense. HRO is a practical logic and logic of operations to be adapted to the disruptive situation.

Reasoning: Deduction, Induction, and Abduction

Our scientific education biases us toward deduction; facts guarantee our hypothesis. This "guarantee of truth" also gives us a strong sense of security. It causes us to "see" only information that supports our initial hypothesis or idea (confirmation bias) and to be "blind" to disconfirming evidence (motivated reasoning). As a result, we search only for specific facts. Under uncertain and ambiguous conditions, however, facts may not exist. The time-compressed state then further limits both our capacity and ability to evaluate information for its factual basis.

Because deduction identifies what is known from known premises, it does not really create information. Induction, however, does increase information by inferring a new conclusion from the present evidence through the continuing process of accepting or rejecting the changing strength of each piece of evidence. It is the nature of the HRO process that we will then test this new information as we initially develop it and throughout the event.

Inductive reasoning also makes real-time information testing easier, because we constantly evaluate the strength and weakness of our evidence, incorporating new evidence in real time. As our evidence changes, so does our conclusion, which produces a dynamic approach of information processing and conclusion refinement. "Doxastic" logic (discussed later in this chapter) is a modal logic for revising beliefs and supports a dynamic structure for inductive reasoning. Coincidentally, active inductive processes are congruent with the process of disrupted rationality in the updating, revision, and correction of information.

"Abductive reasoning" describes a process of expert reasoning to quickly explain a situation or event. This is the identification of a best reason or explanation from inferences (the process of logic) of current information. While useful for the rapid development of a hypothesis, such reasoning also supports and maintains errors when expert reasoning is good but the hypothesis is wrong.

"Bayesian estimation" refers to the use of subjective information and interpretation to revise conclusions. This subjective reasoning has many sources, including experience and knowledge, and is applied in a subjective manner to events.

Deductive reasoning is the science to use for evidence-based medicine; inductive reasoning is the science for uncertainty.

Possibility

The unexpected is a measure of possibility: (1) the ease with which an event can occur while we are more accustomed to a probabilistic model of risk or (2) the percent chance an event will occur. For example, a common maxim in healthcare is that "if you hear hoofbeats, don't think of zebras, think of horses." Zebras bite and are more dangerous than horses. Movie productions have used all manner of large predators, but because of their aggression, few movies use zebras. If there is a possibility of zebras—even if a low probability—then we might want to keep alert. In the HRO, we are attentive to the possibility of events and work to make those events less easy to occur.

The Limits of Logic and the Logic of Practice

We strive to be logical. This is the understanding that, following a linear series of steps, we can arrive at a conclusion that is objective and derived from what we know. "Logic" describes the method of inferring new information from existing information. We typically learn the rules of classical logic without realizing how much our daily experience tempers its use. We may not recognize how we follow a logic of practice in our routine operations and life, particularly work routines requiring judgment or for encounters with the unpredictable.

Critical thinking incorporates classical logic with recognition that human thinking may corrupt the processes of logic and objectivity. Conceptually, metacognition allows us to think of the numerous thought processes we integrate. Classical logic, critical thinking, and metacognition all have limitations in the logic of practice.

Classical (Scientific) Logic

Classical logic, also known as scientific logic, is binary and linear: something "is" or "is not," and its value or characteristic determines the next step. Classical logic has three elements: (1) there is only one correct answer; (2) truth values are either true *or* false, never a little of each (this is the "law of the excluded middle"); (3) the universe is knowable.

Classical logic underlies the scientific method. Items are categorized into discrete sets defined by the presence or absence of specific characteristics. Categories are further combined or connected by specific differences or commonalities. Statements are either true or false, and truth-falsity is independent of the statements' existence in the world. Arguments are either valid (they are accepted) or invalid (they are rejected). Philosophers recognize the limits to this type of logic. For example, we may have to use an expression such as *necessary* or *possible* to qualify the truth of a judgment, which is not allowed when the statement is *either* true or false, not a little of both.

The Limits of Logic

What is rational and logical in structured, predictable environments may be harmful when the environment becomes unpredictable and loses its structure. This is where we find that the internal logic we expected does not exist. (See chapter 2, "What Problem Does HRO Solve?")

Something may appear irrational solely because we do not recognize the system's internal logic, or we have continued our use of classical, scientific logic when the system's internal logic has changed. *The type of logic we need must help us infer reliable information from the unreliable state.*

In the most severe case of a disruptive event, we create information through interaction, and we trust that information only after observing the response to our actions. What we accept as reliable is only what acts as expected, and such reliability will change with time. This describes a practical logic for continuous operations.

Other Logics

Several other types of logic may be used. The most easily understood is "informal logic," the type we use in daily life: "Does it follow?" or "Is it legitimate to infer/assume?" These other logics allow values we need if we are to understand the VUCA-T environments and the indeterminate problem (i.e., time compression, uncertainty, and threat). In informal logic, (1) multiple adaptive answers are possible; (2) many-valued and partially valued logics are used, (3) more than one truth, and partially true values all exist; and (4) the universe is *not* knowable.

Classical logic is static. Because something "is" does not mean it drives an action—that is, we "must" or "ought to" act on the information. This is the *is-ought* quandary of logic; its static nature does not connect a premise to action. "Deontic logic," however, takes us from "is" to "ought to"—that is, if an event occurs, then an action may be either *obligated* or *not permitted*. Deontic logic is the logic of norms or accepted standards.

Logic can also be modified for concepts of time. While the past is fixed and already determined, logical processes can account for the branching of time in the future. "Temporal logic" addresses problems of causality and mechanism, continuous change, planning actions, concurrent or discontinuous events, and the persistence of a fact rather than the truth of a fact.

Logic develops valid arguments that are sound and complete. Logical validity is defined by truth tables, something not available in these other, "modal" logics (discussed below). What is used, instead, is "possible worlds"—that is, the statement is valid for each of the possible worlds that could exist. Through Weick's concept of *enactment* in High Reliability, we create, or enact, *toward* a possible world, thus lending the necessary validity to our logical inferences despite having imperfect information and the influence of time and change.

It is not that we will necessarily use these various types of logic; instead, we have several ways of inferring new information from qualified or changing information, and that information can drive action—all from logical inference.

Logics for High Reliability

The sciences and liberal arts expose us to scientific, or classical, logic. Few of us have come across the other logics that have greater applicability in VUCA-T environments and that support HRO. These logics, some of which are used in computer science, include modal (qualities), epistemic (knowledge), doxastic (belief), temporal (time), and deontic logic (duty), as shown in table 1.

Logic	Propositions & Operators
Classical	Deductive argument AND, OR, NOT If..., then... If and only if...
Modal	Modes of truth Ways and degrees things are true "It is necessary that..." "It is possible that..."
Epistemic	Reason about knowledge as propositions "x knows that..."
Doxastic	Reason about belief (Probably, not necessarily, true) "x believes that..." Accurate, Inaccurate, Consistent, Reflexive
Temporal	Time qualifies propositions Until, Next, Future "It is always the case that..." "It will be the case that..." "It was the case that..."
Deontic	Duty or obligation Drives action Necessary, Contingent, Impossible "It is obligatory that..." "It is permitted that..." "It is forbidden that..."

Table 1—Logic vs. propositions and operators

Modal logic refers to *modes* or qualifications of truth: the different ways in which things are true. Modal logic allows degrees of truth and encompasses a group of logics about time (temporal logic), morality and duty (deontic logic), belief (doxastic logic), and knowledge (epistemic logic). Modal logic concerns necessity and possibility (Garner 2016).

Epistemic logic provides reasons about knowledge as propositions, which may be compared to epistemology, which is the nature of knowledge—the justification and rationality of belief. (Epistemology can also be considered in two aspects: as the definition of knowledge and as the dynamics of "epistemic knowledge logic" and "doxastic belief logic.") Epistemic logic is also found in game theory, robotics, security, and cryptography. Here, knowledge and belief are attitudes, and one's possible world is evaluated as being compatible with or incompatible with the possible world. Epistemic logic allows shared logic and belief. Groups of people who share the same attitudes toward these possible worlds have a form of acknowledged and shared *common* knowledge (Hendrichs and Symons 2015).

Doxastic logic, a form of epistemic logic, provides reasons about belief rather than knowledge, the difference being that a belief is probably, though not necessarily, true. When we are not careful, we may collapse knowledge and belief into the same system, thus making our beliefs refractory to disconfirming evidence and subsequent motivated reasoning. In the worst case, such logic strengthens cognitive dissonance. Doxastic operators capture belief change, as "belief revisions" or "belief updates," when they receive conflicting information or encounter a discrepancy or disruption.

- A *belief update* refers to accounting for a change in the situation and the acquisition of new, more reliable information; this requires us to change our inaccurate old beliefs to a more accurate, new belief.
- *Belief revision* occurs when we identify the old information as being less reliable and we use new, more reliable information to revise our older beliefs; we keep the new belief as close as possible to the old belief while accepting the newer, accurate information.

Temporal logic reasons how time qualifies statements and propositions with two basic operators, future and past. The asymmetry of time describes how the past is fixed, yet the future is branching and open to influence and change. A deterministic view of time requires the use of linear time for the future (Goranko and Galton 2015).

Time, in terms of logic, is discrete, occurring as intervals, or continuous, continuing as instants. Scientifically, we assume continuous instants for scientific logic, computer programs, processes, protocols, and algorithms. But any real-world operation, scientific or otherwise, has a duration that occurs within intervals, and these intervals can overlap or be embedded within other events, run parallel with other independent or interdependent events, jump to other events, or depend on the initiation or completion of different events. (Intervals are used in artificial intelligence and computer science.)

Deontic logic guarantees a system of obligations for action. It provides reasons about duty or obligation and drives action from states. Every proposition exists in one of three mutually exclusive states in this logic: necessary, contingent, or impossible. Things that are possible are either necessary or contingent. Things that are non-necessary are either contingent or impossible (McNamara 2014).

Critical Thinking

Critical thinking is the logical, objective analysis and evaluation of an issue or argument to form a judgment. It is philosophical, without influence from psychology or the neurosciences. Whereas rhetoric (see below) seeks to *persuade*, critical thinking seeks to argue (philosophically, not emotionally). An argument is a system of propositions, a set of premises advanced to support a conclusion. Validity and soundness are used to analyze and assess deductive arguments. For the inductive argument, we use inductive force, inductive soundness, inductive inferences, and degrees of probability.

Our use of the term rhetoric for use in the philosophical form of argument derives from Aristotle's three types of rhetorical appeals: logos, pathos, and ethos (reason, emotional appeal, and morality). Aristotle also described five canons of persuasive speech: invention, arrangement, style, memory, and delivery.

The goal of argument is to produce a clear and completely explicit statement of the argument. If we hear rhetorical ploys, fallacies, or sham reasoning, we will reject an argument without applying critical thinking analysis or evaluation. Implicit propositions, an intentional part of the argument that is purposely left out, are also not accepted. Vague and ambiguous terms must be eliminated.

While critical thinking for analysis or evaluation is an important part of any program, the system has inherent severe limitations in conditions of time compression, uncertainty, and threat. In these conditions, a person may have to use subjective judgment to provide valuation or meaning to information. It then becomes necessary to use overlapping categories and a continuous spectrum of values, which conflicts with the law of the excluded middle (as noted earlier, an item must be in one or the other category), thus interfering with the use of classical logic.

Rhetoric is the art of persuasive speaking or writing by relying on command of the language: the way words, figures of speech, and compositional technique are used. We use the tools of rhetoric in HRO to persuade others of our circumstances and plans. Heuristics, in rhetoric, are used as aids to learning and understanding. (Heuristics, in decision-making, refer to shortcuts or rules of thumb. The aforementioned Nobel laureate Herbert Simon introduced heuristics into decision-making with his concept of bounded rationality. Some researchers, such as Amos Tversky and Daniel Hahnemann, believe heuristics can impair decision-making, while others, such as Gerd Gigerenzer and Wolfgang Gaissmaier, believe heuristics can increase accuracy and reduce cognitive bias.)

Metacognition

Metacognition is a meta-level cognitive process—a form of cognitive monitoring of cognitive processes—often described as "thinking about thinking." *Meta* means "beyond," so metacognition describes the cognition beyond traditional cognition; this distinguishes metacognition from the object-level cognition of basic operations and traditional information processing. Metacognition, through feedback regulation, is a process that *monitors* and *controls* thinking and behavior (Flavell 1979).

John H. Flavell (1979) presented metacognition as a model of cognitive monitoring to explain the change in cognitive abilities in children as they mature. Educational research at the time had suggested that young children were limited in "their knowledge and cognition about cognitive phenomena" (1979, 906). The stored knowledge, experience, and beliefs of older children are thought to improve their cognitive abilities. Metacognition also monitors and controls learning, thus giving it a critical role in deep and meaningful learning." Cognitive strategies are invoked to *make* cognitive progress, metacognitive strategies to *monitor* it" (1979, 909)

Over the following decade, metacognition spread from learning in the field of education to the disciplines of cognitive psychology and social psychology. Stanley Schachter and Amos Tversky, working from their respective fields, studied how people think and how they interpret what is happening in the situation, making "cognitive psychology social and social psychology cognitive" (Mischel 1998, 84).

Stanley Schachter, with Jerome Singer (1962), developed the concept that emotion is the cognitive labeling of physiological arousal. That is, an external stimulus arouses the individual, and the individual, from environmental and internal cues, then labels the emotion.

Amos Tversky, with Daniel Kahneman, studied cognitive bias and risk. Their work on the "availability construct" laid a foundation for the development of metacognition. We find the availability construct to be one of the four most applicable biases and heuristics in HRO. The other three are representativeness, confirmation bias, and overconservative revision. Their prospect theory led to Kahneman receiving the Nobel Prize in 2002. (Tversky died in 1996; the prize is not awarded posthumously.) At the time of his death, Tversky was working on ambiguity aversion (as compared to uncertainty aversion).

It is important to appreciate metacognition in terms of interaction with environments and how people interpret their environments and surrounding context. To enter isolated, austere, hazardous environments requires an adaptive, pragmatic, and resilient mind-set. Though we have not identified the characteristics of metacognition for doing so, we often see that metacognition, as monitoring and control of thinking and behavior, is necessary.

Having an awareness of uncertainty allows us to take appropriate action, which could involve evaluation of the level of uncertainty, knowledge of how to acquire the information, and the use of alternative actions if the uncertainty is insoluble.

The processing style of the individual can influence one's processing strategies in metacognition. The monitoring of memory, comprehension, and cognition are necessary components of communication and oral persuasion. These concepts within metacognition appear to overlap with social learning theory and cognitive behavior modification.

Feelings provide relevance and value to information. Feelings play a significant part in the science of metacognition. For example, how we feel can influence our search for, acceptance of, and value that we give to information we gather from our environment. As described elsewhere, we do not include "feelings" in the physiologic fear or threat response. In the neuroscience of emotion, "feelings" are considered a lay term that is different from emotion.

The Logic of Operations

The logic of operations, as a process, describes the maneuvers and actions used to create the information necessary for the next sequence. We find a distinct logic of operations at each level of analysis. For example, a line worker in production generally will follow a script, deferring to the authority of an immediate supervisor. The executive will use information from the internal and external milieu of the organization—at times seeking council from trusted experts or colleagues—to make adaptive decisions.

Crossing the liminal threshold into the uncertain, time-compressed, and threatening event exposes us to a distinct logic of operations where the environments have greater influence. One could say that the event has a vote in your plan.

A different logic of operations also exists between control operators and emergency responders. Control operators, with more of an engineering mind-set, use a rule-based system to prevent system failure, with standards, practices, processes, and protocols. This is a combined prospective approach that anticipates the worst and uses retrospective learning from the immediate past. Emergency responders, who deal with the completely contingent, dynamic, and evolving threat, entwine themselves into the situation. They use an approach of "interactive, real-time risk assessment and management" (Robert Bea, personal communication).

The logic of operations is asymmetric (or noncommutative). That is, what works in the unstructured environments can work in the structured environments, but what is designed for the structured environments is unreliable with the loss of structure. A structured logic of operations can perform well in the loss of structure, by degree, if the change is not great. This unstated dependence on context will mislead people, particularly leaders, to believe their program will work during a major crisis.

In an HRO, the logic of operations includes (1) how we treat and accept beliefs and knowledge, (2) our reasoning (inductive rather than deductive) and use of rationality, (3) modulation or regulation of the threat-fear response, (4) acceptance of unpredictability, and (5) decision-making guided by feedback loops (see below).

The Logic of Operations in Other Fields

The logic of operations, as a concept, is used to explain the application of mathematical principles to logic, a specific phase in the intellectual development of children, and to order actions for computers to communicate with one another. The following fields use a logic of operations.

Boolean algebra—George Boole first identified the importance of the order of logical processes. "Uniformity in the logical processes of reduction being desirable, I shall here *state the order which will generally be pursued* [emphasis added]. By (VIII. 8), the primitive equations are reducible to the forms...under which they can be added together without impairing their significance" (Boole 1854, 264).

Child development—Jean Piaget (Inhelder and Piaget1958) identified the concrete stage of development as the turning point in the child's cognitive development. This marks the beginning of logic or operational thought. Upon reaching that stage, the child now can *use operations and rules to develop new knowledge* [emphasis added].

Computer programming—Computer programmers (1970s) needed a standard order of actions for computers to communicate with one another. Computers used NOT, AND, and OR, which are common terms in symbolic logic. These operations in computer science are called gates, or "logical" gates, such as the NOT gate, the AND gate, and the OR gate. To direct the order for different computers to act on these strings, programmers began to use the term "logic of operations."

The Logic of Operations in HRO

We consider HRO as being unique for its recognition of the need for a different logic of operations. This is where and how this handbook differs from other approaches to HRO. People will *always* do what makes sense to them at the particular moment and will make decisions based on their sensemaking efforts. All beliefs and behaviors in complex, dynamic environments are logical at the time they are used. What we are doing in this handbook is *changing* your logic from what you may have learned as well as reframing the sensemaking you have been using. If we can do this, then HRO will become a natural method of organization during emergent and unstructured events.

Epistemology

This is knowledge as justified belief. In the absence of facts, we can only work with belief. How we justify our belief determines our actions. When information is uncertain and ambiguous, that information is then a state that we can change through interaction. People in an HRO give credence to real-time information and information gained through interaction, which differs significantly from the structured environments where information is independent of the environments (i.e., context-independent). In unstructured environments, the environments themselves contain salient information, modify information, and give meaning or relevance to information. This is critical in the development and evaluation of information during an event.

Inductive Reasoning

This refers to creating information and refining beliefs in real time. Because of the limitations of facts and factual knowledge, we must use evidence and infer new conclusions. Our efforts are directed toward strengthening our evidence, reducing uncertainty, and resolving ambiguity. Events within the incident have disrupted scientific rationality, but that does not mean our actions are not rational.

While creating information, we are also ensuring safety and bringing control to the situation. Negative feedback and the acceptance of disconfirming evidence paradoxically increase our safety. We form a new reasoning, or rationality, when we direct coherent actions toward strengthening the system while achieving the goal of safe resolution to the more desired end-state.

Modulated Threat Response
Also known as regulation of the threat-fear response, this response prevents panicked, unthinking responses while at the same time motivating action in the face of incomplete analysis. Regulated emotion provides greater clarity in thought and increases the absorption of environmental information.

For the purposes of this book and HRO in general, we follow the convention of Joseph LeDoux and Daniel Pine (2016) in the use of "threat response" for normal, expected physiological responses that can be modulated for effective and adaptive performance. Threat in this condition increases vigilance and motivation, directing actions to control or mitigate the threat. We use "fear response" for the normal, expected mental state that is *not* modulated and that cause consequential performance decrements and maladaptive behaviors. Threat in this condition directs actions toward self-protection and self-interest.

Unpredictability
Unpredictability is expected. Possibility—the ease with which an event can occur—has greater influence than discrete, numeric probabilities. If something has happened in the past, no matter how unlikely, then it can happen again. And it can happen in a manner that will create even worse circumstances. This describes the power, or "Pareto," distribution. As one author, Daved van Stralen, has said, "If it happened once, it can happen again; if it happens again, it will happen worse." Even with the probability distribution, the stochastic nature of events describes how probability distributions themselves can rapidly change. This is the logical possibility, not probability.

The use of the normal distribution and descriptive statistics can also be misleading, because things can share or have overlapped characteristics. Events and things are not discrete. There is the cliché, "If it is predictable, it is preventable." Embedding a predictable event into various environments with its context-dependent information may confound our best efforts to prevent the predictable. Therefore, whether or not an event is predictable, it may still not be preventable. The temporal nature of events, alone, with its ability to branch into new streams of activity, can prevent the ability to carry out plans and predict the near future. Our mindset must also be prepared for the predictable, because "The predictable is not always preventable."

Feedback (or Loop) Decision-Making

This form of decision-making is guided by feedback loops in real time through interactive and real-time risk assessment and management. Negative feedback marks our boundaries for safe operations. This is discussed further in chapter 6, "The Boyd OODA Loop."

HRO as Practical Rationality

A consequentially different level of analysis exists between conventional, lower-tempo, and deterministic situations and severely adverse or unexpected emergencies. The combined characteristics of time compression, imperfect information, and threats interfere with any objective analysis and categorization of events. The threat response, triggered by chaotic or dangerous situations, creates a complete separation between the logic of analysis necessary for these situations and the scientific logic used with conventional deterministic and linear events.

The impairment of cognitive function from these severe threat reactions must be identified and mitigated in real time. Oddly, this may best be achieved in the affective domain. When not mitigated, the standard logic of operations can contribute to failure while at the same time appearing reasonable to those who are not conditioned to work in these circumstances or these environments. Those who have received conditioning for this experience can resolve the situation in a more controlled and favorable way through the affective domain, which is a rather counterintuitive finding. Modulation of the threat response requires synthesis of the cognitive and affective domains of decision-making and reason.

High Reliability operators are vigilant for discrepancies and disruptions, either unexpected or out-of-place observations, events, or responses. These are investigated through observation, interaction, or discussion with somebody who has more knowledge or experience. With practice, the arousal from these discrepancies will drive actions toward reaching the more desired end-state.

When discrepancies cause aversive behaviors, anxiety, or fear (such as anger, frustration, avoidance, confusion, or freezing), we sense a lower-reliability system. But simply sensing degraded levels of reliability is not enough. It is incumbent upon those who discover the degradation to convey their observations and concerns in a clear, concise, and solution-driven manner to members of their teams while simultaneously intervening to rectify the situation.

One problem in healthcare is the profound presence of "silos." We discussed in the preface how implementation of new models of organizing can create silos. Normal human behaviors, such as territoriality, self-interest, and terror management theory, also generate silos. (1) Territoriality describes the drive to protect workspace from incursions by others in the organization, not only physical work-space but also work itself. Hall (1966) coined the term "proxemics" for the cultural expression of territoriality, something we recognize in the cultural influence of how close to another person we can stand without causing discomfort. (2) Self-interest describes the drive to act for the benefit of the individual or the work unit, even at the expense of the organization or those served, such as patients. (3) Terror management theory (Greenberg and Arndt 2011) originally described the motivation to assert group authority but, unfortunately, asserting this author-ity promotes an "us-versus-them" response toward others in the organization. This impedes interaction and the flow of information between work units.

A misplaced sense of duty contributes to silo generation and support. Duty as a value describes the obligation to others, the organization, and to the community (see "HRO as Specific Values" in chapter 1, "What is High Reliability Organizing?"). When individuals collectively consider duty to their unit or program to take prece-dence, then not only will a silo start but it will seem correct once established.

Leadership tone from the top directly or indirectly supports silos within an organization through the use, tolerance, or acceptance of fear (see "Fear as Attitude" in chapter 5, "Cognition and Affect"). In these situations, the group functioning as a silo has created an external adverse environment for those oper-ating as High Reliability.

We can reduce the silo effect when we identify, interpret, and translate salient information. We identify information within its context, interpret its meaning from our knowledge and experience, and then translate its salience and meaning for others who are less familiar with the situation and events. Information must flow as objective, articulate, and succinct descriptions.

Authority migration permits people to act immediately within their levels of knowledge and experience. This facilitates interactions to give meaning to and create information in real time. The presence of an authority gradient, an impediment of communication and information flow between the subordinate and the superior, impairs the effective use of practical rationality.

Summary

It is the structure of a particular problem or situation that allows us to use scientific logic, scientific rationality, and critical thinking. During the loss of that structure, we find these methods wanting, if not placing us in jeopardy. In environments where failure is consequential, the organization must look beyond "preoccupation with failure" to develop a program of vigilance and engagement.

The limits to scientific logic can be addressed by the modal logics: the different ways, or modes, that things are true. We must learn how to use these logics to infer reliable information from imperfect information, understand our changing beliefs in a dynamic world with uncertain information, appreciate how time changes the truths and information with which we work, and comprehend how situations create different, but logical, duties and obligations.

Simon (1957) described bounded rationality as the limits of scientific rationality, bounded by the limits of our cognition and perceptual abilities. Sandberg and Tsoukas (2011) advanced bounded rationality to describe practical rationality in order to explain the gap between the rationality of science and planning with the practical reality of routine operations. Van Stralen, during his early experience in healthcare (1982-1990) identified how threat disrupts rationality to not only impair cognition but also to drive self-preservation and self-interest, which is the unrecognized effect of fear. Hope is not lost; people for generations have modulated their threat responses to overcome these maladaptive fear responses in order to effectively respond. HRO emerged from this modulated response as an effective and logical response for operations within hazardous environments.

HRO may be counterintuitive within the limits of scientific logic and rationality; we also conduct our discussions across different levels of analyses. The program that makes sense to middle-aged, professional executives with graduate degrees may not make sense to a young worker with little or no advanced education—the typical dynamic in the market of change, education, and consulting services. Most significant in appreciating HRO is horizontal analysis, i.e., moving from structured environments with the comfort of binding rules and predictability across the threshold to unstructured environments where rules conflict, compete, or do not apply, and we cannot predict the results of our actions. While we think of this as a rare, catastrophic event, the dynamics and the human mind are the same for a newly hired administrative assistant walking into the office on the first day of work.

We have presented here our argument for HRO as a logic of operations, one that the organization can use for routine operations that rapidly expand during unanticipated emergencies where a suddenly identified discrepancy or a disruption of processes or operations occurs. We present five elements of this construct:

(1). *epistemological* change, where the things we know to be true are only the responses to our actions;

(2). *inductive reasoning*, where we constantly update information through real-time and interactive evaluation of evidence;

(3). *modulated threat response*, which is the paradox of threat-fear—threat drives motivation and action without fear, thus creating self-preservation or self-interest, which can perforate the fabric of our program;

(4). *unpredictability*, which we describe as something that is expected;

(5). *feedback loop decision-making*, which is done during interactive and real-time risk assessment and management and identifies areas of least friction (positive feedback) and the borders of safety (negative feedback).

The hallmark of an HRO is the rapid and agile shift between structured approaches *preventing* system failure to unstructured approaches *responding* to system failure. In the former, the lessons learned from failure were developed into effective rules and processes; outliers are not disregarded as random, independent events but are responded to or explained as discrepancies or system disruptions. In the latter, lessons are learned from real-time interactions; as a discrepancy or system disruption, the outlier may herald the initiation of a process that we must attend to.

The HRO is situational; it shifts rapidly and agilely between prevention and emergency but also utilizes the strengths of each system in the "opposing" prevention or emergency environments. Prevention and emergency may even be attended to simultaneously. In the emergency-response system, outliers include mindless or rigid adherence to the rules and processes that moments before ensured safety through prevention. This creates the HRO paradox that "what helps us can hurt us, and what hurts us can help us." That is, helping and hurting are situational in place and time, with small shifts in space or time causing disproportionate changes in safety margins.

This knowledge is within reach of all members of the organization and can become intuitive to the leaders within the organization, although HRO can be perceived as counterintuitive for those who are not experienced in uncertain, time-compressed, threatening environments. HRO is resisted by those who find security in control.

Conclusions

(1). The logic of operations in HRO adapts to the VUCA-T environments, which differentiates this form of logic from the more commonly used scientific logic.

(2). HRO reduces false debates created by arguments across analysis levels.

(3). Context and time compression can alter the logic of operations within an HRO.

(4). HRO has logic and rationality, but it is a logic of practice and practical rationality.

(5). The prevention of system failure and emergency response to system failure create different shifts in the logic of operations.

CHAPTER 4

HRO AND THE ENVIRONMENT

High Reliability Organizing is an effective method for engaging situations that do not have clear structure. The lack of structure defies attempts to design a system for these situations, and plans do not reliably work. The healthcare and business literature describe an HRO as an organization that succeeds when the environment predicts it would fail, originating as it did from US Navy aviation operations, US nuclear power plants, and California electrical grid system. Weick and Sutcliffe (2015) have codified HRO into five principles. Unfortunately, the common tendency to appreciate only the rationality component of HRO often leads to the mistaken belief that we can design an HRO system and bring it to the organization from the top downward. What this situation disregards is the *affective* component of HRO—the need to regulate emotion and modulate fear, the methods for placing value on uncertain or ambiguous information, and the ability to shift values based on the emergent, newly contextualized situation.

What sets the HRO apart is the significance of the environment. The design and structure of many organizations often stand independently of the environments in which they operate. Knowledge and science are objective—independent of the environment and subjective notions of individuals.

Concepts of intentional High Reliability behaviors and beliefs emerged from successful and effective responses to dangerous situations in dangerous environments in which the threat was real, personal, and imminent. For HROs, information is recognized as being time-dependent and fleeting, which requires one to doubt the reliability of information that has not changed or has not been updated. Knowledge becomes context-dependent and variable. The objectivity of information dissipates; its importance becomes one more judgment to make under pressure.

The demand to treat sicker and more complex patients with a larger professional workforce taxes conventional healthcare and organizational theory. HRO helps overcome these challenges. HRO consists of the elements of *cognition* and *affect* in the person (see chapter 5, "Cognition and Affect"), the *context* within which the situation occurs, and the responding *behaviors*. In this chapter, we will discuss the context within which HRO operates, because HRO development arose as a response to VUCA-T environments: volatile, uncertain, complex, ambiguous, and threatening. (See "The Environment" in chapter 2, "What Problem Does HRO Solve?")

The interaction of cognition, affect, and behaviors, in context, creates High Reliability.

The Environment

Environments, from a distance, appear constant. Upon entering an environment, we experience the dynamic, constant self-organizing that takes place over its own time scale. Humans cannot enter an environment without changing it in some way. Even our presence in the wilderness changes how animals move; our passage leaves marks on the ground and disturbs brush. We become part of the self-organizing activity. Though we are inconsequential in some environments, we still have left a mark.

When the environment becomes adverse or unsafe, we act. This action Weick describes as enactment: we are acting into something that is already dynamic. We shape and create within multiple changing elements. In a sense, an HRO works, not from organized external commands, but from within multiple simultaneous changing environments.

HROs have the elements of self-organization: local responses to local events, internal forces and processes, and nonlinear interactions. What is different in an HRO is intention. People bring intention into the environment. People in an HRO are able to use intention to change environments.

Fire Rescue Ambulance Responses in an Active Gang Environment

When we arrive on scene, we become part of the problem: how we step out of the rig, how we walk up, how we look at people. This is not to say we are causing problems, only that, from the moment we arrive, we are changing the environment and changing the problem. It is different for each one of us. None of us would ever have the same interaction, because our presence is different for each of us, making a different problem.

The fire department sent two Rescue Ambulance (RA) men on a response. The Los Angeles Fire Department used ambulances for medical or trauma emergencies, what is now called an EMS response. During this period, the RA responded without fire engine company or Law Enforcement officer support unless it was requested *after* evaluation of the scene. We could call for assistance with the phone in the house, or one of us would have to leave to use the rescue ambulance radio. It was not uncommon to have some argument and an occasional physical altercation on scene. Every year a few rescue ambulance men were injured in these fights and placed off duty.

Knowing this, you use every faculty of your senses and movements to influence the scene and the people around you. Your countenance, your tone, and the words you use can calm, soothe, and control. They can also incite and anger people. What helped you on the last call may hurt you on the next call. Because you will not know which, until the word is said or the movement is made, you watch every face and listen to every word and detect the tone in which it is said. You are always part of the problem.

You are part of the problem for the system. Help from the cops ranges from them standing aside at a close distance, adding a few words, or immediately restraining an assailant. Each method also becomes part of the problem—a new problem.

From the moment we arrived until we drove away, as ambulance men, we continuously worked a problem we were a part of. We entered an environment that we became a part of.

—Daved van Stralen

We exist within, but apart from, the environment. Because we can separate ourselves from the environment, we too easily see the organization in the same context. Organizations, however, are enmeshed in the environment, with an unclear boundary separating the organization from suppliers, resources, the marketplace, regulators, and customers. The organization can both define, and be defined by, its environment.

Problems and situations likewise exist in environments as amorphous boundaries separating the issue and the environment. If it were not for the environment, we might not have as many problems or difficult situations. But if it were not for the environment, we also would not experience growth and development.

Environments contain information and provide meaning to information: information that we can use, which is the basis of HRO. It is not enough to know where the problem is, the fact that we are in a difficult situation, or where we can locate certain information. The HRO knows how this information will hurt, how it can help, and, likely, why it is there.

It is common to assume that we have rational minds at all times, just as we assume that environments are rational and can be understood at all times. We often assume a greater degree of predictability than is warranted, yet people act as though linearity is the norm, that all actions and responses, whether originating from the environment or us, are proportional. This is the key defect in the non-HRO organization: the overreliance on one's interpretation of the environment while failing to recognize the environment's dispassionate independence of our wishes. The environment is an apathetic, random determinant toward our fate.

For research purposes, controlling all but one or a few variables means that the environment must be controlled as much as possible. This creates an objective and rational, though artificial, environment within which the researcher can experiment. Inadvertently, academic researchers have given preeminence to the rational domain and support the view that environments are rational.

The individual, operating *in vivo*, when outside of such controlled environments experiences a subjective environment through the affective domain: one of attitudes, values, and meaning. Two people operating side by side will experience the same environment in different ways.

The rational domain is universal—that is, general or generalizable—while the affective domain is situational, specific to the particular incident and particular person. Rationality covers reason, patterns, and prediction, while the affective domain covers attitudes, situational evaluation, situational values, and regulated emotion.

HRO environments have their own internal rationality, whether we can detect it or not. Though we believe we are purely rational beings, our response to the environment is affective. A strictly rational response to a dangerous situation is not possible due to the need to place subjective value on information and to interpret responses, which is the virtue of phronesis. (See chapter 1, "What Is High Reliability Organizing?") An algorithmic approach to hazardous complexity, no matter how desirable, is also impossible. HROs not only respond to environments; HROs change environments.

Context

Context comes from the environment; it gives salience and meaning to information and forms the patterns we detect. We must first learn this information (which was the goal of our formal education) without forgetting that it represents an ideal world—one easily studied but nonexistent. Knowledge without context is sterile and nonproductive. Done well, we achieve the competent level of skill performance of the Dreyfus model of skill acquisition briefly mentioned in the previous chapter, capable of generalizing universal principles. Some programs may require novices to have the ability to apply principles to a particular situation. The Dreyfus level of proficiency is achieved through internship training.

This situation creates a problem for healthcare education. Learning concepts and theories independent of specific environments in the process of formal education prepares one to understand experience yet not fully entwine into an undefined situation. Generally, initial educational programs produce people who are competent to solve generalized problems when given sufficient information and resources, thus forming an ideal world that is easily taught to students and discussed in the abstract.

The real world, itself, is the context. Students will discuss going out into the real world, when they are actually in *their* real world, just as their faculty have a different real world of college, hospital ward, clinic, or operating room. Whether blue-collar, professional, academic, subordinate, or superior, we each have a real world in which we function that differs from other real worlds. The difference is in the context.

We produce "possible worlds" (see chapter 3, "The Logic of Operations") as part of our planning, an approach that expresses possible end-states and necessary situations. In a real-time situation, these possible worlds are what we think of as being immediately accessible. They are the form and direction of our effort and change. These possible worlds are compatible with our attitudes and help form our efforts. None of this takes away from the concept of an actual world, except that the actual world is impossible to comprehend without the omniscience of complete knowledge. The necessary but limited use of "possible worlds" for education and planning creates a hidden deficit in our ability to identify and interpret context-dependent information.

In art, "negative space" describes the space around the subject. Negative space helps identify and give meaning to context. It is the voids around the central focus in sculpture; in painting, the negative space is less decorated to bring attention to the subject. Negative space gives meaning to information in unstructured environments. When we cannot describe what something is, we may find it more useful to describe what it is not. This is not a trivial idea. Someone who is untrained in art can draw a picture of her hand, but it may not be an accurate depiction. Drawing the area around the hand *that is not the hand*—that is, the negative space around the hand and fingers—provides a much better representation of the hand (Edwards 1999).

Context derives from personal experience and knowledge, physical and mental position, and aspirations. It influences, and is influenced by, sensemaking. Without recognition of context, non-HRO organizations roll out continuous streams of initiatives without considering contextual influences and the environment.

Framing

To organize experience and structure perceptions, we must filter information, know what is *not* important, disregard noise, and build frames. These basic cognitive structures guide our perception of reality.

As an individual behavior, "framing" defines problems, helps identify causes, informs judgment, and suggests solutions. This involves the selection of information as well as the salience of that information. We want to increase the likelihood that all team members are operating within the same contextual understanding of the problem. Framing increases the probability that a novice will perceive subtle information or detect nuanced differences. This is most vital when vulnerability arises from processes, as we must begin the detective process early in an emergency when the event may just as easily be benign (Entman 1993).

"Salience" makes a piece of information more noticeable, meaningful, or memorable. When this is not taught to the novice, what is most noticeable or meaningful may reflect the novice's individual experience rather than what is important to bring control to the situation. Unless we teach the salience and significance of signs and signals, people become more susceptible to fear and misidentify threats, and they tend to confound noise with important signals. Increased salience enhances the probability that receivers will perceive the information, discern meaning, and process and store the information (Entman 1993).

Framing selects and calls attention to particular aspects of reality. The person's internal logic then takes over, and the frame has thus influenced the inference. This acculturation can change the frame surrounding the issue to change the student's perception without altering the actual facts. As a social behavior, framing helps assimilate social, institutional, and organizational knowledge. It renders meaning to allow us to see what others in our group see and to share the importance of certain types of information. Framing gives meaning to perception, organizes experience, and guides actions. Framing embodies the culture of the organization as the novice acquires the organization's values and processes new experiences.

It is important to note that framing is a learned skill, as are many other components of HRO. People who are inexperienced with the organization and HRO in general can find it difficult to articulate what they see in a manner that will be understandable to the team and to the situation. Simply "seeing something" is not enough when the success of the organization depends on each team member's ability to recognize and respond to external stimuli while simultaneously informing the rest of the team to raise collective situational awareness. Every version of the aviation field's crew resource management (CRM, which started as "cockpit resource management" on the flight deck) has focused heavily on training operators to communicate discrepancies across an authority gradient. A cadence is used that is designed to attain the relevant person's attention, concisely state the problem, clearly propose a solution, and persist until an appropriate decision is reached and communicated back to the team. The result has been a marked decrease in avoidable errors where communication breakdown was the primary causal factor.

When we take an action, the situation will change. But which rules change and which rules do not change? Framing contributes to a sense of stability while continually supporting agility. What rule does not change because of an action? This is the *frame problem* from artificial intelligence. When we infer the consequences of change, we often do not address the question of which rules did not change. Framing informs us of how we can expect a situation to change, which rules to continue to follow, and which rules no longer apply.

One effective method of reframing is to ask for the advice or answers from subordinates. Accepting their answer, then pursuing it with the addition of more information or reframing the situation, helps identify if it is lack of knowledge or difficulty with problem solving. Iterations of this process can identify the focus for education and training. It need not be long, if time is short then make larger steps in reframing or the provision of necessary information, to make it collective, ask others on the team for their responses.

Threats

The signs and signals that indicate harm are context and person dependent. A supervisor's sudden approach can be relieving or stressful, depending on the circumstances and the nature of the relationship the supervisor has with his or her subordinates. In a crisis, the supervisor can calm the situation or stir up more stress. A newly hired clerk has as much stress the first day on the job as some may have in a life-threatening emergency. This is not to make light of such emergencies but to point out that we all have the same brain and neurological responses. The brain does not respond in a proportional manner but on the perception of demand and ability to meet the demand.

Sources of Threats

If it's predictable, it's preventable. Anything that can go wrong will go wrong. We too easily fall to cliché or an adage when discussing predictability and inevitability. Just because we can anticipate or declare something in advance does not mean we can avert the event. Causation is far too complex for this. In the most difficult scenario, several causes interact with one another in a disproportionate level to produce emergent, novel properties. These new properties then interact with various people in the organization from whom the crisis emerges. At any point, a small intervention could redirect events, while at the same time, cascading events can bypass our defenses and quickly overwhelm the system. Even a rapid shift from the prevention of system failure to response to system failure—a highly developed maneuver—may not be enough.

Something seemingly insurmountable or difficult to prevent should not drive us to complacency. We really do not know if something is insurmountable except in hindsight. But this knowledge is available only if the organization willingly accepts failure *from* acting as an integral—and necessary—part of engagement, a method to create information and identify safety boundaries, and the initial step of "early error identification and correction." Failure from *not* acting is invisible and contributes to a level of institutional fear in these events.

It is more common to use Murphy's law ("If anything can go wrong, it will") to support the inevitability of failure. Without digressing into the law's origins, we can discuss how Capt. Edward A. Murphy and Col. John Stapp used the phrase. In the late 1940s, the US Air Force conducted deceleration studies to improve survivability in aircraft crashes and, later, rapid-acceleration tests for ejection at supersonic speeds. Capt. Murphy was one of the engineers; Col. Stapp was the flight surgeon and test subject.

It seems that during one such test, a technician working for Capt. Murphy installed a strain gauge incorrectly, which prevented the recording of data. This led to an outburst about the technician's general level of expected performance: if there were any way of making a mistake, he would find that way. Col. Stapp, who regularly risked his life during these tests, attributed their success to following Murphy's law in considering all possibilities of failure. Hence, Murphy's law to some is a resignation to failure, while to others it is a call for vigilance and consideration of various sources of failure.

During these rocket-sled acceleration and deceleration tests, Col. Stapp realized that the belt lashing him into the sled prevented serious injury during the tests. In 1955, he shared these rocket sled test results with the Society of Automotive Engineers. Two years later Volvo installed seatbelts in their cars (C Ryan 2015). In 1966, federal law required seatbelts in all automobiles sold in the United States.

Whether apocryphal or not, the story illustrates that we can resign ourselves to accepting failure or affirm that we can surmount failure. These clichés or adages unfortunately can lead to complacency, shame, guilt, or blame. Hazards and their mitigation are a complex interplay of energy, information, human behavior, and physiology.

Uncontrolled Energy

The transformation and dissipation of energy is a major source of failure. In daily life, we may encounter one of five forms of energy: mechanical (kinetic or potential energy), chemical, thermal, electrical, and ionizing radiation (radioactivity). Energy can transform itself to other forms of energy, and it will naturally dissipate. These are the first and second laws of thermodynamics. Overheating of an electrical device is one example of energy transformation. Energy also dissipates, a process of increasing randomization called entropy. For our purposes, we must understand that it takes energy to contain energy; the greater the energy to contain, the greater the energy necessary to contain it. The transformation of energy to other forms must be considered when containing energy. Energy *will* transform or dissipate.

Corrupted Information

Claude E. Shannon discovered that information dissipates much like energy; it has a similar equation (called Shannon's information entropy equation), shown below. In the same manner that thermodynamic entropy increases disorder, information entropy increases disorder in a process Shannon defined as uncertainty. Certainty has a similar range as the entropy in a physical system: from the tight order of a crystal to the completely random disarray of a gas. Noise interferes with the transmission of information by increasing the information's randomness or uncertainty. This is not a trivial discussion, as Shannon's information theory forms the basis of all today's digital communications and electrical equipment.

$$C = 2B \, \mathrm{Log}_2 \left\{ \left(1 + \frac{S}{N}\right)^{1/2} \right\} = B \, \mathrm{Log}_2 \left\{ 1 + \frac{S}{N} \right\}$$

Information is encoded at one location, transmitted, and then decoded at a second location. The corruption of communication can occur in any point in the sequence. This corruption can be decreased with various methods, but it is important for us to appreciate that communication, alone, is a corrupting influence of information and a contributor to system failure. We must not blame the individual person for communication failures. *Communication corrupts information.*

Uncontrolled Behavior

We cannot predict how someone will behave in a confused situation or under threat, our own response or the response of others. Throughout this book, we discuss threat responses and unrecognized fear. We also must deal with everyday human behaviors and subclinical, undiagnosed, or untreated psychological traits—some of which are adaptive. Briefly, these are affective processes of emotion or mood—processes about belief or perception, such as psychotic disorders—and personality traits or disorders such as antisocial, narcissistic, or psychopathic disorders.

We will encounter these issues from outside the system when dealing with our patients and the public. It is not our position (nor do we recommend doing so) to make such a diagnosis in the heat of the moment or to use this information to dictate a response. Be aware that some people do not react as expected for a number of reasons; one reason may be a subclinical, undiagnosed, or untreated mental condition. More appropriate for our discussion is the presence of unrecognized fear or a threat response from someone outside the system. One would interact with this person differently compared to within the organization.

Within the system, maladaptive behaviors may have become institutionalized, particularly if modeled by senior staff, administrators, and executives. These include instrumental anger, motivational fear, gratuitous stress, intimidation by countenance, and criticism as motivator. Some people use *instrumental anger,* a strategic use of anger that does not come from the fear response but is calculated to create a fear response in others. People use this type of controlled anger for an extrinsic purpose, as a means to an end that is separate from the emotional reaction to the current situation.

Motivational Fear

Motivational fear is effective. It changes behaviors and it limits questions. Unfortunately, the leader cannot choose the behaviors, and the reasoning for the fear is entirely beyond the leader's control. People will give their own meaning and explanation to the fear stimulus to create new, unintended behaviors. Fear of discipline for not filling out forms leads to "euboxia" (see chapter 5, "Cognition and Affect"), with staff mindlessly filling in the blocks for information, thus ensuring a completed form at the expense of information. Fear of being sued—liability as a threat—leads to the overuse of "third-party" studies such as laboratory or imaging studies, the use of consultants, or delayed decision-making at the expense of well-thought out actions (see chapter 5, "Cognition and Affect"). Similar to euboxia, mindless documentation occurs at the expense of articulate description.

The advice that "to learn how to work under stress, you must be placed under stress" is sometimes a sincere belief, sometimes almost sadistic, but either way it produces *gratuitous stress* that is counterproductive if not destructive to success-fully operating in chaotic, threat environments. This idea may be true to the degree that the person is connected to a supportive other and is given the tools to deal with stress. (This is discussed further in marine recruit training in chapter 12, "Leadership, Authority, Command, and Team Formation," and chapter 14, "Culture"). Too often in healthcare, this becomes an excuse for gratuitous stress, excessive burdening, or unsupportive leadership.

> "Leadership is not about gratuitously inducing stress simply because your mentor induced stress for you. Leadership requires that stress be understood for what it is: a part of the High Reliability reality that can induce enhanced team performance if properly modeled by the mentor and understood by the staff."
> —SPENCE BYRUM

We often hear things like, "If I compliment you, then you will not work as hard. My criticism motivated you to improve" (personal communications with numerous nurses and physicians who trained students and residents to van Stralen). Daniel Kahneman, working with Israeli Air Force flight instructors in the mid-1960s (Kahneman and Tversky 1973), identified the belief that praise leads to performance deterioration, while punishing criticism improves per-formance. Some people believe that praise leads to complacency (even lazi-ness) or overconfidence because, from their experience, they have observed deterioration in performance following praise and improvements following criticism.

What Kahneman and Tversky identified was regression to the mean, misinter-preted as the students' responses to the flight instructor's comments. When the students had performed well, they exhibited regression of performance to the mean, the appearance of skill degradation. When the students performed poorly, similar regression improved the students' performance. The flight instructors interpreted regression to the mean to be a response to their praise or criticism. This interpretation, common to all of us, exposes us to "a lifetime schedule in which we [as teachers] are most often *rewarded for punishing others* [emphasis added], and punished for rewarding" (Kahneman and Tversky 1973, 251).

Kahneman and Tversky (1973, 251) describe performance of flight maneuvers as not perfectly reliable, and "progress between successive maneuvers is slow." Also, complex skills are learned in steps that the student must amalgamate to create a smooth flow for the procedure. Within this amalgamation are memory phases of skill *acquisition,* the *consolidation* of memory (cognitive and behavioral), then *retrieval* when called upon to perform the skill (Sandi and Pinelo-Nava 2007). At any point, stress can release cortisol or adrenaline, thus confounding memory and skill to create variance in performance. The result is a sinusoidal skill-performance curve, as described by Kahneman and Tversky, with continual regression toward the mean, but the mean has a positive slope of steady, regular improvement. With knowledgeable instructors, conditioning during training brings this stress effect under control.

Attribution tells people what they are; persuasion tells them what they are not (Miller, Brickman, and Bolen 1973). This is the reason people are more likely to change when you describe the end-state you desire. For example, rather than saying, "You are always late on assignments," you might say, "I know you work hard to get the assignments completed on time. That's how we work here."

The confusion inherent between preventing failure or responding to failure can lead to distinct differences in thought. *Deference to expertise* is a foundational principle of HRO, referring to the application of local and specific knowledge in preparation for or during an event. ("Deference" here means to defer, as in regard or consider. It does not mean defer in the sense of yield or submit. Deferring to expertise, in the context of the situation, may mean rapid or lengthy consideration; it does not mean mindless acceptance.) The behavioral differences between prevention and response can be found in the same person, but more commonly we may see someone who has more expertise in one over the other. Misunderstanding behavioral differences or styles or not recognizing their expertise can lead to labeling their behaviors as difficult or disruptive rather than insightful, anticipatory, and loyal to the organization. We must distinguish between difficult people and disruptive people.

People see and think differently, which creates a potential source for positive variability in the organization. During a response to a crisis, some of these people may not be able to objectively or articulately express their point, which should not take away from their point's validity. Focusing on the discrepancy that is produced can illuminate gaps in people's thinking, thus improving their performance, or within the system, thus improving the overall program.

This situation differs from the disruptive person. Disruptive people are those who place greater emphasis on themselves and their point of view. From their viewpoint, the goal can only be achieved in one way. Here, the goal is for the disruptive person to have his or her own way while disregarding discrepancies in the environment.

Uncontrolled behavior creates an environment that HRO operates within; we can readily see this in both healthcare and law enforcement, where uncontrolled emotions, behavior, and irrational thought processes are routinely encountered. These people who are outside the organization force personnel to adapt their behaviors to gain the desired goal.

Uncontrolled behavior also occurs *within* the organization. A few types of these uncontrolled behaviors include instrumental behaviors, maladaptive behaviors, and unrecognized fear behaviors. These behaviors, in effect, make the individual part of the crisis environment. These uncontrolled, distracting, and dis-balancing behaviors functionally place these people outside the organization. This is most immediate when the team falls apart during an emergency, or distractions cause maladaptive responses in the leader. A more effective strategy in these situations is to consider these team members as belonging to the external environment rather than being part of the team or organization.

Instrumental anger and instrumental fear describe the creation of fear in members for an extrinsic purpose. We differentiate instrumental anger, a form of intimidation to attain a desired or planned goal (Dodge 1991), from instrumental aggression, which Rule (1974) described as providing some reward or advantage to the aggressor. We base this difference not only on these definitions but on the differences between anger and aggression and instrumental anger versus reactive anger.

Anger is a negative emotion accompanied by physiological arousal and hostile thoughts. Aggression is intentional behavior to harm for the purpose of dominance and control. For our purposes, this makes a distinction between a sudden-onset emotional response (reactive anger) and a pattern of behavior for gain (aggression). Anger, in this approach, is a form of the threat or fear response of fight or flight, while aggression is closer to a strategy for personal gain.

A small group of physicians and nurses were discussing a proposed program to teach mask ventilation to emergency responders not affiliated with the hospital. They agreed on the need and benefit to the community. Hospital legal counsel attended the meeting and struck up a friendly conversation with a nurse. The counsel then asked several questions about the program and described how he had protected the medical center from a similar program years ago. Suddenly he began shouting that there was no benefit to the medical center for this new program and challenged others that they would benefit personally. He rose to his feet and continued the tirade, stating that "this was over before it started." Walking to the door, he calmly turned and quietly said, "What we have is failure of leadership."

—Anonymous witness

Instrumental fear describes the presentation of a conjured but possible threat to change behaviors. This type of fear can be in the form of the threat of liability ("We can be sued") or failure. The extrinsic gain is to stop an action or to obtain a desired behavior not intrinsic to HRO.

Recurrent fevers and repeated positive blood cultures in a critically ill patient with a central venous catheter led physicians to question if a blood clot located near the tip of the catheter could be seeding the blood stream. The injection of contrast material during a portable chest radiograph was inconclusive. The removal of the catheter, if the clot was attached, could send an infected embolus through the circulator system. The radiologist recommended transporting the patient for fluoroscopy. The bedside nurse had been resistant throughout the day to any patient transport; finally, the nurse asked, "Are you sure it's safe?"

This created a dilemma for us: answer yes, and she might have reduced her vigilance; answer no, and we became responsible for any complication.

—Daved van Stralen

The normalization of maladaptive behaviors does not stress the program until it is tested by unexpected crises. Long periods of limited environmental demand or modeling by respected leaders makes this situation possible. The clearest example is rigid hierarchy or the absence of any authority migration for local decision-making. This becomes normative behavior for the discrepancy, disruption, or crisis.

During team formation in an emergency response, some members will exhibit unrecognized fear responses. Other team members who recognize such a response must support the member to bring the person back into the team. It is the mark of good leadership in these convergent teams, formed for the functional purpose in a local system failure, to maintain vigilance and early recognition for these changes.

We cannot predict how someone will act when under immediate threat.

Uncontrolled Physiology

Uncontrolled physiology, the ultimate threat in healthcare, can be acute or chronic. Acute uncontrolled physiology relates to the oxygen-delivery equation (oxygen delivery = cardiac output X oxygen content of the blood). In the chronic state, uncontrolled physiology occurs in debilitating or disabling diseases.

The complex medical patient is a high-risk patient in healthcare. For example, physician billing for a patient with multiple chronic illnesses and one acute exacerbation is similar in high-level decision-making to a patient who receives cardiopulmonary resuscitation. This situation is not necessarily wrong but is a reflection of the fact that chronic illnesses rob the body of the physiologic reserve necessary to fight an acute illness. The acute illness can affect chronically ill organs in unpredictable ways and can lower the threshold toward death.

Healthcare education understandably teaches about individual diseases, since this is necessary to produce competence in healthcare graduates. What remain untaught are the nonlinear interactions between diseases and the emergence of novel properties, presentations, and responses to therapy. Age (at either extreme) acts as a disease, increasing complexity. All complex medical patients have early heralds of acute illness that healthcare providers who have not learned about complex medical patients will not readily recognize.

Complex medical patients may have undiagnosed, undertreated, or unrecognized pathophysiology completely independent of presenting complaints. The hidden severity of illness contributes to delayed diagnoses and more severe illness. In this manner, the resource demands of the complex medical patient may become an unrecognized threat to the healthcare system.

Overall, threats in the healthcare system have the same sources as threats in all industries and environments, including

1) uncontrolled energy that can transform or dissipate unpredictably;
2) information uncertainty from detection, decoding, transmission, encoding, and communication;
3) uncontrolled behaviors from inside or outside the system because of
   a) expected limitations on cognition and perception (bounded rationality);
   b) unrecognized fear and threat responses;
   c) subcriminal or criminal behavior;
   d) subclinical or clinical psychopathology; and
   e) deficits in command, leadership, or team formation;

4) uncontrolled physiology from acute disturbances in
   a) tissue oxygen delivery;
   b) chronic debilitating illnesses;
   c) the complex medical patient;
   d) multiple interactive diseases of an acute, chronic, or exacerbated nature.

System failure is predictable; it is too complex to be preventable. Anything that can go wrong, will go wrong, so be vigilant.

Response to Threats

The commonsense nature of the duality of safety and operations, one is only possible because of the other, became clear to van Stralen when RAdm Mercer, during a discussion, said, "We achieve safety through operations and operations through safety." This was nearly a direct quote from van Stralen's fire captain, William J. Corr who, after risky fire operations would say, "Remember, it's safety through operations and our operations are through safety." Mercer is a veteran of US Navy aerial combat over North Vietnam and Corr was a US Navy World War II veteran in the South Pacific Theater. Both men embody this duality of safety and operations as the means to respond to and engage threats.

HROs developed within hostile, limiting environments. From the individual level to the organizational level, members are problem-oriented, process-driven, and sensitive to vulnerability. Safety and operations are intentionally integrated to create unity, if not duality, of safety and operations. While HROs have also formed in safe environments, the codification of High Reliability Organizations came from organizations operating in high-risk environments or that conducted high-risk operations. What they have in common is their pragmatic nature.

Problem-Oriented

Solving a defined problem can be straightforward, because it is familiar and follows universal principles. The indeterminate or undefined problem is a complex blend of events, the environment, individuals, and the organization. This requires specific evaluation of more of the information available and generation of problem-specific information. General rules and guidelines, well-accepted protocols, and more specific rules may create error rather than contribute to success: what Reason (1990) called "the strong-but-wrong rule."

This is not to accept unrestrained "freelance" behavior or anarchy but to have the pragmatic freedom to focus on problem-solving with improvisation.

A respiratory care practitioner (RCP) was assigned to the pediatric subacute care facility from another unit. During discussions of how to manage a respiratory emergency, the RCP continually said he would follow the rules. When pressed, he used the standard Heart Association resuscitation rules and guidelines. When pressed further to describe what he would do if the patient did not respond, he continued with following the rules. He would not provide any therapy in a life-or-death situation unless it was in the rules, and he said he would follow those rules even if the patient did not respond to therapy.

My frustration was relieved when a bedside LVN [licensed vocational nurse] heard the conversation and advised how she would treat, by watching for response. She mentioned several treatments that were within the rules but that the RCP thought could only be ordered by a physician. A passing RCP assigned to the facility joined the conversation and agreed that it is the duty of the RCP to hand-ventilate the patient until he or she finds a pattern that works.

This is what we mean by being "problem-oriented" in HRO: you solve the problem (phronesis) versus following a scientific principle that is not working (episteme).

—Daved van Stralen

Operations on the edge of failure cannot prevent all error or failures; some will cause injury or impede operations. These events take resources away from the purpose of the organization. Therefore, response to failure is built into routine operations, mitigating to the extent possible the consequence of the error and allowing continuous performance toward the desired end-state despite the event. It is the duty of all members to identify errors early and begin corrective actions (i.e., leader-leader rather than leader-follower).

The high-risk event starts within routines and mundane happenings. As activity accelerates and draws energy and resources, the threat grows and the consequences become unrecoverable failure. Early in this course, it is likely that the least experienced and least knowledgeable people could have taken action to stop the progression. To seek permission to engage (or to wait for the threat to become better) defined will allow the event to move closer to cataclysmic failure. Wishful thinking that it may not fail sometimes works by buying time for the event to self-resolve. When thing is wrong, failure is extreme. For this reason, every member of an HRO has the unwritten authority and duty to engage the situation and lead efforts until relieved of duties. This is leader-leader action for a problem-driven response.

The abstract nature of formal education, science, and planning cannot account for the granular nature of the local environment at that moment of failure. HRO emerged from these local interactions at this finite, granular level.

Process Driven
The HRO relies on smooth performance in its operations. Any interruption or disturbance is immediately engaged. The logic of operations rapidly changes when the process changes from preventing system failure to responding to system failure. The strict adherence to procedures of the control operator gives way to problem-solving in real time. This requires a shift in attitudes and values as well as discernment of the salience of the information.

Sensitive to Vulnerability
Vulnerability at the edge of failure places the whole operation at risk. Because these are processes, vulnerability develops over time, but at some point, elements of vulnerability become visible. All members of the organization are vigilant for these elements. From the Yerkes-Dodson law, as shown in figure 2 below, we can see that an HRO maintains itself at the peak of the curve, with optimal arousal and optimal performance. High-risk situations have a narrower distribution, thus requiring greater experience and insight into these operations.

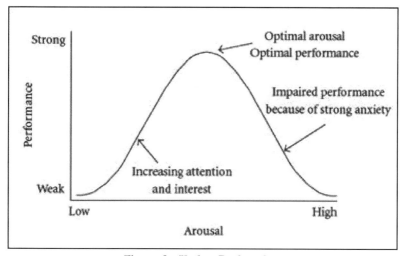

Figure 2—Yerkes-Dodson law

The Yerkes-Dodson law highlights one interesting aspect: it helps organizations dispel the notion that all stress (arousal) is "bad" for the organization. As seen in the figure, arousal actually causes an organization to raise its performance to a fairly well-defined point. HROs will recognize that point and proactively take mitigating actions for the stress, while non-HROs will not recognize what we call the "point of no return" and will subsequently fall off the back of the stress/performance curve and suffer suboptimal performance (or worse). The law, and the relative push/pull associated with remaining within the bounds of manageable stress despite a potentially life-threatening event, both help HROs recognize, manage, and train for scenarios associated with the stress/performance relationship.

Pragmatism

HRO is pragmatic rather than objectively rational or reasoned. In the HRO, the logic of operations in dynamic times is modified toward the subjective and affective, such as regulated emotion, situational values, and evaluated information. This shift to the pragmatic, subjective, and affective impairs the acceptance of authentic HRO processes. HRO is not a structure you bring to your organization; it is a process that contributes to adaptability in the face of sudden events. The misunderstanding that you can design your system to "be HRO" has impeded efforts to achieve High Reliability.

Liminality: The Threshold

There are many types of rites of passage. It may be a transition into adulthood or a membership in a tribe. (An example is military recruit training, such as for the US Marine Corps, as described in chapter 12, "Leadership, Authority, Command, and Team Formation," and chapter 14, "Culture.") During the middle stage of a rite of passage, the participant enters a period of ambiguity, disorientation, and stress. Often this is during the night, when perception is limited and human support is lacking. In effect, the experience mimics death as the person passes from one life stage to another. This middle stage is called the "liminal," after the Latin for threshold, and liminality is where that quality of disorientation and fear one feels resides.

The danger of crossing the liminal threshold can be seen in military pilots who have flown between one hundred and three hundred hours. They have been rigorously instructed, have accomplished much, and have been conditioned to be confident in their abilities, but they are significantly hampered by their lack of experience outside the training environment. An inordinate amount of confidence, coupled with a limited experience base, produces a fatal combination if the pilots are not trained to recognize the approach of the liminal boundary.

—Spence Byrum

This disorientation, as well as the fear it evokes, occurs when we are under threat and do not know how to respond. Once we learn what works, we begin to become oriented, and the fear dissipates. The dissipation of confusion and fear is experienced to some degree by those who are learning HRO methodology. The disorientation is also a significant source of resistance, negative judgment toward the methods used, and distrust in relying on this approach by those who have not experienced these results.

Transitions at the Threshold

This liminal threshold can occur in expected or unexpected ways. Transitions to a new position or situation, though expected, have a threshold, as does the unexpected High Reliability situation (HRS). Whether expected or not, the person experiences a new, unfamiliar internal logic at best, or disruption of internal logic at worst. (See chapter 2, "What Problem Does HRO Solve?")

Other than internal logic, people are most disrupted by *overload* during transitions (Weick and Sutcliffe 2008). Overload is a state induced when the amount of input to a system exceeds its processing capacity, or a mismatch occurs between information processing and information loads. As Weick and Sutcliffe argue, the traditional conception of capacity is a finite amount: too much information and information is lost, missed, or interferes with processing. Overload is physical and perceptual. Weick and Sutcliffe (2008) further argue that enlargement of understanding will *decrease* overload. The organization can evaluate the existing repertoire of practices and desires.

We can rapidly reduce some of the effects of overload and disrupted internal logic by identifying the effect of the availability heuristic (Tversky and Kahneman 1973), representativeness heuristic (Kahneman and Tversky 1973), and grouping elements in like clusters. Our natural tendency is to place greater value on what we think of first (digital data) and precise information. Accepting all data and information as discrete elements leads to overload, as described above.

The HRO principle *reluctance to simplify* also corrects the drive to accept what first comes to mind (availability heuristic) and the assumption that what we see is what is happening. When we accept our first impression, we have inadvertently simplified the situation and will likely stop looking for more structure. Consultants, colleagues, and other participants will offer advice from the availability of information in their minds. This is likely associated with their identity, meaning that rejection of their first impression may be taken as an assault on their identity.

We can reduce the effect of availability during routine operations by listing four to seven elements (treatments, causes, and the like). The first two to four are the most available to our mind and likely the least significant. The others are more difficult to bring to mind but also carry more information.

> During patient care rounds. Ron Perkin (MD, FAAP, FCCM) routinely asked for five of almost anything—diseases, medical conditions, causes, therapies. For example, if a child had low urine output, he would ask for five ways to increase urine production, whether related to the immediate problem or not.
>
> I would work with the team to make a list and would insist on seven items. Sometimes I would ask the group, and each person was required to think of one item. As a group, we discussed the nature of the first three and learned that they carried little information and would contribute less to the care of a child than the last few, which were always significant for our operations. As a routine, the staff began to recognize the risk of using our first impressions.
>
> —Daved van Stralen

What we see is what we think. When rapidly evaluating patterns, we too easily form judgments about the underlying structure. In reality, we observe the topography of the HRS, not the underlying forces and transformations. Combine representativeness with availability, and we are at risk of believing we know what is happening upon first view. Unfortunately, this will contribute to overload on individual people, the system, and the organization.

The representativeness heuristic responds well to making lists. As a practice during routine operations, we spend some time thinking of what else can cause or contribute to the event. Processing data into meaningful groupings is not simplification but identifying the underlying structure. A redundancy in data easily occurs when we measure the same process in multiple way. A bias also forms for precise measurements that are reproducible over a narrow range but may not represent underlying processes. This bias toward precision continues even against descriptions that are accurate when near the target. Also contributing to this bias towards precision is the nature of some accurate descriptions, they may be vague or fuzzy.

Grouping like data—that is, data representing a similar process—can "debulk" our load of information. We often find that we are working with three to five processes rather than thirty independent events, and of those processes, several are connected by cause and effect.

> The first day of patient-care rounds in the pediatric intensive care unit, the pediatric residents often present a patient they've had difficulty understanding. The amount of information overwhelmed them. We would go to the whiteboard and make a list of all problems, no matter how insignificant. The first items on the list were always fluids, electrolytes, and nutrition. ("FEN" are the active tasks for all patients in the hospital and are always given first.) They would list mechanical ventilation but not the indication for its use. If anyone mentioned this, it was always in connection with why the child was placed on ventilation. We always had four columns of seven to ten items.
>
> As a team, we grouped the elements together. This required us to determine if increased heart rate was related to cardiovascular problem, respiratory problem, pain, agitation, or some other cause. We usually had four to five groupings. We then identified what could kill the patient if left untreated, what needed to be resolved to transfer the patient to the hospital ward, and what needed treatment regardless of the patient's status.
>
> We now had only one or two life-threatening problems that we must discuss in detail, then one or two problems we had to treat in order to transfer the patient out of the unit. The rest would be resolved during routine care.
>
> —Daved van Stralen

The Liminal Event

The HRS is the quintessential liminal event. The degree of disorientation is within the mind of the individual; the degree depends on the person's ability to rapidly match personal attributes and immediately available resources with unexpected demands and expectations.

This sense of liminality is not uncommon during a life-threatening event. We can see from HROs that there are effective ways to survive as well as to continue operations. It is often easiest to understand the principles and dynamics of HRO when viewed as effective means to operate when the environment has suddenly lost its structure. In fact, the liminal event is *why* HRO matters, and *when* it matters.

Executives, managers, academicians, and scientists use linearity and deterministic processes for prediction and planning. They rely on an intact cognitive mind and full executive mental functions in all members of the organization. What is missed is the turmoil of the liminal event. We encounter loss of the internal logic of the system that we rely on to react and engage the HRS. The immediate world becomes nonlinear and indeterminate. Our minds shift to self-protection, our behaviors reflect unrecognized fear, and we miss that this is happening, as our thoughts and actions all make sense at the time.

The liminal event is an event such as a community disaster or an internal hospital disaster. To the bedside nurse, however, it could be an unexpected cardiac arrest. To the physician, it could be the report of a patient evaluated in the morning who is transferred to the ICU that afternoon. The liminal event is "macro-cosmos" to the organization and "micro-cosmos" to the individual.

Some organizations perform well and develop people who converge jointly to enact a preferred end-state. Studying these HROs and their response to the HRS matters. Studying how people within the HRO respond to not only the dramatic event but also to the benign or mundane event is when HRO matters.

Raindrops Keep Falling on My Head

[The Dude Fire in the Tonto National Forest, Arizona, started by lightning on June 25, 1990. Responding to the fire was a fire crew from the Arizona State Prison at Perryville consisting of inmates certified as Type II wildland firefighters. Type II crews have less experience than Type I Interagency Hotshot crews. During a fire blowup on the second day of the fire the Perryville crew tried to escape but the fire entrapped 11 crewmembers. Despite deploying their fire shelters, six of the members died and the remaining five suffered burns, two crew members critically burned.]

In my briefcase is a map that's never really been discussed in all the years of analysis of the fatal Dude Fire. I'd intended to give it to one of the training hosts for use in the first Dude fire staff ride to assist in the discussion of fire spread before the blowup. I didn't give it to him, though, because he had his own map.

During a critique session the day after taking a hundred students back through the Dude fire, it occurred to me how well the training hosts had described the dramatic events surrounding the fire: the downhill run the night before; the downburst the next afternoon, which drove fire over the Perryville crew; the sustained crown fire through the next night.

While driving home from the critique session, I suddenly realized the significance of the map in my briefcase. The most significant fire activity for training purposes was not any of the dramatic events that we had focused on. It was the fact that the fire had hardly spread at all near the Perryville crew from 8:00 a.m. to 2:00 p.m. that fateful afternoon. I pulled the map out of my briefcase and studied it again. Instead of focusing on the lines representing the dramatic fire activities, I focused on the lines representing a slow fire with short flame lengths, backing into the prevailing winds, backing down slope, hour after hour, from 0800 to 1400. No problem.

Yesterday at the Dude staff ride, Dick Rothermel had wondered aloud, for the benefit of the group, about the significance of raindrops to the decision-making processes of firefighters. I had fought lots of fires in the rain under the Mogollon Rim in central Arizona. No problem. But what if the raindrops were coming only from the convection column of a large fire? This morning, Bob Mutch also wondered aloud, for the benefit of the group, about the significance of raindrops to the decision-making processes of firefighters.

When I remembered the map in my briefcase, I concluded that it would have been more useful to the students to discuss the *lack* of dramatic events before the blowup. Why do we always focus on the dramatic events when the subtle events may hold the answers to our inquiries?

Well, my map's in my briefcase, and raindrops keep falling on my head.

—Mike Johns, assistant US attorney, former wildland firefighter

---

People can have liminal characteristics, and liminality can have temporal or spatial dimensions. This handbook describes the liminal human characteristics of an individual in the liminal dimensions of time and space for time compression, uncertainty, and threat. It is instructive to identify when the environment is crossing the threshold, though, more commonly, these limiting edges are a spectrum ranging from the mundane to the alarming. Experience also has a spectrum, for what is a liminal threshold for one person might not be for another, and what is not liminal for someone with a specific set of coworkers might be liminal with a different set of coworkers.

Every environment contains information. When the context changes, so, too, does the value of information; you have then crossed a threshold and have entered a liminal space. Each environment operates on a separate system of logic (a logic of operations for that environment), and these logic systems are asymmetric. The logic system for the irrational environment can operate in the rational environment; the logic system of the rational environment, however, cannot operate in the irrational environment.

HRO is counterintuitive to those who have not been exposed to a high-risk environment. The new liminal space directly influences framing but also forms a pattern for acculturation and culture shift toward HRO. This means more than having one frightening situation; it means working in such an environment, having modeled the necessary attitudes and behaviors. For those who have experienced these situations, it is necessary—and better for future threat response—to have successfully processed this information rather than operating on false assumptions and psychological scars.

These events change the threshold of detection of information, becoming more sensitive to threats while enabling the practitioner to become more responsive and effective.

The Particular

We deal with the particular, whether it is a problem, situation, or event. This means that we do not deal with the routine or normal, which limits our ability to use statistics, probabilities, and the normal distribution curve. In the universe of the normal distribution and random, independent events, an outlier is unlikely to recur because of randomness, therefore it can readily be disregarded because it is independent of other events. In other words, the outlier is unlikely to cause any effect.

The particular makes HRO different, because each event is new and unique and may easily cause an effect. When the particular occurs, if unnoticed, disregarded, or unattended, it can quickly cascade out of control. We must adjust our values to the situation. This does not mean that we become self-serving or operate out of self-interest because we have a duty as an obligation to our colleagues and organization. We improvise, but it is constrained improvisation. We have the independence and freedom to act, but it is action within discipline. This is the virtuous nature of HRO.

It is important to note that HRO is *problem-driven*—that is, the environment, and the problem within the environment, is our source of vulnerability and drives our action. We must also evaluate information in its context, no matter how fluid the environment becomes. This means we value information based on the immediate situation and change that valuation if necessary throughout the process. Rigid adherence to prior norms and values, and the evaluation of information from an abstract perspective or from initial events, quickly become dangerous.

HRO is problem driven. The codification of HRO by Karlene Roberts (La Porte et al 1988) and the elucidation of HRO principles by Karl Weick and Kathleen Sutcliffe (2015) are descriptive principles rather than prescriptive measures. Daved van Stralen identified the significance that specific attitudes have for influencing behaviors when under stress. These are important to bear in mind, because attitudes are modeled by senior members of the organization and are learned from experience. Later, with Tom Mercer, van Stralen identified five values that give an HRO authenticity; Weick later expanded that number to six.

Emery Rowe and Paul Shulman (2015) identified how the logic of HRO operations differs between preventing system failure and responding to system failure. This involves differing actions and operations. HRO is not a system of rules or a formal, rigid structure. HRO is a way of thinking: a belief system and mind-set that encourages specific behaviors. HROs are vigilant for vulnerabilities, engage problems early to enact better end-states, and support people in this process in a manner that will permit the continuation of the organization's routine processes *while* engaging the unique or cascading event.

You can see in this section that resilience, reliability, and safety are all integral parts of operations. The HRO operates in hazardous situations, either by intent (such as with military operations and wildland fire) or by exigency (as in caring for medical emergencies, critical care patients, or in the operating theater). This explains why opposing means of achieving HRO appear to be possible—one to prevent system failure and another to respond when the system has failed. The concern of the "control operator" is the lessons learned in hazardous situations that are later codified into rules and procedures. If we deviate from these lessons "written in blood," we increase risk and begin the movement toward failure. On the other hand, when a failure has occurred, rigid adherence to rules and procedures becomes increasingly risky and impairs the inability to respond to, and contain, the failure. This is the approach of the "emergency responder." This ability to move smoothly between different logics of operations is the hallmark and strength of High Reliability Organizing.

HRO in Healthcare

Though the healthcare field developed through inductive and deductive reasoning, it now has a tendency for the linear and deterministic. That is, if the physician is able to make a diagnosis, then he or she has a greater chance of predicting the course of disease. With the improvement of medical and surgical treatment, a precise diagnosis would allow a more specific treatment that would be more effective and have fewer complications. This has led the culture of medical care to have greater respect for the diagnostician, an experienced physician who can make a difficult diagnosis when other physicians have failed.

Knowledge of particular information for the disease, such as is found with medical specialization, became more prominent in healthcare during the early twentieth century. For example, in the 1920s, the creation of specialty neurosurgical units reduced death and complications following neurosurgical procedures. Nevertheless, medical and surgical care remained linear and deterministic.

The thoracic surgeon Dwight Harken introduced prolonged anesthetic and surgical care of an unstable patient in 1951 at Peter Bent Brigham Hospital in Boston. After open-heart surgery, it was standard at the time to admit the patient to a bed in a regular hospital ward. Harken reasoned that continued monitoring of electrical heart activity, electrolytes and fluids, and oxygenation would permit real-time treatment overnight, thereby reducing these deaths. He and a nurse created a special unit, later called an intensive care unit, and found that the death rate dropped dramatically. This was the first hospital unit named an intensive care unit.

During World War II, Harken had performed the largest series of open heart operations to retrieve shrapnel without a death: a total of 134 patients (Harken 1946). He built on this experience by performing the first closed mitral valvuloplasty for mitral stenosis in 1947 and continued these operations at Peter Bent Brigham Hospital. To reduce postoperative deaths, Dr. Harken and a nurse colleague created the first ICU to continue anesthesia care and monitoring after the operation. Some authorities consider the neurosurgical unit in the 1920s or the polio respiratory units to be the first ICUs. The neurosurgical units appear to have been for the care of specific surgical complications, rather than monitoring for unstable physiology. Polio respiratory care units housed cohorts of patients in iron lungs, a type of negative pressure ventilator. Patients in iron lungs can be cared for at home with minimal monitoring.

Whether cardiothoracic, neurosurgical, or respiratory, the movement toward intensive care and resuscitation did not have significant impact on the structure of medicine or its logic of operations. Healthcare historically developed to diagnose and treat disease under the direction of a physician or surgeon. As we improved our ability for the early identification of serious illnesses and the treatment of trauma, we encountered greater ambiguity. The use of discrete clinical criteria to diagnose serious diseases is a century old. With success, clinicians identified patients earlier in the course of diseases; doing so added to the clinical signs but increased ambiguity, as several diseases were found to have similar antecedents. Cardio-respiratory arrest, the final common pathway in critical and emergency care, is now being identified earlier in the course of the process. While laudable in reducing mortality, the increased ambiguity has added to recognized (and unrecognized) fear among caregivers that they may have improperly triaged a patient, thereby burdening the system or possibly sending a patient home to die.

Until the 1960s, decision-making relied on scientific rationality and tended to be subjective and performed in real time, though protocols and algorithms did exist. Decision trees did not appear until the 1960s, when they were first introduced for capital investment and later applied to healthcare. Complex problem-solving and the science of decision-making did not become academic pursuits until the 1970s.

Many organizations other than those in healthcare have found effective problem-solving approaches, some of which could benefit healthcare. The approach we use in this handbook is the High Reliability Organization, codified from naval air operations, military operations, wildland firefighting, nuclear power generation, and the electric transmission grid. The danger comes in context-independent translation of this approach (with the attendant HRO culture) to the healthcare field without awareness of, and allowance for, the cultural tradition of healthcare. Initiative, which is valued in HROs, can appear to be unconstrained freelance behavior within the culture of healthcare.

A rigidly structured hierarchical culture with a deterministic approach designed and organized to prevent failure has some of the characteristics of the control operator HRO. (See chapter 1, "What Is High Reliability Organizing?") Everything learned by HROs revolves around the desire to have members of the team contribute to the decision-making process. HROs recognize that even the people with the highest levels of competence and associated experience can make an error or miss an indicator. It is therefore incumbent on the supporting cast to contribute in a manner that would be precluded by the presence of a steep hierarchy. The sole reliance on scientific rationality, such as with evidence-based medicine, impairs the responsiveness necessary for dynamic problems. The focus on error and poor outcomes can impair the initiative necessary to effectively engage an unexpected emergency.

HRO represents the intersection of the rational and the pragmatic, of the objective and the subjective. While this may appear counterintuitive or even confounding, experience demonstrates that healthcare professionals are willing to adopt this approach. Most people who are accomplished with the HRO mind-set learned it at an early age. In the 1970s, the average age of a sailor on the flight deck was nineteen to twenty years old, yet aircraft carriers were becoming, at that time, exemplars of HRO principles. The reason is because carrier commanders like RAdm Thomas Mercer became virtually obsessed with the notion that, despite the inherent risks of carrier aviation, crews could operate safely as teams. Members of those teams regularly reported incidents in an effort to preclude them from becoming accidents. Further, the teams allowed their young sailors to speak up when they saw indications of unsafe operations, thereby gaining their engagement in the process and ensuring that the fleet would remain combat ready despite a plethora of human factors that conspired to limit their collective success.

One problem associated with learning HRO is the belief that it will prevent or mitigate error, solve specific problems, or be implemented in a turnkey manner where, once instituted, executives can then turn their backs on it. Rather, HRO is not only a way of thinking that a logic of operations may be found for all members of the organization, regardless of position in the hierarchy; it also permits the flow of information and the migration of authority to act in dynamic situations of uncertainty, time compression, and threat.

Five Principles of HRO as Environment

The following constitute the five principles that Weick and Sutcliffe (2015) discuss in their book.

- When approaching adversity, one does not want to fail. This drives a continual search for potential failure points (anything that might contribute to failure). This is *preoccupation with failure.*
- Uncertainty is always more complex than it first appears—nonlinear interactions of basic principles create new and unexpected properties in the system—therefore, one does not simplify to the first answer, the easiest answer, or the apparently simplest answer. This is *reluctance to simplify.*
- Because events are continually changing, one must be sensitive to changes in the situation and the performance of those in the immediate vicinity while maintaining strategic efforts toward the desired end point. This is *sensitivity to operations.*
- No matter what happens, one must persevere by constantly reevaluating and sensemaking until events become contained. Stopping means failure, which could mean death. This is *commitment to resilience.*
- People also realize that some of those around them may have a better understanding of the situation or may have special knowledge related to the operations or situation. This is *deference to expertise.*

In real time, we will experience and observe disruptions in our processes and discrepancies in our observations and expectations. These disruptions will guide us closer to sources of the problem and possible solutions.

Adaptive Selection for the VUCA-T Environment

Parsing the elements of HRO with consideration of adaptiveness and environmental context is difficult. What makes this almost impossible is a changing threat environment and selection for and loss of these elements. High Reliability Organizing is often defined by an outcome in relation to a dangerous environment. Today, because of the HRO characteristics, these organizations operate in a safer environment than when they first developed. This makes it more difficult to identify which characteristics provide the adaptiveness and resilience of HRO, as some characteristics have become remnants and some are lost, since they are no longer needed.

How, then, do we identify HRO behaviors when the selection pressure is relaxed and the advantage of having these behaviors has been removed?

Trait Selection from Adversity

Because we may think that our beliefs and behaviors naturally fit our circumstances and the situations we encounter, we tend not to ask where these beliefs and behaviors come from. Beliefs, behaviors, team formation, and organizational structures are traits that come from our education and training, scientific or academic studies, or culture, or they develop as a response to the environment.

In the High Reliability Organization, these traits developed in response to (1) adverse or hostile environments and (2) the proximity of hazards to people, production processes, or organizational systems. High-risk environments place selection pressure on people and the organization, which results in traits that contribute to survival and effectiveness. An HRO trait is a behavior, belief, attitude, or structure that contributes to the adaptive fitness of an HRO.

In an operant manner, the environment and these interactions also act on the HRO and individual people. This means that we may not be able to completely identify what makes us reliable or safe.

HROs developed to effectively enter adverse or hostile environments by maintaining system performance (preventing system failure) and overcoming environmental adversity (mitigating threats and hazards). For this to occur, the HRO interacts with the environment at the level of the individual. Beliefs do not change the environment, which makes behaviors preeminent. A belief represents High Reliability to the extent that it supports a behavior to maintain operations or reduce threat. For this reason, most discussions in this book focus on behaviors or connect specific beliefs to behaviors. We do use concepts and models, but we do so in support of situational and contextual operations.

Various behaviors and beliefs reinforce one another through interaction: repeated behaviors will change beliefs, and strongly held beliefs will influence behaviors. We learn through the consequence of actions—reinforcement learning—to a greater degree than from what is explicitly taught. Actions are selected from past experiences (exploitation) by new choices (exploration) and observation of negative feedback (safety). Environmental responses must be observable and salient if they are to reinforce behavior and lead to learning. This is HRO trial-and-error learning. In this way, the environment acts upon the individual and organization.

Cognitive dissonance and motivated reasoning obstruct this operant type of learning and change. When faced with an experience or an environment that disconfirms one's strongly held beliefs, some people will continue to hold their beliefs. This happens even as catastrophic failure commences. The further one is from the situation, the sharper concepts seem and the more fuzzy and ambiguous the situation (i.e., reality) appears.

The organization that is in the process of becoming HRO will adopt beliefs, behaviors, and structures that have developed within HROs. Some HRO traits correlate as a suite, or "behavioral syndrome" (from behavioral ecology), that buttress one another or maintain a focal trait. When taking an HRO trait out of context, the developing HRO risks selecting a trait that is salient or attractive to leaders in the organization but has lost the important focal trait.

For example, many HROs have what appear to be rigid hierarchical structures, with obedience and conformity. Taking this situation out of context, the developing HRO assumes this rigid hierarchy without the concomitant values of initiative or engagement behaviors. Then, when plans do not run as expected, line members will continue to follow a plan that needs updating and may not advise their superiors of unplanned or unexpected changes in the situation.

A resident physician placed an intravenous catheter in the femoral vein during treatment a patient in severe cardiogenic shock with very low blood flow. During the night, the nurses told the attending physician and resident physician that the leg had begun to swell, a known complication of having a large catheter in a small vein. The attending and resident physician instructed the nurses they can reduce the leg swelling by following standard treatment of elevating the leg. This

> maneuver uses gravity to assist venous return flow through the impeded vein or by way of accessory venous pathways. The nurses were asked to report the response to elevation of the leg. The next morning, they observed that the leg was pale, with very weak peripheral pulses. The catheter had been placed in the femoral artery, which had low pressures due to the weak heart function. The nurses had reported information they thought would bring a physician to evaluate the situation, not the accurate information of what they had observed. They had learned not to report information they believed their regular attending physician did not want to hear. As a group, they would create information they believed would lead to a response from the physician without the anger.
>
> ANONYMOUS PHYSICIAN

Hierarchy and obedience have a place in HRO, but in support of the focal trait of standardized, coordinated responsiveness. Hierarchy and obedience come in a "suite" of traits that provide coordinated fluidity to standardization.

Loss of Adversity and Relaxed Selection

"Relaxed selection" is the absence of selection pressure. When an environmental demand or threat is removed, the HRO trait no longer has an adaptive advantage. In studies of evolution, this is called *relaxed selection*, which leads to the disappearance of traits that once were necessary for survival. These traits eventually disappear, but some break down quickly, while others linger (Lahti et al. 2009). Traits that were once key to survival and performance may erode when the selection pressure is no longer present.

Loss of selection pressure not only occurs from a change in environmental adversity but also because of a change in the nature of the selection pressure. For example, the demands of a supervisor who has not operated in an adverse environment will create arbitrary selection. In such situations, the supervisor may not obtain the wished-for behaviors; subordinates develop protective behaviors rather than productive behaviors, which is the distinction between natural and artificial environments. This is similar to animal domestication, the introduction of domesticated traits that, while attractive and productive in a protected space, are unsuitable for survival in the wild condition (Post 1971).

For example, behaviors and attitudes that developed in an environment of large-scale wars and economic losses over a thirty-year period (i.e., several generations) creates behaviors that create attitudes and then beliefs. Follow that environment with another thirty-year period (another several generations) of decreasing warfare and economic growth, and we have "relaxed selection" and changes in behaviors, attitudes, and beliefs. This is the risk of losing what we need for crisis, because crisis has gone from daily routine to rare events. We can see this "experiment" in world history from 1915–1945 and 1950–1980, respectively.

Behaviors are not necessarily lost quickly when selection pressure relaxes; the speed of loss is related to costs. Lahti et al. (2009) differentiate between constitutive and contingent costs of traits. *Constitutive costs* are automatically incurred to maintain or express the trait; these costs are independent of all environments. *Contingent costs* are incurred only if the trait is expressed due to particular features of the environment; these are environment-dependent costs. Constitutive traits, even though they once had important functions, have a cost to maintain. They are most likely to be lost with relaxed selection. Contingent traits, however, only have a cost when expressed, and thus are more likely to be found as remnant traits.

HRO traits may remain despite relaxed selection pressure from a safer, less adverse environment. We would like to know if (1) the behavior is maintained, even though it has no role; (2) the behavior assumes a new role (and can be misused, since the reason is gone); or (3) the behavior had an additional hidden role that becomes apparent only when the trait is lost (after Lahti et al. 2009). Bruce Spurlock has asked the question, "What causes a behavior to drift?" He has observed adaptive behaviors, well integrated into an organization, drift over time to weaken or transform to become less adaptive (personal communication).

Some of this loss or drift from adaptive HRO behavior may occur in an operant manner. The strength of a behavior is modified by the behavior's consequences, such as reward or punishment. In operant conditioning, stimuli that are present when a behavior is rewarded or punished come to control that behavior. The loss of HRO traits can occur when people escape the adverse situation—a trait that is strengthened, though by negative reinforcement.

Organizations operating in a familiar or less-adverse environment do not have constraining selection pressure. This permits greater variation in operations for the same function and adoption of traits attractive to people but with limited function. This can make these organizations poorly suited for severe adversity.

Loss of Behavior

When selection pressure relaxes, we can expect traits to fade—more rapidly if the trait carries a cost. If HRO traits persist, their existing function may continue to be adaptive, or the trait could acquire a new or secondary function.

A trait can be lost if it reduces reliability, safety, or the competitive fitness of the organization. Keep in mind that reliability and safety may appear to contribute to fitness *only* in adversity or the face of hazards, but if their costs reduce the competitive fitness, then they will be lost, so long as adversity and hazards are rare or not severe. But they can serve a dual function: traits for adversity and hazards may also increase competitive fitness. Although these are the more valuable HRO traits, as noted above, it is not uncommon for HRO traits to come in suites to buttress one another or to focus on a more critical trait. This provides two scenarios for the retention of HRO traits: either they contribute to competitive fitness or they are necessary because adversity and hazards are severe and/ or frequent.

Conclusions

(1). HRO is a response to the environment; HRO enactment changes the environment.

(2). Framing the situation brings focus to salient information and filters noise.

(3). When entering an unstable environment, the organization must maintain vigilance to threats, which is a duty of all members of the organization.

(4). Because of the VUCA-T environment, HROs must maintain vigilance to threats.

(5). The VUCA-T environment is inevitable, because energy, behaviors, and physiology cannot be completely controlled.

(6). The HRO responds to threat pragmatically through engagement.

CHAPTER 5

COGNITION AND AFFECT

I n a crisis, decision-making, action, and operations are most effective when our thinking and emotions work together. Our cognitive abilities contribute knowledge and reasoning, while our emotions provide focus and drive decisions and actions. Unfortunately, the majority of work to date in cognition, sensemaking, and decision-making has focused on objectivity, reason, and rationality.

We rely on our objectivity, cognitive abilities, and rationality to provide medical care to our patients. We use logic, reason, and facts for clinical decisions. This is the what, where, and how of scientific thinking in healthcare, as shown in table 2. This is such a strong belief that we become unaware of any influences that weaken our thinking and we reject influences that can strengthen thought and operational performance (which is the affective domain). Cognition and affect can battle each other or work in synergy.

Cognitive Domain	Affective Domain
What Objective—outside ourselves Related to reality and truth, unbiased; Descriptions of physical phenomena that are unchanged despite observation under a variety of conditions	*What* Subjective—within the mind Feelings, ideas, opinions, of a sentient subject Personal perspective and experience
Where Cognitive—mental process Evaluation, reasoning, and judgment; The mental processes of perception, memory, judgment, and reasoning	*Where* Affective—emotional process Volitional process; the will to act The emotional processes of attitudes, values, and beliefs
How Rational—the possession of logic, rules, facts, and reason	*How* Arousal, attention Sympathetic nervous system

Table 2—The cognitive and affective domains

Our valuation of objectivity in the sciences, to the disparagement of subjectivity, makes it hard to achieve any success in dealing with the combination of uncertainty, time compression, and threat. In the interests of being scientific and to further our studies using good research design, we have come to depreciate subjectivity, disregard context, and deny stress-impaired cognition.

Subjectivity of our thought and evaluations are difficult to justify to others. Their idiosyncratic characteristics, unique to each of us yet also shared to some degree with like-minded people, make them difficult subjects for research. This is the affective domain of experience, feeling, and emotion. "Affect" includes attitudes, social and personal values, subjective valuation of information and action, and the ability to regulate emotion (the modulated fear response). The subjective qualities of affect are necessary determinants in High Reliability Organizations (HRO.) In fact, it is the very subjective nature of these qualities that breeds success in dealing with uncertainty, time-compression, and threat.

When the situation presents itself as "simple," we in HRO are reluctant to accept it as simplicity. We often find complexity in the simple situation, because complexity is often where information lies. This reflects a combining of the objective, subjective, and context: a way of finding complexity in what, objectively, readily appears to be simple. Making the High Reliability Situation (HRS) complex is a way of finding answers.

Context gives meaning and value to information and circumstances. A moderate wind refreshes on a hot day but is miserable when it adds wind chill to the bitter cold. Context informs us of whether we may have support or obstruction in performing our tasks. Context shifts our general knowledge to the particular and demands higher-skill performance of proficiency, an expert level, or even mastery. Context demands judgment.

We judge our cognitive ability with our own cognitive ability. In effect, we use our judgment to judge our judgment. One consequence is the inability to identify cognitive performance decrements within ourselves. In cold-weather mountaineering, the climber constantly evaluates the judgment of others on the team. The first sign of hypothermia is loss of judgment, which the victim will be unaware of. The military demonstrates the loss of cognitive abilities at altitude with the use of decompression chambers and stresses the importance of monitoring others on the team. "Time of useful consciousness" (TUC) describes the amount of time people can perform their duties after sudden depressurization in a plane. This is the reason flight crews instruct air passengers to place oxygen masks on themselves before placing the mask on a child or disabled person—otherwise, by the time the passenger uses the mask, unrecognized hypoxemia will have caused loss of judgement then unconsciousness. Physical, physiological, or emotional stress *will* impair cognition, and we will not recognize the condition in ourselves.

One distinction of crossing the liminal threshold into a dangerous environment is the value placed on affective judgment. Cognitive skills, rationality, and scientific logic, to the exclusion of affective decision-making, will cause us to miss the rare, lethal threat and the salience of the early herald. Our goal is to identify system failure in the covert, compensated state that we have missed due to the compensation. Cognition and rationality risk waiting for certainty, but by then, the system is entering the overt, decompensated state.

The Cognitive Domain

We commonly consider decision-making to be a cognitive process of logic, reason, and rationality. These processes inform our education, training, planning, and leadership style. Cognition describes the mental processes we use to acquire knowledge and to understand what is around us; it forms the basis of the scientific rationality we use in research, planning, and for daily operations. Cognition consists of our objective perceptions, thinking, and experiences; it is how we make sense of the world, and it constitutes our knowledge, decision-making judgment, and problem-solving abilities.

Cognition consists of our symbols and language skills, our ability to manipulate symbols, our grasp of concepts, our understanding of relationships, and our flexibility in thinking. Rasmussen and Vicente (1983) matched categories of performance with types of situations and then identified the type of information used. Skill-based behavior uses *signals*, a term that refers to sensory input that communicates information. Rule-based behavior for routines that come from a stored rule or procedure uses *signs* to indicate the state of the environment. Signs convey meaning and are used to start or modify predetermined actions. Knowledge-based behavior, for causal functioning and reasoning when we encounter something novel, uses *symbols* to represent the abstract thought used to describe what we have never before, or not yet, encountered. The higher the level of performance, the higher the cognitive level and the greater the risk of impairment under stress.

Signals	Sensory input, communicate information
Signs	Convey meaning
Symbols	Representations of abstract thought

Table 3—Signals, signs, and symbols

In an emergently dangerous situation, levels of cognition are highly influenced by factors we may not yet recognize or control. Below are a few basic cognition-related definitions we can use without entering into a deep philosophical discussion on the subject.

- *Cognitive science* examines how we acquire knowledge and understanding through thought, experience, and our senses. This knowledge is accessed, remembered, and processed by operations within the human mind.
- *Cognitive capacities* describe our capacities for reasoning, our mental representations, and the models we share.
- *Cognitive knowledge* or the cognitive domain of knowledge (from Bloom's taxonomy of learning) describes the processes, theories, and principles of science. Cognitive knowledge is our knowledge and intellectual skills; this is how we know.
- *Scientific logic* describes the *linear* process of making inferences to create new information from existing information. Information must be discrete and categorized—that is, in one group or another without overlap or ambiguity. (Compare this to other logics, such as the modal logics, which can infer action, duty, or value or can infer new information from imperfect information; see chapter 3, "The Logic of Practice and the Logic of Operations.")
- *Reasoning* describes conscious thought, which creates a sequence of mental states to form explanations, judgments, and conclusions.
- *Rationality* is the use of reason in accordance with reality.

The Limits of Cognition

Certain limitations to our perceptive and cognitive abilities create *bounded rationality*, which Herbert A. Simon has described. These limitations deceptively affect our cognitive ability to make judgments. Because we use our judgment to judge our judgment, judging when we have lost our judgment becomes tricky.

Cold-weather or high-altitude operators and mountaineers monitor the judgment of their partners. In this same way, when operating in high-risk situations, we have a duty to monitor one another's judgment and performance.

Unrecognized or hidden limits to our cognitive function *due to* the environment alone are well known to those who operate in extreme environments. Cold-weather or high-altitude operators know that one of the first signs of hypothermia or hypoxemia is loss of judgment, something of which the affected person would be unaware. These operators watch one another for changes in judgment and, if identified, initiate the proper intervention. Judging your partner's judgment is not to criticize or be critical; it is meant to save lives.

Logic, reason, and rationality assume the ability to place objects into discrete and distinct categories; otherwise we would reach several conclusions with the same known values. Reliance on logic, reason, and rationality create a conundrum when, for any reason, we encounter a situation where we cannot separately categorize things. Uncertainty prevents the inference of new information. A value must be placed on existing information, and stress impairs our cognitive abilities. Cognition and rationality do not place value on things. The value of concrete and abstract things in these environments changes based on the situation and the moment. These are the limits of cognition.

Unfortunately, uncertainty, time compression, and threat in the VUCA-T environment—volatile, uncertain, complex, ambiguous, and threatening—impair cognition and limit rationality. Though we often describe this situation in the extreme, the same principles apply whenever we are in a novel situation, for example the first day on the job. We have discussed the limits of rationality and logic and described the logic of operations in chapter 3, "The Logic of Practice and the Logic of Operations." We will discuss unrecognized fear and the threat responses in chapter 9, "Threat Responses and Unrecognized Fear." In this chapter, we will discuss the synthesis of affect and cognition.

High Reliability operations *qualitatively* differ in reasoning and modulating emotion; the difference creates a threshold between the logic of operations of the routine, deterministic environment and that of VUCA-T, high-hazard, stochastic, indeterminate environments. The identification of thresholds between environments, the characterization of the logic of operations for stochastic events, and the conditioning necessary to modulate emotion better enable the translation of HRO methods to industries that have not yet operated with hazards at such close proximity.

The Limits of Knowledge

Knowledge consists of the facts, information, and concepts we have acquired through experience and education. We tend to consider knowledge as explicit and objective—something we can bring from memory to our immediate attention. Michael Polanyi (1958) distinguishes this *explicit* knowledge, information that can be readily transmitted to others, from *tacit* knowledge, information we know but find difficult to describe. (Tacit knowledge is subconsciously understood and applied, difficult to articulate, developed from direct experience and action, and usually shared through highly interactive conversation, storytelling, and shared experience; explicit knowledge, in contrast, can be more precisely and formally articulated.) "We can know more than we can tell" because effective operators "do more than they can know" (Polanyi 1966, 4). We know more than we can tell because we integrate most of the particular information of our situation without attending to them. Because we do not attend to them, we do not notice them. HRO represents an effort to make visible this invisible tacit knowledge.

Though we may view knowledge as objective and opinion as subjective, they are actually similar, separated by degree of belief and whether others share our belief. Epistemology describes the study of knowledge; for our purposes epistemology is the value we give to our belief. This is an important distinction, because HRO relies on local, situational knowledge that may rapidly change in time. In contrast, medical knowledge has other characteristics interfering with its reliability, including the prospective, randomized, controlled trial; the preferential bias for quantitative studies and numbers-driven information over qualitative studies and descriptions of experience; the rejection of anecdote; and the preference for the reductionist approaches used in complex situations. While these approaches have many benefits, the fact that healthcare professionals constantly seek to quantify, reduce, and simplify is in direct contrast with one of the core principles of HRO: the *reluctance* to simplify (Weick and Sutcliffe 2015).

The notion of "reluctance to simplify" guards against our tendency to pay greater attention to those things we know or can control or those things we think we know or think we can control (Weick, personal communication). This does not imply a duality between simple and complex—or that we can toggle our thinking back and forth between them—but that "simple" has different degrees. When we simplify from the complex, we risk losing information as we categorize, disregard signs and signals in the environment, or consider complex information as extraneous or environmental noise. The danger is in using our knowledge to limit the obtaining of new knowledge from the uncertainty and complexity of the situation. "Reluctance to simplify" is reluctance to make things simple and reluctance to accept simple—in this mind-set, it is in complexity where we find valuable information.

The foundation of scientific medicine is the prospective, randomized, controlled trial. The unexpected nature of the events to which the HRO responds makes any prospective study nearly impossible. Randomization cannot be done, because these events or processes emerge from nonlinear interactions occurring at the local level. (As noted earlier, "nonlinear interactions" describe those interactions that occur in differing degrees to produce a relationship that is not a straight line on a graph.) They will not form the normal distribution necessary for statistical analysis. The HRO operates in environments that can lose structure; therefore, any information from a controlled environment is less likely to apply in the uncontrolled or unstable HRO environment. It would also be unethical for any experimental trial to place a normal, healthy human into a dangerous or potentially life-threatening environment.

Even with this standard for knowledge, we may later find that these findings are false. "A finding from a well-conducted, adequately powered randomized controlled trial starting with a 50 percent pre-study chance that the intervention is effective is eventually true about 85 percent of the time" (Ioannidis 2005a, 2005b). We seriously undermine our reliability and safety when we base high-risk interventions on knowledge that we might later find to be false. The dynamic qualities of HRO can increase the possibility of self-correcting any unidentified false knowledge.

> Referring to an article about HRO in a medical setting, a patient safety officer said, "The article seemed descriptive rather than numbers-driven. Unless there is some specific data, it will be met with skeptical responses" from members of the quality improvement committee.
> —Patient safety officer at a university medical center

This rejection of qualitative and descriptive research has impaired the ability of healthcare to incorporate the safety and reliability methods that have been developed in other industries. Though some people in the "hard" sciences may depreciate qualitative research, they use its products from the fields of human behavior, decision-making, and ethnography, to name only a few. The sciences of psychology, sociology, and social psychology have developed the use of qualitative research to develop theories, including the evaluation of validity and statistical analysis.

We've heard numerous physicians say, "That's anecdotal!" The rejection of the anecdote is not uncommon in healthcare, yet the anecdote is a primary source of safety and reliability knowledge in high-risk industries. (In general, anecdotes deliver social knowledge to maintain or change a culture.) This seems an odd belief in healthcare, considering the publication of case reports in the medical literature and the reliance of physicians on these presentations for the odd or rare patient.

Members of an HRO use anecdotes to share their lessons learned from unique or novel situations. Anecdotes also impress on the novice the effects of poor decision-making skills and the need for vigilance against the early signs of a crisis.

In general, the use of "reductionist" approaches for complex situations is necessary to identify or create processes and protocols that prevent system failure and to create decision trees for use by inexperienced members. Unfortunately, reducing complex situations to a few simple elements that can readily be taught through cliché and metaphor sets everybody up for failure when things do not go as planned or predicted. Reducing knowledge to general rules and universal principles—the basis for the Dreyfus model of competence and Rasmussen's rule-based processes—fails when the particular is encountered or when an exception occurs. It is here that proficiency or expert performance (the Dreyfus model) and knowledge-based processes (Rasmussen's work) come into play. This is where the organization moves from the conventional approach to HRO.

Anecdotes, shunned in healthcare, describe particular situations in context, which is a higher demand than universal truths or generalizable concepts.

Catastrophic situations rarely go as planned, because team members actively seek to avoid those very situations, thus delaying appropriate response or notification under the erroneous assumption that the decision-makers must know what they are doing, when in fact the decision-makers are not even cognizant of the increasingly dangerous situation. Having a non-attributional setting is critical to allow more junior members of the team to speak up when things are not going as predicted and the team is entering extremis.

The Affective Domain

As noted earlier, "affect" describes how we experience feelings or emotions. Generally speaking, affect consists of valence (the subjective positive or negative value), arousal, and intensity of motivation. Affect is the term psychologists use for emotion, but it is more than emotion as the sense of basic emotions or how we feel. While cognitive science studies the objective, affective science studies the subjective. This includes our personal attitudes, values, motivations, and mood as well as our emotions. For our consideration, we will discuss the affective domain as (1) attitudes and values, (2) the value placed on information (evaluation), and (3) the regulation of fear responses and modulation of threat reflexes that impair cognitive capabilities.

The concept of emotions is complex and dependent on the specific field of study. Emotions can be the state of feeling—a description of the level or feeling of arousal. For the neuroscientist, emotion is more commonly thought of as the fear response; in everyday discussion by the public, emotion is the feeling we experience.

Emotion is both a feeling and a physical expression. As a physical expression, emotion is recognized in the right hemisphere and amygdala. The right hemisphere is more adept at discriminating emotion than the left. The amygdala is triggered by the expression of negative emotions in other people, particularly through facial expression. This facial expression of emotions has been documented in scientific research; for example, those primates without facial hair express emotion through blushing in the face. More recently, researchers have revealed that dogs have a genetically determined behavior to respond to humans' facial expression of emotion.

Emotions, rather than interfering with decision-making, are indispensable for rational decisions. It is our emotions that give value to information and motivate us to act. Knowledge and cognitive abilities, the basis of planning, make up the cognitive domain. Our emotions and feelings, however, motivate us and drive our actions; this is the affective domain. We believe we use our cognitive abilities when we plan and conduct business; we depreciate the part emotion may play but actually incorporate the affective domain in all our activities and decisions (Damasio 1994).

A fourteen-year-old girl described this quandary of reason and emotion as "the valley where the two mountains of reason and emotion meet and twine their efforts together in winding streams that quietly defy your logic" (Mack and Hickler 1981, 103).

Attitudes and Values

Attitudes influence *and* follow behavior. According to a medical ethnographer we spoke to, copious research from anthropology, sociology, and organizational psychology shows that attitudes follow behavior (personal communication, 22 May 2012). We replied that our current thinking is that attitudes derive from repeated behaviors reinforced by modeling and mentoring; those attitudes are preselected and targeted because they are the attitudes that influence behavior when the supervisor is not present. These are not opposing views. The social psychology research is quite clear that repeating behaviors will create attitudes. The same medical ethnographer replied that this summary of current thinking seemed 100 percent correct.

Research has inadvertently moved away from the purpose, or utility, of attitudes and does not address the reasons that certain organizations, particularly public safety and the military, select specific attitudes. Attitudes are how people express their beliefs and values through their words and behavior. Values are more specific, deeply held attitudes that reflect the importance someone attaches to something.

Attitudes and values are shared across a culture and, for the most part, are visible during routine interactions. Just as the stress of an extreme situation reveals the hidden attitudes, biases, and values of individual people, HROs include similar attitudes and values that the public does not often recognize. Mostly, this is because these attitudes and values only become apparent in the tension of the moment during actions to prevent system failure or, in emergency operations, when the system has failed. At these moments, the layperson or academic researcher is either not present, is distracted by the events, or does not recognize what is happening.

Relativity

Einstein described relativity through the story of a man bouncing a ball in a train. To the man inside the train, the ball bounces straight up and straight down. To the observer on a hillside who is watching the train and the man bouncing the ball, the course of the ball takes more of a sinusoidal curve. Because he is being carried forward with the ball, the man inside the train does not see the forward motion of the ball caused by the movement of the train. The man outside the train does see the forward motion of the ball's trajectory, and he sees that it creates a sinusoidal track.

We experience an emergency through our own perspective. We evaluate risk from our experience and abilities compared to the nature, degree, and proximity of the risk. Others cannot help us in evaluating the threat or our response. It does little good to tell somebody to "be calm" or "do not get excited." Once a stimulus is perceived, the course of the stimulus within the person's brain is beyond our control and possibly beyond the control of the person. Some consider this situation the weakness of subjectivity, while others see this as the strength of HRO.

The attitudes and values of an HRO are directed to adaptive sensemaking and adaptive responses for these intimate encounters. Relativity is relative. HROs contextualize relativity and rely on the team's collective sensemaking to raise the level of awareness so that HROs function as teams despite widely varying levels of experience and knowledge.

Objectivity

Having objectivity in our plans allows for use across a wide variety of people. The consistency of standardization makes responses consistent, and we can predict the actions of others to let us rely on their responses.

Physician detachment allows a physician to reliably care for a patient without being influenced by the patient's feelings, pain, or emotional distress. This is not to say that the physician ignores these things but that they do not influence clinical decisions about medical treatment. In the extreme, this may seem like a loss of empathy. The physician must find a balance between treating the disease and treating the patient who has the disease.

Scientific objectivity, like scientific rationality, reflects the belief that particular perspectives, values, personal interests, or specific needs of the community must not influence scientific thoughts or processes. This belief can lead to the inordinate influence of evidence-based medicine and the application of information derived from deterministic, linear sources to volatile, complex situations. While the certitude of this knowledge provides security, the response by the environment will be unpredictable. Scientific objectivity limits our ability to use judgment and adapt our actions to the particular situation.

Such is the contradiction found in medicine, as providers typically feel substantial reluctance to embrace some of the standardized processes of HRO. Alan Reider, senior partner of the preeminent law firm Arnold and Porter, puts it this way:

> Heightened litigation risk in medicine—both from the regulatory/ enforcement and malpractice perspectives—has prompted the need to develop standardized protocols to promote regulatory and clinical compliance. Following the protocols not only reduces the potential for noncompliance, but it also demonstrates a commitment to compliance, thereby reducing—if not eliminating—potential liability in the case of a bad result. Failure to follow the protocols, however, increases the risk and level of potential liability, as it can be used to support a disregard for the standards of practice that are accepted by the medical community.

Meaning

Our purpose, or what we intend, may be known to us but not to others. In ambiguous situations, meaning may come from the context of the situation, our experience, or our knowledge. Others who have different experiences or knowledge or different perceptions of the context will give different meanings to the same information.

Attitudes and values influence the meaning we give to uncertain or ambiguous information. HROs strive for consistency of the attitudes and values necessary to prevent crises or respond to crises. Giving meaning to information is found in the affective domain.

Attitudes

According to Banaji and Heiphetz, "Attitudes are preferences, 'the predisposition to treat entities with favor or disfavor'" (2010, 350). Petty, Wegener, and Fabrigar write that "attitudes have been defined in a variety of ways, but at the core is the notion of evaluation" (1997, 611).

The affective, or feeling, component has great influence in evaluation. At one time, researchers thought that attitudes had three components—affect, cognition, and behavior—with the affective component more pronounced. In fact, attitudes summarize and integrate the cognitive and affective reactions (Crano and Prislin 2006). When it comes to evaluation, the cognitive and behavior components have less influence than affect.

The lack of consistency between cognition and affect has a bearing on cognitive dissonance. Unexpected stimuli during HRO events can elicit unexpected behaviors and reveal implicit undesired attitudes. When this occurs, the person must deal in some way with the discomfort from the resultant cognitive dissonance. Anger, justification, defensiveness, or becoming adversarial or averse to engagement are common reactions to reducing this discomfort. Paradoxically, Weick (1964) found that expending effort while performing a task reduces cognitive dissonance, an early academic description of one of the first tasks taught to public-safety novices: "Engage. Always engage" (van Stralen). This engagement with the problem aligns affect and cognition which then supports attitude change (Cooper 2007; Harmon-Jones 1999, cited in Banaji and Heiphetz 2010).

Cognitive dissonance, the source of the biases "confirmation bias" and "motivated reasoning," is a major threat to establishing reliability and safety. The discomfort arises from several sources, examples of which include "known" reality versus perception; universal knowledge versus the particular; personal perception and meaning versus that of subordinates, colleagues, and superiors; and experience in the event versus more centralized authority. The gravest danger is the dissonance across the liminal threshold between the VUCA-T environment and conventional business operations. Reducing the discomfort by diminishing or denying evolving reality and human response is a prelude to failure and an unrecognized but critical cause of error.

Attitudes are weak predictors of behaviors. While they do not *predict* or *cause* behavior, they do have an influence on behavior. The attitude-behavior relationship depends on the person, the situation, the attitude (for example, how much knowledge people have about the attitude object), and the measurement match between attitudes and behavior. What is not clear is whether researchers measure specific attitudes and *specific* behaviors or if they measure specific attitudes but *general* behaviors. This ability to influence behavior *dependent on the situation* strengthens such behavior's use in unexpected HRO events. It is in such cases that the organization or leader has no control over someone who is faced with uncertainty, time compression, and threat. At such times, all the person may have is the attitudes embodied from training, modeling, and the organization's culture (Banaji and Heiphetz 2010).

We can become bogged down with definitions of attitudes and whether they *cause* behavior. For our purposes, attitudes are combined cognitive and affective interpretations or reactions to something, whether a thing, situation, or event, and they influence behavior. The affective component *influences* behavior to a greater degree than cognition does.

The Function of Attitudes

Attitudes, pervasive and measurable across humanity, have functions. We will use the four functions of attitudes proposed by Katz (1960): utilitarian, knowledge, ego-defensive, and value-expressive.

- *Utilitarian attitudes* are directed toward rewards and punishments but also foster group identity. In this function, the attitudes we have observed in a person may indicate whether that person has the necessary attitudes to prevent emergencies in a high-risk-environment respond to emergencies during a system failure. This use of attitudes is fairly common among military and public-safety personnel.
- The *knowledge function* supports our understanding of situations, particularly for novel information or sudden, unexpected events.
- *Ego-defensive attitudes* protect us from psychic threats; in that sense, they support our self-esteem. While these attitudes are a source of prejudice, they can support us during a crisis and can contribute to our resilience. On the negative side, ego-defensive attitudes impede discovery of the sources of failure when people become self-protective and begin to justify their actions or blame others.
- *Value-expressive attitudes* express our core values and beliefs. Though these are foundational aspects of the individual, some specific attitudes are foundational for an HRO and are shared with people as value-expressive attitudes.

In addition, *engagement attitudes* are key to HRO culture. The effective modulation of attitudes precludes unanticipated events from overcoming the collective decision-making of the team. Complacency cannot exist in an HRO.

Attitudes are adaptive reactions to environmental demands, particularly hazards. Attitudes for High Reliability developed as successful responses to dangerous events, modeled and taught to later generations. If the frequency of hazards continued, we would see continuation and stability of the attitudes. As the environment becomes settled and safety increases, we may witness the extinction of the adaptive attitudes caused by this shifting baseline (discussed below).

A novice who enters the industry during this period of settling and increased safety may not learn the reason behind specific attitudes. As the novice becomes experienced, the reasons behind specific attitudes will be lost, which extinguishes the attitudes necessary for the rare event. The inability to support these attitudes while mentoring and teaching new novices can shift the baseline of attitudes. Daniel Pauly (1995) first identified such a baseline shift in fisheries science, where he noticed that new researchers used their initial observations of the fish catch as a baseline of fisheries productivity and change. Over time, the change in fisheries appeared smaller than when measured over the span of several careers. The loss of High Reliability attitudes is a danger over long periods of high safety achievement.

The loss of knowledge has not been lost because of poor translation. Most likely, knowledge is lost when it is no longer used or necessary. In the early stage, this loss of knowledge may act through complacency; as complacency becomes institutionalized, knowledge is lost.

Safety in some industries has maintained a prolonged state of improvement. HRO developed from high-risk activities where failure can harm, or even kill, the participant or operator. With experience, we may have learned how to do things safely, though the risk never completely disappeared. This increase in safety permits people to enter programs or hazardous environments who did not have the mind-set to engage high risk in a safe manner. A gradual change of baseline occurs, and what was once considered unsafe begins to appear safe—if performed correctly by the identified rules. In the worst case, what was once considered safe and heavily relied on is now considered unsafe, if not irresponsible.

What once was the source of safety and prevention of failure then becomes considered the source of failure and considered unsafe. HRO, itself, seems to focus now as a means to prevent failure rather than as a method of engaging danger and entering adverse, hostile, or dangerous environments. Error, once a sign of action and immediately correctable by further action, has become a sign of poor performance, and the behavior is corrected later through training. HRO has moved from protection through engagement—moving forward—to protection by process—sheltering in place.

Acquisition or Embodiment of Attitudes
Attitudes can be acquired through life experience, social learning in the organization, mentoring, didactic lectures and counseling, and modeling from others who embody the desired attitudes.

The attitudes of an emergency response HRO come from training and socialization. They are also developed during an emergency response; some members may possibly have the selected attitudes from previous life experiences, or they may have learned them within their family of origin. (Family of origin is a psychology term that refers to the family in which a person grew up.) The military and public safety select for specific attitudes. Recruits or trainees internalize these attitudes from repeated behaviors under the direction of a drill instructor and from social learning during their initial field assignments. Senior members of the organization embody and model these attitudes. In civilian life, we must accept the attitudes that members of the organization bring.

Civilian organizations that change attitudes risk their programs being misconstrued as controlled indoctrination (or brainwashing). A more passive approach of modeling by senior members who embody desired attitudes, values, and behaviors is not only more effective but will also be more socially accepted.

The Principles of HRO as Attitudes
We can state the principles of HRO as attitudes, which makes the concept of HRO and the five principles more understandable and accessible to most people. Attitudes influence behaviors; in this way, attitudes can create a bias for action for immediate engagement, even if that engagement takes the form of observation or notification. Those five principles are as follows.

- Preoccupation with failure: What is your attitude toward failure or the system vulnerability? What is your attitude toward a discrepancy or system disruption?
- Reluctance to simplify: What is your attitude toward working with complex situations? What is your drive to investigate?
- Sensitivity to operations: What is your attitude toward changing your work priorities without notice? What is your attitude toward maintaining normal work assignments during a large disturbance?
- Commitment to resilience: What is your attitude about giving up? What is your attitude toward working a problem until it is solved or you reach an acceptable end-state?
- Deference to expertise: What is your attitude toward the knowledge of those who have less experience or are lower in the hierarchy than you?

Additional Attitudes

We have found that the fundamental principles of Weick and Sutcliffe (2015) work well as attitudes. In making HRO operational, however, we have identi-fied several additional attitudes and values that contribute significantly to High Reliability operations.

Acceptance. During an emergency (or in preparation for one), responders can become quite upset with the circumstances and the victims. The responders may believe that the victims contributed to the situation. This attitude will have an immediate effect on people's performance as well as the performance of those around them. This is more than simply passing judgment on whether an event ought to have occurred or on someone's culpability in the affair; it can turn into anger that the event should not have occurred or that someone's incompe-tence led to the event. Mixed in with sensemaking, decision-making, and tactical maneuvering is the sense that the event should not have happened.

We often see this situation arise in safety presentations, where someone dis-cusses an unsafe behavior that led to a tragedy. Comments by the presenter might include, "What were they thinking?" or derisions of people's intelligence or com-mon sense. The result is that, since we are not like those people, we do not learn from their failure.

It is important to accept that an event happened and that we should now work on the problem. Instead, people often seem to believe that it is important to have, and express, their opinions that events were preventable and then make comments during the episode.

> When I worked in emergency services in the 1970s, I noticed we often responded to calls late at night from people who had been experiencing or struggling with some kind of medical condition all day, yet they were calling for help late at night. When I asked my colleagues about this, they told me, with an air of resignation and acceptance, that this was the "sundown effect." They believed it occurred because whatever sources of support people had throughout the day were no longer available late at night. Television stations stopped broadcasting, so there was no longer anything to distract people. Lacking distraction, they now focused on the pain they'd had all day and called emergency services, feeling much more worried about their condition than they were earlier.
>
> I heard the same story in the 1990s, now accompanied with anger about these responses. People seemed angry; they felt it was wrong to call so late because it represented an abuse of resources. The responders and

caregivers did not know (or did not understand) the dynamics behind these late-night calls.

I always think it helps to explain to people why this happens. Understanding why is important. In the absence of other facts, people tend to explain the circumstances from their point of view. Having an understanding of why things can happen can be very helpful in getting people to accept the information that's coming at them.

—Daved van Stralen

We have identified several types of acceptance attitudes: (1) accept the problem and don't intervene; (2) accept your partner's action, even if you don't agree with it; and (3) accept the information as it is given. (Some people disregard this information if it disconfirms what they think they know.) In the military, this is usually a bigger problem in the beginning of the training cycle, when people are new. This is especially so for people who have had additional experience in another industry or field. Early on, you can ask them what surprised them. If you do not intervene, they will become accustomed to things being the way they are.

Some police officers can manage two conflicting descriptions of the same incident. Different officers have different patience levels for this kind of conflict and ambiguity. Some officers take the view that they cannot change it; they could probably predict what people are going to say, because they've heard it many times before. It then becomes built into the nature of the work that "this is what we do."

As an example, after 2001, when police departments went on heightened alert, they used to do vehicle searches before they got to the local airport; they narrowed lanes to slow the vehicles. A team of six officers was dispatched to the airport to work at night. Drivers became frustrated about possibly missing flights, and officers became frustrated at the drivers not understanding what to do. One officer decided to walk back to see what drivers would see as they approached the narrowing lanes; he looked at cone patterns and lighting. The officer then understood that it was not clear to the drivers what they should do. He told the other officers to get the same view so they would understand why the drivers were not doing what the officers wanted quickly—because what the officers wanted could not be done. The officers calmed down and communicated more clearly after that. The drivers responded to this change in the officers' behavior.

Communication style is sometimes taught, but it is more likely gained through experience. Going into a situation, police officers know that, with the high emotions people have, they will probably hear the same person tell the same thing many times over, even though they only need to hear it once. The officers don't have time for the repetition. There is a way to interrupt people without being rude: you can move forward and let them know that you understand them.

You have to be careful when you start saying "I've heard this already," because you can pick up new information through the repetition. In the dispatch tapes for an airplane crash, for example, the dispatchers kept saying, "If this is about the airplane crash, we have it," and not listening to the callers. They started radioing to the chief officer on the scene to ask if a second airplane was involved in the midair collision. There was a second plane, but it was at a different location. The dispatchers did not know that, though, because they were shutting the callers off.

—Steve "Pappy" Papenfuhs, Sergeant, San Jose, CA, Police Department, retired; educator law enforcement human factors and Constitutional use of force

People often cannot imagine all the ways in which things can fail. Explaining the nature of the various things that intersect in healthcare—people, adaptive behaviors, complex adaptive systems, and uncertainty—challenges people's understanding of the system. Some people have trouble accepting the conclusions. What they are really asking is whether they can *trust* the conclusions. We can show staff what happens in actual cases, but healthcare professionals are not typically trained that way. Rather, they are trained on rules, procedures, and processes. We want people to recognize problems that need earlier engagement and then to seek assistance. If people wait until they don't know what procedure to apply, then things will become a lot worse. It will then become harder for others to provide support, because the flexibility will be gone. A new approach to strive for zero harm in healthcare might make people less likely to act during conditions of uncertainty.

When you take a navy ship or airplane into a dangerous situation, it's often hard to discriminate between the danger you're putting yourself in and the danger of not intervening. You want to invent a system that gives people credit for reporting problems. If you openly discuss error, those discussions can be a learning experience. You have to make a decision about how to balance the risks and benefits. Some people I knew thought it was important to distinguish between not committing ("sins of omission") and engaging with a lot of uncertainty ("sins of commission") and doing the wrong thing. I know of many cases where not engaging earlier allowed things to escalate and get much worse. We had a lot of discussions about the unintended consequences of "zero harm" or "zero accidents" leading to less reporting, even though errors would still happen.

  —Capt. Ralph Soule, USN (retired)

Neutrality. Acceptance and neutrality are related attitudes. Neutrality is more than the opposite of bias. Being neutral means to investigate without passing judgment, not only of a moral nature but also of the causation and people's attempts to justify their actions. Neutrality reduces defensiveness and increases information flow. It may be that neutrality has greater importance than we recognize in gaining information and investigating (1) situations where error is attached, (2) anything with a moral basis, or (3) cases where judgment (versus decision-making) is involved. For example, the members of SAMU, the ambulance service in Paris, wear white to show their neutrality from the police, military, and fire services (Pierre Carli, MD, medical director, SAMU of Paris, personal communication).

When I worked in an economically poor area as a paramedic, the more experienced paramedics taught us that biker gangs would always protect us, because we took care of them. We were neutral. I noticed this in the paramedics I worked with—actually career ambulance men who'd started work in the 1950s. They had opinions, but on scene, with only a few exceptions, they passed no judgment. With the Crips and Pirus (later called Bloods) moving north into South Los Angeles, we would often encounter adolescents who, as we approached them, would look and act like gang members. We remained neutral, so we could quickly discern from their behaviors different classes of adolescent: those who were protecting themselves and were actually frightened of gang members (and appreciated the protection we could provide); those who wanted the cachet of gang membership, though they did not belong; those who wanted to impress others so that they could become gang members; and actual gang members. Had we not remained neutral, it is unlikely we could have discerned these differences.

  —Daved van Stralen

Disagreements and "going to school." As retired rear admiral Thomas A. Mercer, commanding officer of the USS *Carl Vinson*, said during HRO studies, "Maybe

I need to go to school on this." This is a common phrase that naval aviators use when they do not understand (or disagree about) something. Starting the discussion with "I need to go to school on this" can diffuse the situation, because it is a neutral statement that reflects one's receptivity to personal learning. The statement effectively asks to delay resolution until more information becomes available and emotions subside, thus putting a pause to arguing. The phrase helps people understand what they are missing; it's a way to say "I need to learn more about this" or "There may be more information out there" instead of saying "I'm wrong." By moving the focus from the other person to asking how we think, we can then seek understanding rather than being right. A similar expression is, "We are at cross purposes."

Expectations. Expectations, in HRSs contribute to, if not create, fear and anxiety within people. Rather than focusing on their performance, people may focus on responses to their actions and the eventual outcome. When this happens, every "failure" is a sign of their quality of care. If we believe we are good people because of our successes, then we will readily believe that we are bad people whenever we fail. Expectations for a good outcome shift the mind-set, and unrecognized fear responses begin to appear.

> Early in my ambulance career, whenever we responded to a call, family, friends, and bystanders would step in, unsolicited, to assist us. Sometimes they were excited, but our presence and demeanor would calm them enough that they could capably assist us. They didn't know what we'd do, nor did they know how to help us.
>
> Over a short period of time, I encountered a new type of person. These people watched us. They stood back. They did not participate and were unsure of themselves when they did help. Some expected us to do things or say things that seemed odd or out of place. Same neighborhoods; it all happened in a short time period. I asked around, and other medics told me to watch a new television show called *"Emergency!"* That explained my experience. I could now tell who watched *"Emergency!"* Those were the people who had an *expectation* of what we would do and what would happen.
>
> Then I went to medical school, and by the time I reached my fellowship in critical care, expectations had become onerous. Even physicians in charge had expectations, and they expected us to meet them. When I became a physician in charge, expectations now came strongly—from families, nurses, other physicians—that I would do everything correctly, that I would do e-v-e-r-y-t-h-i-n-g, and anything bad or unexpected or

unwanted was, well, was my fault or a deficiency on my part. The expectation of a good outcome influenced the team's thinking and their own expectations. They did not say it, but it was there. In fact, I could sometimes tell the types of movies or television shows people watched by their actions and expectations.

I saw good people leave the field. Good, caring, intelligent people left. Many who stayed soon developed a knack for justification. They no longer learned as much from their experience. The worst thing had happened: the environment had lost its vote. The brutal audit of our system had disappeared. All sensemaking and actions had become context-free and were now done in service of meeting someone's expectations.

Expectations—sometimes spoken, often unspoken, always denied—had ruined emergency performance, in my estimation, and they brought with them the importance of 1) justification of actions, or protecting yourself defensively, 2) the concept of blame and error, or protecting yourself by taking the offense through finding fault in others or the system, and 3) the loss of learning from mistakes. It is this hard-won education through knowledge creation that ultimately protects us the best.

—Daved van Stralen

Fear as an Attitude

Fear as an attitude has two manifestations—as a response to threat and as a method of control. As a threat response, fear can strengthen the organization by motivating action, vigilance for vulnerability, and preoccupation with failure. It hurts the organization when fear impairs thinking and actions, remains unrecognized, or contributes to situational cognitive distortions. Some people, at various levels in the hierarchy, will use fear as a method for control. We cannot predict or control how the person will respond to fear; we may well see maladaptive or dangerous responses. As a method of influence or control, fear has no place in an HRO.

The threat response is a physiological response. Because of the moral weight placed on the concept of fear, we urge caution in calling this the fear response, even if it is physiologically correct. In fact, this moral judgment may be what causes many fear responses to remain unrecognized. These responses include anger, aversion, and avoidance, among others (see chapter 9, "Threat Responses and Unrecognized Fear").

The fear response interferes with our early engagement of the problem. Rather than denying or hiding this fear, we must articulate what it is that is causing us concern. Some people may simply say what their concern is, or where the solution or program will fail, without offering suggestions. They believe it is their duty to identify any and all possible failure points. Where this situation differs from the discussion of fear is that these people only state what failure would look like (or where the system will fail) and then say nothing more. They offer no suggestions or insights and do not participate in discussions to overcome their objections.

People use fear as a method of control. At the point of action, it may be *intimidation* by stance or countenance—the quiet, piercing stare when someone does *not* respond to communication. Actually, the stare *is* the response and can quickly elicit nervous, defensive responses from people. (One woman described how she handles this form of intimidation: "Simple. I'm a woman, so I'm used to being stared at. I just stare back.") This is not command presence, even if the person uses it as such. Rather, it is a hollow command presence that is used either for intimidation or to mask the person's own fear. As a command presence, countenance and stance will bring calm. This form is differentiated from the hollower form of command presence by being "other" centered rather than centered on self.

Instrumental anger or aggression is the aggressive use of anger, or the appearance of anger, for an *extrinsic* purpose. This can be done to achieve power, to intimidate others into a desired action, or for the prophylactic prevention of disagreement. In this third case, people agree with the person to avoid the discomfort of witnessing what appears to be an emotional, angry outburst, which might be confused with emotional anger. Though tolerated and even accepted as an effective practice and desirable leadership trait, instrumental anger is quite dangerous in the VUCA-T environment. Compare instrumental anger to reactive anger, which is the immediate emotional response to a fearful event. Reactive anger is situational rather than a constituent of a person's personality or habit in social discourse. This type of anger is often unrecognized as one of the fear responses, but it should be addressed in real time (see chapter 9, "Threat Responses and Unrecognized Fear").

Instrumental fear (fear for motivation) works rapidly, because it operates at the level of emotion, thus bypassing cognition. Further, fear impairs cognition and the slower cognitive processes, just as it would during a bona fide threat. The intentional use of fear—fear for an *extrinsic* purpose—to bypass cognition is similar to instrumental anger; it coerces others into a desired action or to prevent disagreement. Fear, which operates on the affective level, blunts the use of logic, reason, or rationality by both parties.

While the use of instrumental anger is more likely directed toward subordinates, instrumental fear can also operate in any direction. Every member of an organization has the duty of vigilance to identify vulnerabilities. In a rational system, this creates the HRO principle "preoccupation with failure," and the organization can attend to, and resolve, a source of failure. Instrumental fear uses vague threats or risks with delayed consequences as a rubric to control actions toward a different, extrinsic purpose.

Intentional fear provides power. While a person who is extremely fearful can occupy resources and the attention of others, the use of fear for power refers to the use of fear to control resources for an extrinsic purpose. Rather than building system strength or adding to organizational knowledge, intentional fear rapidly places people into defensive or offensive postures (see *liability* below). People's actions are no longer directed toward the problem but toward protection; this is a never-ending process, as one can posit that the system cannot be too safe.

> The hospital's patient safety reviewer (PSR) asked the team in a procedure room if they must monitor room temperature and humidity, since this was done by other services in nearby rooms. (They did not do this monitoring.) They answered that they didn't know, which is a phrase people often use to avoid creating false answers because of their good intentions and a desire to help. This situation was reported as a safety breach to the supervisor: the staff should also know which rules from other services they *didn't* need to follow. The supervisor therefore had to prepare an educational presentation.
>
> This room had long had a problem with maintaining sterility while opening cans; devices could only be used once before being sterilized in a room on a different floor. The staff relied on reciting a short song to time their procedures; this made the system vulnerable when time pressures for deliveries unconsciously drove the staff to sing faster, but their requests for timers went unfulfilled.
>
> The discussion focused on the importance of rules and knowing which rules to follow and not to follow. That is how the hospital keeps patients safe. One would not want to lower safety standards—thus the need for the educational presentation.
>
> The safety person demonstrated productivity by identifying a problem (without knowing specific rules) and blunted any disagreement by the use of the fear of patient harm. Breaching rules often seems to be more of a safety problem, as doing so crosses units in the hospital—compared to one room's problems with opening cans and timing procedures.
>
> (A federal regulator of an agency with a long history of increasing safety once provided the insight that regulators are at risk of showing

productivity through lists of rules breached, fines administered, and educational presentations created; it is far more difficult to demonstrate productivity by what did *not* happen.)

This particular supervisor was problem driven (i.e., phronesis): the supervisor achieved safety, reliability, and productivity by identifying problems and then developing solutions. The creation of educational presentations to teach rules from other departments takes time from addressing more immediate threats.

The patient safety reviewer was rule driven. In a rule-driven system, which is an easy administrative approach, risk comes from broken rules. In a problem-driven system—which uses practical wisdom and an HRO approach—risk comes from unsolved problems or following the "strong-but-wrong" rule (James Reason). It is difficult to respond to vague but real "safety" concerns about broken rules, as breaking a rule is immediate and visible. It is easy to disregard specific problems when the breach is less common and consequences, even if more dire, are delayed. The use of instrumental fear prevents discussion in order to combine or prioritize goals.

-Anonymous hospital manager

Expression of internal fear. People, either individually or within a system, may have *hidden hostility* or put up *quiet resistance.* We will not use the terms "passive-aggressive" or "passive resistance" because, as categories, they do not allow us to address the problem as situational, a group dynamic, or happening along a spectrum of behaviors.

People in the HRO may have to engage a daunting situation or overcome some idiosyncratic aversion, either recognized or unrecognized. They desire to avoid confrontation and disagreement while not revealing the internal fear they are experiencing. Characteristic behaviors and traits reflect this redirected or indirect anger from this internal fear.

When faced with an immediate demand for action, they may pretend ignorance, or during the event they may allow failure to occur. Disagreement may occur through sarcasm or through questions such as "Are you sure this is safe to do?" or "Do you know what you're doing?" When we encounter expected errors during the activity, rather than describe the situation and correct the expected error in an honest manner, they use justification, alibis, and blame. Their negative attitudes and passive resistance can be such that their behavior ensures that we will remove them from potentially being in similar situations in the future.

Leading up to an event, people may manipulate and procrastinate, presenting their actions as simple prudence or their dedication to safety. They will put up resistance to learning new knowledge or the lessons learned from previous experience. This resistance differs from motivated reasoning (i.e., overscrutiny due to strongly held beliefs), because they do not offer a deeply held belief that can be discussed. This stubbornness can also be hidden as overzealous attempts for safety. They generally have a pessimistic outlook, along with a cynical or bitter nature. Found in the individual as a constellation of traits, this cynical nature may represent the improper placement of that person within the organization, or even the person's improper choice of industry or career. Found in varying degrees throughout the organization or within a system, this nature may represent poor education, training, or leadership. Tone does come from the top, but poor leaders interfere with that tone to create a climate of fear, where the only protection people feel they have is in this indirect expression of hostility and resistance.

On walk-arounds as a supervisor or someone new to the organization, you will notice this climate by guarded discussions and choice of words. What you will find missing are open discussions and communications. People substitute phrases or clichés in place of honest judgment and select safe words that will distance people from consequences or keep them from presenting their own decisions.

The HRO, in contrast, has free, open, and almost aggressive communication and mutual respect among its members. People are free to fail, because failure is always an option. This underscores the point of walk-arounds: the leader does not "show the flag" but participates in meaningful discourse.

Negative Consequences of Fear as an Attitude

Organizations that operate in the VUCA-T environment must openly address five specific areas, or domains, of fear: legal, risk management, financial, human resources (HR), and administrative. These domains may flow in a top-down manner, but they can also develop at lower levels of managers and line staff. From above they reflect the fear of consequences, and from below they result from lack of information and knowledge.

Liability. Probably the most common concern in an emergency environment is liability, which leads both to failure from *not* acting and to overzealous attempts and distracting protective actions. Liability consists of specific legal elements: duty to act, breach of that duty, proximate cause (the link of breach to the harm), and damages (harm) to the plaintiff. Because of the difficulty in measuring harm, the concept of damages takes the place of harm. The damages reflect the amount of money the harm costs the plaintiff.

The VUCA-T environment presents strong possibilities for liability by the organization. Uncertainty and ambiguity allow a harmed person the freedom to fill in the blanks and to give different meanings to ambiguous information. This can be followed by inductive reasoning to reach a conclusion that participants in the emergency could never have foreseen. Time compression forces the hand of people to make decisions and act before they can obtain complete information. This clearly shows the importance of having systems for documentation and having *articulate descriptions* of uncertain and ambiguous information, along with evolving conjectures used by individuals or the team.

We know fear impairs cognitive abilities; it is probably unwise to describe actions as a fear response. It is vital to characterize the impending threat that justifiably distracted attention and resources, but it is equally vital for the organization to disabuse people of the idea that the fear responses (anger and avoidance in particular) are adaptive.

> A medical center administrative committee was considering a quality-improvement study to identify the risk of bacterial infection versus length of time for a specific procedure. There were no published guidelines or studies of incidence of infections. It was fairly straightforward to do: obtain serial cultures every four to six hours and identify when bacteria became evident. The study had unanimous committee approval.
>
> A senior executive officer attended the next meeting and advised the committee that this could open the hospital to liability if bacteria were shown to become evident during the procedure. The committee began to back away from evaluating the risk of bacterial infection, despite their discussions that infection in a patient could lead to greater liability. One committee member then asked, "What duty are we breaching by conducting this study?" The executive could not answer. The evaluation was never conducted.
>
> -Anonymous physician

In the face of threat, individuals and organizations are justified in protecting themselves. Throughout this book, we may discuss the behavior of organizations as a corporate entity. While this has legal standing, it is also true that corporations do not go to jail. In that same vein, organizations do not feel fear; only individuals can. The same human responses for fear—in fact all the behaviors discussed in this book—are found throughout the hierarchy, from executive to management to the line level. Their manifestations may differ because of responsibility or personal background, but the mechanisms are all the same. Unwarranted defensive or offensive actions are evidence of fear as a driver.

Defensive actions are important to resist active attacks on the organization's integrity or ability to operate. On the individual level, unwarranted defensive actions appear as justifications and alibis to not act or decide. Excessive concern can lead to guarding against imagined threats and the organization wasting resources while making preparations or missing opportunities.

Offensive actions are outward, aggressive movements made for the purposes of controlling the situation and are usually carefully planned to attack a problem away from the organization. Unwarranted offensive actions, when impulsive, become chaotic, thus increasing the probability of unexpected and unwanted consequences. On the individual level, they occur as blame and instrumental anger.

Unwarranted defensive and offensive actions greatly decrease the quality of communication within the organization and impair the organization's ability to respond to threats.

Strength is the third option for protection. In healthcare, strength comes through the use of knowledge and wisdom. In the course of this book, we will demonstrate that knowledge is both cognitive and affective. We will also demonstrate that wisdom develops from experience in applying the sciences to particular situations (such as with anecdotes). For liability, we would be better served to focus on breach of duty rather than generalized fear of litigation.

Duty to act is likely the greatest vulnerability of the organization regarding liability. But hidden sources of liability that can be readily corrected lie in poor descriptions, miscommunication, rigid and nonadaptive decision-making, and the influence of unrecognized fear. Zealous emphasis on documentation can lead to a focus on completion of the form at the expense of accurate descriptions.

I read in an article that a team of paramedics had delayed transport of multiple patients from a motor vehicle collision because the hospital staff needed certain information to complete their paramedic contact forms. After reading this article, I started to notice the prevalence of filling out forms taking precedence over descriptions of patients or situations. People would vigorously seek out information if it matched a box on the form, but they would disregard important and salient information if it had no place on the form. I coined the term "euboxia" to describe the importance of filling out all the boxes. Of course, there are degrees of euboxia, such as primary euboxia, where the boxes are filled in with

desirable values, secondary euboxia, where the boxes are filled in but with less than desirable numbers, and so forth. This story helped the staff focus on the importance of the information, how it would affect medical care, and the importance of providing useful, articulate descriptions. We also described those who were overly focused on forms as having euboxia, and their patients as being "euboxic."
    —Daved van Stralen

Risk management is the process of identification, analysis, and acceptance or mitigation of risk or uncertainty. While initially developed for financial investment, the term is also used for any risk that can harm the organization's operations and survival. The International Organization for Standardization (ISO) has published standards for risk management known as the ISO 31000 family of standards (see chapter 11, "Other Systems"). (The ISO intentionally adopted initials that don't match those of its three official languages.)

    Sources of risk come from human-factors variables (human performance, mental states, and decision-making), technology, and infrastructure. Sociotechnical systems (STSs) describe the interaction between people and technology. Jens Rasmussen looked at STS from an ecological view of a human working in an environment of technology. From this he identified the "skill, rule, knowledge" framework in human factors, which forms the basis of James Reason's structure of error analysis (for example, skill-based error, rule-based error, and knowledge-based error).

    It is through human-factors variables that risk management began to influence HRO operations and why engineered solutions appear attractive to executives and managers. The methods used for voluntary entry into a dangerous environment across the liminal threshold become a trade-off in the risk-management approach. That is, the decision to act in the face of danger is risk of harm versus increased value to the organization. Human factors are one set of processes that decrease the risk of a dangerous entry or action due to human performance.

    Risk and value will increase or decrease as explicit, tangible values that can be defined, categorized, and measured across fields. Risk managers in the business field may find it difficult to grasp risk as implicit, tacit, and intuitive. For business leaders, the methodology that HROs use to reduce risk and enable operations in dangerous environments are counterintuitive and would appear to bring ruin on a business working in a financially risky but physically safe environment. Risk aversion has different meanings and contexts between risk management and HRO operations.

Risk management, through ISO, has a well-defined vocabulary and methodology. Risk managers identify and characterize threat, assess the vulnerability of assets from *specific* threats, determine risk as a finite probability factor, identify methods to reduce risk, and then prioritize various risk-reduction measures.

It is important to note the use of *probability* in risk management. Risk is calculated value from a *measured probability* multiplied by the *cost of failure* and is an indication or suggestion of how much the organization should, or is likely to, spend on risk mitigation. An HRO, on the other hand, views risk as *possibility* and mitigates risk based on threat to life or property. This is the difference between creating value, conducting exploratory business, and saving life or property.

The purpose of a business organization (and the function of risk management) is to protect assets and create value with business actions to minimize risk. The purpose of an entrepreneurial organization that operates in an adverse financial market is to create value in uncertainty by balancing risk with the *possibility* of value creation. These businesses enter adverse environments for exploitation (to grow markets) and/or exploration (to identify new markets); catastrophic failure is unlikely but possible.

HRO developed to enter dangerous environments, where catastrophic failure is possible. The purpose of the HRO is to save life or property while operating in risky situations or dangerous environments, which was the goal of the original HROs. Healthcare today amalgamates value creation, asset protection, and risk spanning healthcare organizations that take high-risk patients and those that do not. Regardless, healthcare has innate risk that is more similar to the environment where HROs developed. For example, US nuclear power generation and US commercial aviation demonstrated that the approaches of risk management and HRO can work in unison.

Because the purpose of risk management is to identify and mitigate the vulnerability of the organization, such management has a place in discussions of fear as an attitude. That is, risk is balanced with financial return; some organizations are more risk averse than others. At the extreme, risk aversion has the same characteristics as fear responses. Risk is not accepted without some promise of return commensurate with that risk. In contrast, HROs developed to actively engage threats and reduce risk through operations interactive with the VUCA-T environment. The financial benefit to the original HROs went to other organizations. For example, military operations do not increase the financial value of the military, and wildland firefighting does not increase the financial value of the firefighting service. Instead, these dangerous operations are conducted to protect the value of people and property outside the HRO.

This situation makes it difficult, but not impossible, to use the principles of risk management for HRO operations. As the civilian nuclear power industry learned, HRO operations allow for the use of dangerous technologies. In the United States, commercial aviation found that HRO operations not only increase safety but also decrease cost (Christopher A. Hart, chair, NTSB, personal communication).

Administration. HRO operates in a high-trust environment in which operators are some distance from administrators and other authority figures. Trust is easier to develop and maintain when people work closely together. This distance has led to the development of several approaches to delegate authority. One way, used in HROs, is to develop skilled decision-making and judgment. One method of delegation of authority is through the development of protocols, which is more common in lower-tempo organizations working in more stable environments.

There is nothing wrong with either approach, unless those people in central authority do not trust the operators working in the unstable environment. Uncertainty and ambiguity have the greatest effect in the immediate vicinity; from a distance, it may be difficult to discern how little somebody might be *able* to know. This can lead to second-guessing and unfounded criticism of decisions, particularly the belief that people nearest the incident have poor judgment. To enforce authority from a distance, weaker leaders and managers rely on fear.

Finance. Similarly, to risk management, finance is concerned with lowering costs and increasing income. While it is laudable to lower costs, the redundancy necessary for high-risk operations will increase cost. If this increased cost is not of value to the organization's leaders, then the operations themselves should be reconsidered. It is appropriate to educate people on waste and the cost of items, because it is possible to take actions during an emergency to reduce that will have little or no effect.

We should not use the finance department, sometimes called the bean counters, to reduce the staff, training, and equipment necessary for safe and effective operations. The difficulty here is that the training and the benefit of that training do not occur in the same fiscal year. Regardless of these arguments, fiscal constraints are real, but fear does not belong in the discussion.

Human resources. The attitudes and values of HRO are not shared with society and become critical elements only when a crisis develops. Someone who resists—who does not, cannot, or will not embody these attitudes and values—does not cause danger during low-tempo times. Cognitive defenses from principles, rationality, and scientific logic are well-accepted defenses. It may be difficult to remove such people from the organization, but the articulation of the affective domain as a standard may assist in keeping these people further from crisis operations. That is one of the purposes of this book.

Personnel. Earlier, we discussed safety climate and how tone comes from the top. What is often left out is the fear of being wrong, making an error, or expressing an honest concern that will lead to retribution from supervisors. Whether well-founded or not, these fears support an environment that suppresses initiative and the values of HRO. The fear produced is not clearly identified, acting almost as an ether through which people move and perform their work. One value of good leadership is to identify this hidden fear and intervene: not to suppress it but to eradicate it.

Fear as an attitude can be intentional, instrumental, or a byproduct of human nature. Its intimate qualities sometimes make it difficult to identify. Its prevalence in society can give fear acceptance as normal. After one experiences a workplace that is devoid of fear, consisting of high trust, respect, and delegated decision-making, fear in the work becomes easily recognizable and its detrimental effects clearly understood. This is a major stumbling block to organizations seeking HRO status.

Vulnerability. This is the risk awareness that Karlene Roberts describes. What do people do about it? This is more than simple acknowledgment; it is doing something to engage the risk in order to enact a safe circumstance. In most of us who routinely work in high-risk environments, vulnerability became a normative behavior, with the belief that safety comes from vigilance and proactive actions, then interactive behaviors when crises emerge. In an organization, Weick and Sutcliffe termed this preoccupation with failure "never assuming infallibility"; we call it accepting your vulnerability.

I worked on the fire department rescue ambulance in an area that was highly influenced by gangs and drugs. The department staffed the units with two medics; we did not have portable radios, and a fire engine did not respond. Nor did police unless the caller said the words "gun" or "shooting." As we talked with people on scene, we knew that a word, term, or phrase that relaxed tension on a call could initiate a fight on the next call. As we talked, we watched the faces of everyone in the room to see which way we were headed. I have bandaged a patient while the patient punched me. A number of my friends had to go home for injuries from fights. These experiences develop specific behaviors and beliefs: a culture for providing medical care in an austere, unpredictably hostile environment.

As I moved from fire EMS to healthcare, my workplace went from threat (criminal, gang, and drug behavior) to safety (hospital wards, ICU, and the OR). My behaviors and culture did not fit, and it was hard to explain to people what I was thinking and doing and why, though some seemed to catch on. Over ten years passed before I recognized who would understand this approach and who could not—it was based on vulnerability and the response to vulnerability. If people recognized vulnerability from high-risk situations, then they understood and accepted this approach.

—Daved van Stralen

A Barbeque for Subacute

I once volunteered to take the position of medical director for a subacute care facility that was having difficulty with state licensing. As a pediatric critical care physician, I had no background in long-term care, though I had managed the ventilators for a home mechanical ventilator program.

Walking around, I asked the staff if they provided high-risk care. They all provided the same answer: "No, we're a nursing home." After a few weeks of hearing the same answer, I decided to provide a picnic for all staff at the end of the week—outside and for two to three hours. For several days I walked around the facility inviting people. They had little discussions between themselves. When I asked them what they were talking about, they told me of their plans to assign time periods during the picnic to make sure someone was in the facility at all times. "But didn't you say the care here is not dangerous or high risk? We'll all be together for two to three hours."

The staff told me that some of the kids would have problems; at least one child might die. When pressed, they told me how a child could die. This gave me the presentation information I needed. They realized that the care they provided was high risk; a child could even die. They told me how the child might die, which was their area of expertise in the care they provided. Then I pointed out that, in the last three hours, no child had died, so they had saved a life. We just didn't know which child had been saved. In fact, during each typical twelve-hour shift, they saved the lives of four children.

—Daved van Stralen

Discrepancy. It is too easy to think of HRO as something that is related to risk, safety, resilience, or danger. When these things happen, we can call on the principles of HRO, but will we be able to apply them as an individual, or as a group, when the time comes? Our plans, based on HRO, may not apply to that given situation. Our plans may not even work. We know our beliefs and desired outcomes, but during our response, a discrepancy will develop between the actual and the intended: our beliefs do not seem to be working, and our desired out-come moves out of reach. We must identify the point of discrepancy as early as possible. Subtly, the beginnings of failure may lie hidden in the fluctuations of daily events, visible only as an incongruous observation or discrepant response to our actions. How do we develop the ability to identify discrepancy, and how do we develop in the novice the possibility of, and awareness for, discrepancies? This is the problem of sustaining HRO in an organization.

Do we know why (causation-action-justification)? When we operate with uncer-tainty and ambiguity, we create a hypothesis or have a conclusion of what is occur-ring and how it may have come about. We act, observing the response to our action. How can we know the cause of the situation, the *cause of our behavior,* and did our action cause the result? For this discussion, we would like to focus on what causes our behaviors, and how this cause can become known. After the behavior occurs, do we know the cause, or are we justifying our behaviors and beliefs to reduce the discomfort from cognitive dissonance? Causation may remain unknown to us, and we may create justification for our own purposes.

Wildland firefighters do not know if their actions kept a fire that grew to one hundred acres from developing into a two-thousand-acre fire, or if they could have stopped the fire at five acres. This is the same problem we face in healthcare: Did we stop the patient from dying, or did our treatment cause more problems?

Engagement. The importance of engagement is to identify nuanced and sensitive feedback and to create responsiveness of the situation to your actions. Engagement, as interaction, creates information and helps you gain a sense of control and self-efficacy. Others involved can read the situation from your activity. This is blocked by the ideas of "first do no harm" or "do the right thing." How do we teach engagement in a world that demands to know the situation and act in the correct manner?

Novelty. When we encounter the novel, or "black swan," situation, we first address what we know. Novelty has a basis in the known. Is there an 80:20 rule that all novel events are based in prior experience? As an allegory, the black swan event warns us that things can exist despite our lack of experience or ability to conjure them. The risk is that some people set irrational fears within the story or lay the groundwork to justify a lack of preparation for such an event. Shouldn't we look for the known within the unknown, for it is at the known where we can begin acting? Can we debunk the black swan or, at the least, see it as a distraction? After all, swans are known; only the color is different.

While teaching in the ICU, one reliable method I used to evaluate staff for their ability to deal with emergencies was to tell them an odd, but true, fact or story. It would not be related to healthcare. Some people were genuinely interested, and some feigned interest. Some would be perplexed. But the reaction I had the greatest concern for was with the people who became angry with me. Not angry because I was wasting time but angry because they believed I was lying to them, misleading them, or trying to make fools of them. In my experience, these are the people who do not respond well to novel situations. If they could not think that something would happen, if they did not know the science behind it, or if they had never experienced anything like it, then they would not believe that something new could happen; then they would not accept that it could or would happen. It was as if they had a defined blind spot to new experiences. Maybe these are the people whom the black swan story is good for. Otherwise, my students would always look for the familiar deep within the novel, since this was where they could anchor their actions and begin engagement.

—Daved van Stralen

Complacency can be the enemy of improvement. That is, imposing programs on people to stop complacency will only work in the short term unless we address the underlying beliefs.

When we first created the pediatric intensive care unit, I noticed that the staff made great gains then became complacent, even losing their vigilance, despite my best efforts to draw their attention to what I now know is mindfulness. Nothing worked until a near miss or a crisis occurred. After a few cycles, I asked my senior partner what was happening, and what I could do about it. His answer was, "Sometimes you have to fall apart to fall together." Accepting this maxim made life easier. I let the complacency run its course, but I had to increase my vigilance, using the "fall aparts" as lessons learned to build improvements in performance.

—Daved van Stralen

Complacency, as group belief, must be addressed. The use of complacency to explain people's failure to perform has dangers, as it is too easily used against people when the system created the behavior.

Self-efficacy. Though not clearly defined as an attitude, self-efficacy does motivate behavior. We discuss it further in chapter 13, "Models of Leadership."

When I began working with medical people and teaching them resuscitation, I found that their greatest impediment was hesitancy. They would not engage situations if they thought they might be wrong or might do something that would make things worse. Engagement, early and immediate, was my objective. Looking to Albert Bandura's (1982) self-efficacy concept as an interpretation and explanation, I worked to increase the self-efficacy they needed. These are not little accolades but demonstrations that the person made a difference by acting. When something went wrong, I pointed out that the person had uncovered information that we did not have before, a form of "destructive engineering" that revealed what we otherwise wouldn't have seen. Errors and mistakes, in this approach, became "inadvertent destructive engineering" that made the invisible visible.

—Daved van Stralen

"Un-values" and "anti-goals." What values do we *not* want?

Working in High Reliability systems and low-reliability systems, I soon identified differences in mind-sets and the way of thinking, but of similar significance is the difference in values between the two cultures. I found it easiest to identify the values that appeared foundational to HROs; I could understand the reasons for their absence in low-reliability systems.

More recently, I looked at the values of "low-reliability organizations" (LROs) and wondered which ones were immaterial to HRO—that is, they are present in an LRO but, though not found in HRO, are of little consequence to creating or sustaining High Reliability. This led to the question: Are there values and goals that can block the development of HRO yet appear reasonable, even seem necessary, to the non-HRO person? Most evident is centralized authority and the idea that authority migration has hazards that are greater than the problems the organization faces. Can we identify values and goals that appear reasonable to the lay professional yet prevent the organization from realizing High Reliability?

—Daved van Stralen

Values

A value is a unique attitude, in that its features transcend specific situations and are ordered by importance relative to other values. Value or values have meanings in economics, sociology, and ethics. The field of economics considers value to be the relative worth or importance of something. In sociology, values are the ideals, customs, and institutions of a society. In ethics, values refer to good moral principles. In the field of logic, deontological ethics (the ethics of moral obligation) judge morality as a duty or obligation, linking action to the consequence of a logical conclusion.

We will discuss the value of information later in this chapter and in chapter 10, "Sensemaking of Noise." We discussed values as a moral duty or obligation in chapter 3, "The Logic of Practice and the Logic of Operations."

"Values" in this section refer to the values of a culture. The conceptual definition of values has five features (Schwartz 1994): (1) beliefs that (2) pertain to desirable end-states or modes of conduct and that (3) transcend specific situations; (4) guide the selection or evaluation of behavior, people, and events; and (5) are ordered by importance relative to other values to form a system of value priorities.

After conducting research and reviewing the literature of values in multiple countries, Schwartz et al. (2012) described values as forming a circular motivational continuum (see figure 3). Values that are similar are adjacent to one another, with opposing values placed across from each other (table 4). Schwartz et al. identified "face" as a new value. *Face* expresses self-enhancement and conservation, which are related to *power* (having control through status and prestige) and *security* (avoiding shame or humiliation). Social recognition and respect preserve one's public image and maintain face as a source of power. The idea of face emphasizes maintaining a public image and putting up defenses against threats from attacks on that public image; it emphasizes avoiding shame that undermines security. Exploiting *prestige* enables the control of others and the command of resources.

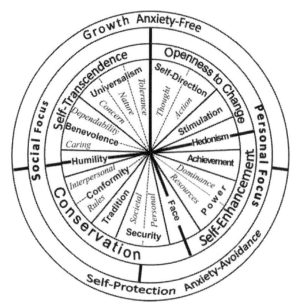

Figure 3—Schwartz et al.'s proposed circular motivational continuum of nineteen values with the sources that underlie their order (2012).

Conservation Emphasizes submissive self-restriction, preserve traditional practices, protect stability	Open to Change Emphasizes independent thought, freedom to decide and act, favoring change
Conformity Restraint of actions, obedient, self-discipline Avoid conflict	*Self-direction* Creativity, freedom, choosing own goals, curious, independent
Tradition Symbols of the group's solidarity, expressions of its unique worth Takes the form of beliefs and norms of behavior	*Stimulation* Variety and stimulation maintains optimal, positive (not threatening) state, relates to underlying self-direction Defying authority: - Conflicts self-direction and conformity - Compatible self-direction and stimulation
Self-enhancement Emphasizes pursuit of personal interests, success, and dominance over others	**Self-transcendence** Emphasizes welfare and interests of others, transcend one's interests for others
Power Social dominance—social power, control over others, social status & prestige Resource control—wealth, material possessions Influence over people, impact on events Avoid or overcome threats by control of relationships & resources	*Universalism* Understanding, appreciation, tolerance, and protection for the welfare of *all* people; Tolerance, Societal concern Universalism values derive from survival needs of individuals and groups. Universalism for the welfare of those in the larger society
Achievement Emphasizes success judged through cultural standards of competence Attain social approval for status and prestige to control or dominate people and resources	Conflicts between specific values (e.g., power vs. universalism, tradition vs. hedonism) are also near-universal. They differ only in the object of concern—all societal members (universalism) or in-group members (benevolence).

Table 4—Values conflicts (opposites in the pie chart from figure 3)

Value Shifting: Obedience-Initiative, Conformity-Creativity

HROs may have different values for different situations while still maintaining the feature of transcendence. For the emergency-response HRO, we can see a conflict between several values that Schwartz (1994) also identified as conflicting values. He found conflict between values that emphasize independent thought and action and favor change (self-direction and stimulation), in contrast to those that emphasize submissive self-restriction, the preservation of traditional practices, and the protection of stability (security, conformity, and tradition).

Public-safety organizations and the military value security, conformity, and tradition during routine operations. During an emergency response, their values shift to self-direction and stimulation. This shift in values has gone unnoticed in many HRO studies, but it is not insignificant. If they did not shift values, then we would see them saluting superior officers rather than engaging the threat.

Physicians and surgeons may deride someone who takes the initiative and is creative as a "freelancer" or a "loose cannon" who lacks the control necessary to join with others and conform to medical practice or follow medical direction. What they miss is the importance of initiative to immediately engage uncertainty and threats and to use the creativity necessary to solve novel problems.

We can see this situation at work in the friction that develops between medical control physicians (who work within the medical culture) and paramedics (who work in the public-safety culture). The procedures performed on a dying patient have a higher probability of failure and may harm the patient or contribute to death, thus decreasing the physician's sense of security during a resuscitation. Any useful procedure in the face of death is valuable to the paramedic to save a life, which increases the paramedic's sense of security when performing a rescue. This conflict often leads to disagreements between physicians and paramedics regarding endotracheal intubation, in particular, one side seeing the risk of death and the other seeing the benefit of rescue. Looking through the lens of security as a value, we can better understand the emotional character of the argument.

> Several critical care medicine experts, sitting on a panel to discuss HRO in the ICU, were once asked how they taught the staff to shift values when the tempo changed. After some embarrassed discussion, the panelists admitted that they had not considered this aspect. The ability to independently shift values, and know when to shift, is a hallmark of an HRO.
> - Daved van Stralen

To achieve High Reliability, leaders in the organization must support this shift toward initiative and stimulation when people encounter discrepancies or disruptions.

Conventional	HRO
Conservation (tradition, conformity, security) emphasizing submissive self-restriction, preservation of traditional practices, and protection of stability (security, conformity, and tradition).	Openness to Change (including self-direction and stimulation) emphasizing own independent thought and action and favoring change (self-direction and stimulation)
Conformity Restraint of actions, obedient, self-discipline Rules, tradition, and security	Self-direction and stimulation creativity, freedom, choosing own goals, curious, independent
Power achievement attainment of social status and prestige control or dominance over people and resources (authority, social power, preserving my public image) Achievement obtain resources for survival	Tradition Traditional modes of behavior become symbols of the group's solidarity, expressions of its unique worth, Traditions most often take the form of beliefs and norms of behavior

Table 5—Conflict in values between conventional business models and HRO

HRO Values

Members of an HRO share a set of closely held values that support operations to prevent or respond to system failures. Several of these values we associate with the principles, inner characteristics, and moral qualities of character. Values, much like attitudes, cannot be effectively taught to the novice but are learned, or embodied, through experience, reflection, and modeling of others who embody the values.

> Infusing HRO values and attitudes into nurse education is a start. Healthcare leadership must also frame the HRO values and attendant benefits for the entire organization's culture to give novice nurses the context they need to appropriately apply the tools of HRO. HRO begins with leadership. Educational and frontline supervisors can convey leadership support to the novices to embody these HRO values.
> —Spence Byrum

When novices want to learn, they do not ask the experts—not only because of the authority gradient but also because they routinely ask those who are closest to them in terms of ignorance. For example, a teenager does not ask an adult about sex. The teenager asks other teenagers. How teenagers embody their attitudes and values toward sex and sexuality, however, can be learned from their observations of their elders. Novices to HRO are equally unlikely to ask HRO experts how to act and what to believe but will model their attitudes and values. Combined with experience, reflection on that experience, the use of mentoring, and observations of these values in respected peers and superiors, the HRO novice can embody the attitudes, values, and ideals of High Reliability.

Organizations often have difficulty measuring values and attitudes. Values have a strong moral element, while attitudes are rooted in morals and philosophies. As a result, many organizations and leaders tend to stay away from character-related values and attitudes (see "Human resources" above). Mentoring is the guidance of self-reflection after a difficult episode or performance. Most difficult and rigorous for the leader is to model values and attitudes; leaders must practice the values and attitudes of High Reliability themselves, particularly when others do not appear to be watching.

High Reliability values form a bedrock for operations in dynamic, dangerous operations. They make the five HRO principles described by Weick and Sutcliffe come alive and become operational. The values we have identified are duty, empathy, dignity, honesty, humility, and resilience, discussed below.

Duty

Duty as a value is expansive and describes the moral obligations of members to their subordinates, peers, superiors, and the organization. Your responsibility for others comes from your humanity rather the line of authority.

Duty is somewhat unique, in that sociological values, as the qualities that make beliefs desirable, tend to be passive and do not necessarily drive action. Duty is both a sociological value and a theory of ethics. *Deon* is Greek for "duty" and lends its name to deontological ethics, the ethics of moral obligation.

Ethical theories tend to describe a state of affairs or beliefs that will lead to what type of person we desire to be. Deontological ethics links this idea to our choice to act or not act, with actions being deemed obligated, permissible, or not permissible. Actions are judged by being "right," which takes precedence over what is good or what advances us to the greater good.

Consequentialism is a theory in ethics that describes something as being desirable by the consequences of actions we have chosen. Moral value is what brings about the greater good. It is not the action that is moral, but the consequence. We may not reach a desirable or "right" consequence because of circumstances beyond the capacities and capabilities of the system. We solve problems for a solution, but an HRO event is not a single problem. More to the point, we strive for a desired end-state but actually work toward the "most" desired and "most" right end-state.

The difference between taking the "right" action or acting toward the "right" consequence may be less important than acting for the greater good. Discussions with effective HRO operators continue to reveal the importance of placing the good of the group or system ahead of one's self-interest. Duty derives from belief; we must distinguish between people's core beliefs with beliefs about the world. While some core beliefs may preclude participating in HROs, beliefs about the world must reflect the world as it is. We must update beliefs as information changes or becomes available, which is a fundamental principle from temporal logic (see chapter 3, "The Logic of Practice and the Logic of Operations"). Motivated reasoning (overscrutiny because of strongly held beliefs) interferes with dynamic response to a greater degree than confirmation bias, because refusal to change beliefs or disproportionate scrutiny can delay effective response or create dys-synchrony between the HRO and the dynamic event.

Strongly held beliefs are more difficult to change to match the circumstances, which can rob an HRO of its pragmatism. This is not to say that our actions are entirely situational but that we have a moral obligation to weigh our personal beliefs with what is right in the particular situation. Duty in the context of values does not refer to job tasks or transactional duties (something more commonly described in the plural form "duties"). These duties are the tasks and responsibilities people have because of their position or role in the organization. *Duty means that people need to know they can count on you.*

Empathy

We are all capable of making mistakes at virtually any time. Empathy means to put yourself in other people's shoes and to see events, or experience operations, through their eyes. This provides people with more intimate contact with the situation. In accident investigations, empathy provides insights into what made people think the way they did at the time they did something. In this regard, empathy is not sympathy, where one may share, in general terms, another's feelings. Empathy means to experience, in a more realistic way, the other person's predicament.

My friend and colleague Kathleen Bartholomew has written a book called *Ending Nurse-to-Nurse Hostility: Why Nurses Eat Their Young* (Bartholomew

2006). In it, she does a masterful job of describing the devastating effect of a culture that has persisted for years despite many people's efforts to have it changed. Lack of empathy for the challenges that those who are new to nursing face must change now lest we succumb to a major contributor to the current nursing shortage. Many highly competent and caring nurses have been driven out of the profession by their peers, who must completely embrace empathy if the culture is to be transformed. Not doing so will put patients in grave danger and will erode the very bedrock of patient safety.
—Spence Byrum

Organizations, as legal entities, lack empathy, partly as a consequence of the need to remain profitable and partly because leaders maintain a greater distance from those who are in immediate peril. Organizations are famous for circling the wagons and "eating their young." This is the sad experience of some beginners and novices when they enter new professions or new organizations.

Empathy, which is sometimes perceived as a weakness, falls into the "touch-feely" category of leadership traits. If you lack empathy and cannot put yourself into other people's situations, then you may reject empathy, but that is more of a fear mechanism. When you put yourself in other people's shoes, it dawns on you that you would have done the same thing. You can no longer say, "That wouldn't have happened to me." Empathy, in this sense, is much like gentleness, a form of controlled strength. Gentleness is controlled strength.

This controlled strength is reflected in the story of a combat veteran. The first commander he went into combat with was very empathetic. The soldier did not realize how much empathy it took to get people into combat. His commander was stern when he needed to get good performance out of people but empathetic when someone failed.

When our lives are threatened, we must band together to solve the problems we cannot solve alone. We must lead with strength but have the humility to look through other people's eyes.

Conducting investigations with empathy, rather than blaming someone, illuminates hidden factors. Knowing the outcome makes it difficult to put one's brain in another person's brain. Looking at what people knew and what they didn't know can bring out what led to their actions, thus making the invisible visible. Empathy helps us to understand the frame of reference of others in an investigation, which is necessary to identify common ground for improvement.

Empathy can build trust; people must have trust to carry out their tasks. To have a trusting relationship, you need trust in each person and yourself. In a crisis, we need every member of the team at optimal functionality. We can lose people when they realize they made a mistake or committed an error. You will hear this when people begin to make excuses or justify actions, particularly when they begin to perseverate about an idea, decision, or action. At that point, you may become firm to keep the team functioning, but you do so with empathy directed toward the person. You do not want to lose anyone on the team.

Empathy is how we offer aid and how we learn from others. Without empathy, we cannot learn from the mistakes of others. *Empathy means knowing that "that could be me."*

Dignity

Every job, every task, is important. The leader must have a good appreciation for this and not make people's jobs harder. What pays the greatest dividend is talking to workers as important people and not making their work more difficult. People need to matter and to feel they are important.

> "One must put him/herself in the place of those whom he would lead; he must have a full understanding of their thoughts, their attitude, their emotions, their aspirations, and their ideals; and he must embody in his/her own character the virtues, which he would instill into the hearts of his/her followers."
> —GEN. JOHN A. LEJEUNE, US MARINE CORPS, 18 JANUARY 1921

Dignity contributes to High Reliability by helping people feel safe in their environment. Dignity separates actions from who the person is. In the heat of the moment, you may view people's actions as who they are rather than what they have done. Even if they need counseling or correcting, at the end of the day, they need to feel they matter to the organization. People may need strenuous counseling, but you must take the time to say how important they are. If you must discipline them, then discipline them without taking away their dignity.

When people know that they can make decisions, they become mindful. When they are treated with dignity, they become even more mindful.

Taking away dignity begins a deadly spiral. When we fail to give people their dignity, it becomes easier to criticize, fail to support, or isolate individual people. We sometimes work with difficult people or those who are on the margins of society. Not recognizing the dignity in these people moves our standards of who deserves dignity and who does not. Dignity is not earned or deserved; it is a part of our humanity.

There is a difference between dignity and respect. You do not have to respect people to treat them with dignity. You can choose whether or not you respect someone and can set your own standards for who to respect. If the person is alive, then there is a supposition that they have dignity. *Dignity means that every job is important.*

Honesty

Trust, like respect, is transactional between two people. Honesty is the truthful representation of the situation, events, and one's capabilities. Transparency is linked to honesty but is more passive compared to the active role of honesty in communication. That is, with honesty, "I deliver this to you," while transparency is created by honesty. *Transparency and honesty are tools to convey truth.*

> "I trust you until I see you putting yourself first."
> —US Army combat medic and Vietnam veteran

Honesty and integrity must come from the top down as core values, supported by system and superiors. There can be no question of retribution, as even the suggestion of retribution will stop the honest flow of information in communication. Honesty leaves one feeling vulnerable; the alternative is self-protection through excuses, blame, or justification. We do not want people to misrepresent the facts because they did not trust the outcome or trust the system and the people working in the system.

Trust can come from beliefs and past actions. Trust, as in a high-trust system, can occur without previous experience; it takes internal strength to trust people to the extent of their capabilities observed in real time. *Honesty means that what you say represents what is happening.*

Humility

Humility is the foundation of learning and is required if people want improvement. Humility is a tricky thing for the HRO, where you want people who know a lot and feel confident, yet at the same time they know that they do not know everything. You must know that you know more than others, yet there are limits. Having humility means being humble enough to listen to different perspectives, different contexts, and the larger picture. Having humility helps open one to discordant information. Ask one question at the end of each discussion—"What do you think?"—as doing so shows that people's opinions are valuable.

Having humility means to have the hubris of confidence while in doubt. Having humility affords you the opportunity to recognize that you do not have the knowledge necessary, but you can still make the decision. Arrogance must not be accepted, as this is the denial of doubt. Doubt is necessary for vigilance against vulnerability and preoccupation with failure. Confidence plus doubt contributes to honesty and moves one toward humility.

> We key in on the Pattons of the world, who do well in the thick of battle. This strategy does work, but when you're talking about developing HRO, you may not be able to act like the general did in the movie *Patton*, which continues to be discussed as good leadership in the nonmilitary literature. Good leaders today have to be more enlightened than that. Some people are superb in combat but are pushed aside in peacetime, and vice versa. But to develop and train personnel, to draw out good leadership for the long term, involves talking about different leadership styles and personalities.
>
> Humility in HROs means that no one person can know everything all the time. It means that a member of your team, regardless of rank, position, or experience, may in fact save your bacon if you, as the leader, listen.
> —Spence Byrum

Humility is adaptation and feedback, which is tied to how often you update your sense of what is going on. The more frequently you update, the more humble you will be. You choose when to vary the frequency of when you obtain feedback. The bold have less reliance on feedback and therefore update less frequently. The flexible person relies heavily on feedback and thus increases the frequency of updates. *Having humility means that we cannot succeed without others.*

Resilience/Perseverance

Failure *is* an option. We continue to work the problem until it resolves itself or we reach an accepted end-state. While failure is not an option, it is also true that quitting is not an option. Once the problem is over, we return to normal operations feeling a bit smarter and a lot stronger. Perseverance is the key to making it through, while resilience is the willingness to do it again.

Perseverance is predicated by ownership: you have to feel like you own the problem (or part of the problem). You have a sense of duty to be involved. When working with others, you'll sense pride in the positive sense. Having the freedom to act—the empowerment that people can act—keeps them persevering.

You must control your emotions so that you won't lose opportunities to achieve success; this also requires maintaining your patience with others. Set things up to reduce distractions so that you won't have the surprises and emotional responses that interfere with perseverance. As the leader, look at what's causing the emotions in others, and then address the causes rather than the emotions or the people.

Self-reflection means that you look back to learn; self-awareness occurs in real time.

Having self-control means to be more aware. *Resilience means that we will get through this together.*

Interactions of Values

Values influence actions, but few values create action as an obligation. Duty, as a sociological and ethical value, describes the obligation to act when given a situation. "Standing in other people's shoes and seeing through their eyes" is not a mixed metaphor but a description of immersing yourself in their experience. The duty to act on this sharing of experience is what uplifts sympathy to empathy, even if the action is merely to stand by and provide the presence of an accepting human being.

Honesty reduces the corruption of information that occurs during communication. Having fidelity of information to the situation supports effective decision-making and action, along with judgment of the situation for engagement and perseveration. Honesty and dignity support deference to expertise; when people are honest about their observations and judgments and we dignify them through acceptance of their decisions, we will experience greater mindfulness on their part.

We can discuss further interactions of the five principles of HRO as attitudes and the six HRO values. We will leave it to your organization to pursue these endeavors.

Placing Value on Information

The objectivity sought in the use of theoretical reason, scientific rationality, and cognitive processes, even when tempered with biases and heuristics, fails in environments of uncertainty and ambiguity.

Theoretical reasoning, which is concerned with matters of fact and their explanations, refers to reasoning about explanations and predictions, whose objectivity and impersonal nature make them accessible to anyone. This is Immanuel

Kant's universal law, where a *principle* is a *maxim* if it is based on someone's desires or a *law* if it applies universally. Pure reason is unconditional; that is, it does not depend on something else. This applies to the sciences and experimentation, where the purpose is to predict and control outcomes.

The problem in the HRO setting is that most things are conditional, because they depend on something else. Events in our environment result from processes. Therefore, the unconditional *pure reason* is of little benefit to the HRO and of little use in the VUCA-T environment.

Practical reasoning is a distinctive standpoint that depends on the person and the situation. This type of reasoning seeks the best alternative for action before any action is taken. We can expect reflection to place value on actions. Time compression limits, if not prevents, any reflective thought. The threat response interferes with the valuation of information when people balance preservation through self-interest or collaboration. Cognitive function, as a linear and logical algorithm, is not only impaired in these situations but can become dangerous. Decisions and actions, whether we like it or not, are distinctly a first-person point of view. Even when decisions and actions are done collectively, people will influence one another, and we cannot predict or control whether the group will rise up or the performance will deteriorate.

Practical wisdom (phronesis), Aristotle's intellectual virtue, aims to make good choices. Unfortunately, the inability to predict masks the results of any choice until after the action is taken. Aristotle considered this a virtue, the first of his four cardinal virtues, because one must think of the greater good. This is the ability to perceive what is required for the greater good in terms of feeling, choice, and action *in particular situations.*

Practical wisdom involves general knowledge, particular knowledge, the ability to reason toward a choice, and the ability to act on that choice. The person must place value on information and actions specific to the situation and the specific time. With uncertainty, we must choose value. With ambiguity, we must give meaning. With equivocality, we must choose action.

We do not know the truth. With experience, we can attain practical wisdom. In theoretical rationality, we regulate our beliefs and cognitive states. In practical rationality, we regulate our intentions, plans, and actions.

Impairment of Cognitive Capabilities
Cognitive decision-making is rational, objective, and instrumental toward a goal. It uses cognitive and logically connected processes and is *independent of context.* We find that cognitive decision-making fails us when we encounter the unexpected

or we are faced with uncertainty, time compression, or threat. Uncertainty robs us of our scientific rationality. Time compression impinges on our bounded rationality. Threats impair cognitive function.

In these situations, we must assign value and meaning to information, our goals, and our actions. Classical logic has the law of the excluded middle, that either the proposition is true or its negation is true. There can be no partial truth. The scientific method relies on discrete measurement of entities. There can be no partial value. Yet the real world does have partial truths and partial measurement values. There are no excluded middles or discrete categories; characteristics will overlap or be continuous.

Unrecognized fear responses (anger, frustration, avoidance, confusion, or freezing up) not only affect people's performance; because these responses are either the witness to or focus of unrecognized fear responses, they also create performance deficits, thus significantly contributing to system failure. Learning to regulate emotion is critical: this is not complete blockage or the denial of emotion but the use of regulated emotion for the purpose of creating motivation and focus.

Cognitive-Affective Decision-Making

Our attitudes and values affect our decisions. From social psychology, we know that attitudes do not determine behaviors to the degree of our beliefs, but attitudes and values do *influence* behaviors. Bloom's taxonomy of learning includes attitudes in the affective domain (as compared to the cognitive domain, with measurable principles, concepts, and facts). Values are deeper, long-standing beliefs we hold. We also evaluate the value of local information; we decide whether to use it to make decisions and we permit local information to change our operations. Finally, HROs evolved in live-or-die environments, and the structure continues to be used in dangerous circumstances.

Translating this model to safer work environments has posed a problem: how to transfer, or translate, the ability to think clearly in the face of immediate threat. We must condition people for this type of thinking, but not by Pavlovian conditioning. (This has been tried in some venues—scare or stress people so they know how to work under these circumstances—but this strategy often fails.) We also may not have the control of the operant response (i.e., how the employee responds) for use in operant conditioning.

A different type of conditioning seems to take hold when we act in the face of threats. People like organization and clarity of cognitive decision-making (biases, heuristics, and the rest), and they take pride in critical thinking, which uses linear and logical thinking, avoids fallacies, and insists that hypotheses are drawn from the facts. In live-or-die situations, threats impair cognitive processes, and we begin to use the affective domain for the valuation of information and action.

These strategies do not work (we repeat—they do not work) when (1) we do not have information; (2) facts do not help us; (3) we unconsciously rely on attitudes to guide us; (4) our values are what motivate us; (5) we must place value (valence, either positive or negative) and degree of value on the information we do have; and (6) we must generate information in real time (Bea's interactive and real-time risk assessment and management) and use our brains, even when stress or fear have hijacked the brain and its higher levels of thinking. What to do?

Separate academic work has been conducted on affective (emotional) decision-making. As stated earlier, we use affect as (1) attitudes and values, (2) to place value on information, and (3) to regulate emotion (or to modulate the threat/survival response). The purpose of emotion is to facilitate adaptive behavior and decision-making in response to salient events. As such, emotion is vital to survival. Emotional expressions play a powerful communicative role, for we convey emotional states to others via the stereotypical posturing of facial features. Emotional expressions are thus a key component of social interactions, since they indicate the likely future behavior of the displaying animal's communicated intentions and desires and they influence others' emotional states (Leopold and Rhodes 2010; Andrew 1963; Davidson et al. 2007).

HRO is not taught; it is learned. This simple, though important, point explains the failure of many organizations to adopt HRO. HRO consists of attitudes—rather than being "preoccupied with failure," consider asking, "What is your attitude toward failure?"—and attitudes are learned, not taught. Attitudes are in Bloom's affective domain of knowledge, a domain of attitudes and practicality: "How will this help?" As Patricia Benner observed in the nursing field, competency, part of the cognitive domain, becomes institutionalized because the generalizable principles can be standardized for a novice workforce. Learning the particular to develop proficiency through the use of specifics and case reports demands more time, training, shared insight, and modeling of senior, more experienced people. It also means that leaders internalize the attitudes they desire in their subordinates.

Rationality is less about being free from error than about not making mistakes that one could avoid by exercising one's cognitive capacities well; thus, evaluations of rationality must be sensitive to the limits of the cognitive powers of any subjects who are evaluated as well as the features of their external circumstances that affect their ability to exercise these cognitive powers to the fullest.

Attitudes are modeled. The public safety field and the military both select for attitudes and internalize them in recruit training; they rely on modeling the attitudes and behaviors by the drill instructor and in training with negative punishment, where punishments are removed as recruits use desired behaviors or demonstrate desired attitudes. In the civilian world, we must take all attitudes, but we cannot realistically do this: as Thomas Mercer (RAdm, USN, retired) has observed, the civilian world considers this brainwashing. We must comment that *you do not learn to work under stress by being placed under stress.* This common misconception in the healthcare field comes from people who believe that the military uses this approach. (When asked, people often say they have not been in the military but saw this idea in the movies.)

On the other hand, when the system has failed, rigorous adherence to processes will limit the fluid responsiveness necessary to bring control to the situation. For our purposes, we will call this dichotomy *control operator* verses *emergency responder.*

People want their problems solved; administrators do not want confusion; executives do not want disruption but instead ask if something will solve their problems. HRO is not a solution, or means to solve, a specific problem; it is a way/means of resolving a situation or event, not a path to a solution or a guarantee of good results. Executives and administrators will look for HRO in structure; HRO is what they "purchase." What you have others do does not matter; what matters is what you do. HRO represents relationships and interactions across the hierarchy. HRO is a verb, not a noun. HRO is attitudes and behaviors, not a script or structure. It is about information flow and authority migration in unstructured situations in order to remain steady during dynamic situations.

Conclusions

(1). HRO utilizes the affective domain of attitudes and values, the evaluation of information, and the regulation of emotion.
(2). The five principles of HRO can be understood as attitudes that *influence* behavior and are learned through modeling the behavior of senior people.
(3). Fear, often unrecognized, impairs cognition and performance.
(4). Risk management, a well-defined discipline, has limitations because of the human fear response and the uncertainty and ambiguity of threats.
(5). "Cognitive-affective decision-making" best describes how people think and perform in an HRO.

CHAPTER 6

THE BOYD OODA LOOP

Most often, the first people to encounter or engage crises are also the lowest-ranked and least experienced people. These are the line staff who are the first to come upon or enter the VUCA-T environment. The models that senior and more experienced people understand may not make sense to someone who is new to the industry, organization, or situation. The OODA loop of Col. John Boyd (USAF) can serve both the novice with the least experience and the veteran expert (see figure 4).

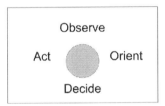

Figure 4—Boyd's OODA loop

The OODA loop is a cycle for rapid, real-time interactive hypothesis development and testing. To create the loop, the person **o**bserves, **o**rients, **d**ecides, and **a**cts, then observes the effect of the action. The action creates the loop for a continuous cycle and gives the OODA loop its power and agility. The importance of OODA cycling is how the response to actions drives the system; we must then understand the meaning of the responses to our actions: for example, the patient improves, is unchanged, or deteriorates.

Note in our figure that we do not identify the starting point and have not placed arrows showing the direction of flow. Weick observed that "one can start this sequence anywhere and move either in a clockwise or counterclockwise direction" (personal communication). Our starting point may be by choice or may be when we become aware we are looping. The iterations, once started, do not end until the end-state is reached.

Weick has described the utility of Boyd's OODA loop (in either sensemaking or enactment) by starting at A, the act phase (personal communication). Acting is the first step in engagement and is the active part of Weick's sensemaking; acting is also the initiator of Weick's enactment, and acting can create failure that is both visible and correctable through the looping. The latter is critical in HRO to oppose failure from *not* acting, which is invisible, not detectable, and not correctable.

We think by acting (Weick 1988), that is, we make sense of the situation by acting (Weick et al. 2005) and gaining information, both positive and negative, and we enact change in the environment by acting (Weick et al. 2005). Acting is affected by immediate past sensemaking, guiding the next decision-through-acting. In a novel situation, whether novice or veteran, we must create structure for sensemaking, but context affects information, time compression affects acting, and threat affects thinking. The OODA Loop and its bias for action assists us in surmounting these problems.

The Novice

The novice makes a slower, more deliberate loop, often getting bogged down in the first "orientation" function and then again in the "decision" function. Speed comes from becoming smooth rather than from thinking faster. Smooth cycling comes from experience, which is the background for our statement that "what you do in an emergency is what you do every day."

Because of lack of experience and training, civilians do not readily engage unwanted or unexpected events in an effective or meaningful way, particularly in circumstances with compressed time. When faced with uncertainty or threat, civilian novices typically rely on algorithmic protocols, consult with (putative) experts, or withdraw from engagement when their independent actions could have prevented calamity. This failure to engage is significant in working environments where early rapid decisions and actions can prevent cascading failure. (The working environment is the place where people engage the organization's external environment, either at the executive or operational level.) More commonly, civilians will fail to act, thereby following the healthcare dictum from Hippocrates, "First, do no harm," which often translates as "Do nothing."

Novices, Fear of Decision-Making, and the Boyd OODA Loop

When working with pediatric resident physicians, nurses, and respiratory care practitioners in a pediatric intensive care unit, I have learned that the use of John Boyd's OODA loop can help these people overcome their fear of causing more harm than good in these situations. They learn the use of the OODA loop by beginning the discussion with the harm that would result if they did nothing and how the OODA loop gives them the ability to (1) sense events through short feedback loops, (2) better read situations, and (3) gain the agility to act effectively and meaningfully. This learning builds a decision frame within which they can use the OODA loop to navigate toward resolution of the problem or control of the situation when protocols cannot help.

We first discuss time scales by asking the questions, "What if we do nothing?" or "What if we wait too long?" They not only describe the consequences of delayed action but also develop the sequence of events that would lead to failure, which creates the attention set for these early heralds. They now have the ability to place themselves along this timeline with some concept of the acceleration of events and the dynamics that can be created. We then discuss the consequences of acting too soon, improperly called "crying wolf." They come to view acting too soon as being relatively benign compared to delaying their actions.

Then we discuss the amount of intervention to undertake; for this discussion we often use medication dosages. They can use too little or too much of a given drug. An overdose causes well-identified findings, but in a seriously ill patient, a smaller dosage of drugs may cause an overdose, the overdose may have different signs, or the patient may require more than expected amounts of the medication. We discuss what this situation looks like and what to do as we near the adverse response. Administering too small a dosage of the medication is clearly unwanted and nearly obvious, but is dangerous as it can falsely reassure the team.

They now have a decision framework of "too soon, too late, too much, and too little," which provides boundaries or limits for decision-making. This pre-event decision framework becomes part of the "orient" function of the loop, which permits more rapid responses to early heralds or changes based on observing the results of their actions. Within this decision framework, they are safe to decide and act, and I can support them. But because this situation then develops a framework that does not have any protocol or outside guidance, they must now rely on their judgment.

The above discussion requires descriptions of interventions and responses. These are not developed as prescriptive actions but as criteria of when to act and the expected responses to people's actions. All actions are described with possible responses of whether it "worked, did not work, or had no effect." Any unwanted or unexpected result is understood as being new and important information; that is, successful decisions bring control, and unsuccessful decisions generate new information (this would be information we did not have before). There is no failure in the conventional sense. The most difficult response to interpret is "no change," as this could refer to the wrong diagnosis, the wrong treatment, or the wrong amount of treatment.

Having the knowledge of what it means not to act gives people confidence to intervene and to use greater effort when situations deteriorate. The OODA loop's focus on response to actions (therapy in this case) supports people in acting more quickly and forcefully. The only other part we need to discuss is the question, "Is this reversible?" Nonreversible interventions are more serious and take greater thought before acting, although that is part of the decision framework they freely work within.

This decision-making framework, with the use of Boyd's OODA loop within the framework, has enabled pediatric resident physicians to competently and confidently engage unexpected and unwanted events, which has reduced the number and severity of resuscitations at the hospital, lowered medical costs, and increased patient safety.

—Daved van Stralen

Novice to Expert: Observe, Orient, Decide, and Act

If there is one focus where fears, threats, problems, hazards, education, training, mentoring, blaming, leading, and following converge, it is the decision. The decision has become the motivation to find organizational design methods to reduce risk and bring structure and predictably to healthcare and numerous other high-risk industries. Executives and managers strive to centralize decision-making removed from subordinates. The decision is a source of blame and is often believed to be the cause of the errors that endanger patients.

Rather than teaching decision-making methods, we rely on lists, protocols, algorithms, decision-trees, and the phone. (When asked what paramedics should do upon encountering novel, difficult situations, numerous physicians have answered, "Call me.") The maxim "First, do no harm" has killed initiative, engagement, and decision-making in countless healthcare professionals and avoids the follow-up question, "What if doing nothing is harmful?"

Fear of deciding and acting becomes institutionalized as organizational knowledge, which Weick described within enactment as failure by not acting, which is undetectable. Not acting creates an organizational knowledge that no one will question, thus preserving inaction over generations. Novices observe the fear of deciding that veterans and their superiors model. We learn, and inadvertently teach, that *not* to decide is a good choice.

John Boyd's OODA loop is an effective approach to teach decision-making to the novice. Decision-making seems intuitively to be a linear process—you collect information, decide, then move on to the next decision to make. If necessary, we can use rational thought and our cognitive abilities to make the difficult decisions. This deterministic model—the information determines the decision, and the decision determines success—fails when decisions must be made with imperfect information, the desired outcome is not clear, and threats impair cognition. An adaptive approach is to use short feedback loops as probes and information generators. This is the OODA loop developed by John Boyd, as shown in figure 4 at the beginning of this chapter.

Of the numerous high-risk industries, healthcare may stand alone as one where centralized decision-making increases as the risk increases. The dictum "First, do no harm" contributes to inaction in critical, time-dependent moments. We have found that using a simple loop decision-making approach can meet the concerns of those who resist authority migration and will increase safety for any decisions that inexperienced people make. It is also the simplest and most effective means of implementing HRO into an organization, since it builds trust within people and between those at various levels of the hierarchy. Decisions and actions develop from the individual's duty within the profession and scope of professional practice. The beauty of loop decision-making comes from its self-correcting nature and the ability to take action in increasingly small increments.

John Boyd and the OODA Loop

In 1968, John Boyd presented his concept of the OODA loop during the Vietnam War for fighter pilots to outmaneuver their opponents (Thompson 1995; Hammond 2001; Coram 2002). He developed this approach after studying air-to-air combat in the Korean conflict to better understand why American pilots in the Korean conflict flying the F-86, a plane inferior to the MiG-15, had better kill ratios than American pilots in the Vietnam War flying in planes superior to the MiG. He found the difference to be the American pilots' better ability to see out of the cockpit and their ability to much more quickly switch from one activity to another. This ability to outmaneuver also contributed significantly to the success of the major tank battles in World War II.

Boyd used the concepts of the OODA loop and maneuver warfare (made possible by OODA cycles), along with several more of his concepts, to create the F-16 (Hammond 2001, 94–98). Despite this use of the OODA loop, the US Air Force did not embrace the concept for formal teaching. The US Marine Corps, however, formally incorporated the OODA loop and the derivative concept of maneuver warfare into its doctrine (Hammond 2001; Coram 2002).

Since both pilots in a dogfight are engaged in continuous OODA cycles, the objective in air combat is to "getting inside an adversary's OODA loops," to outmaneuver another person's thinking, and to disrupt his view of the world (Fallows 1981, 29). In other words, you should maneuver so rapidly that your opponent begins to respond to your actions or becomes confused rather than responding to the situation and understanding events as they unfold. This causes confusion in the opponent, thus leading to over- and under-reaction, followed by loss of situational awareness. Pilots could then act with agility and force rather than using analysis of the situation (Orr 1983, 35–6).

We use the OODA loop in healthcare as a method to outmaneuver a rapidly changing disease state (McConnell and van Stralen 1997). We cannot "get inside the OODA loop" of diseases and inanimate situations, however, because they do not think or have strategies and tactics. This is not trivial, as one of the goals of the OODA loop is to "get into the head" of your opponent while, for us, we are attempting to predict and influence the trajectory of the system through interaction with the system. In addition, we have attended leadership and decision-making lectures where we learned the importance of intimidating your opponent. While this works against human enemies, it does not apply to inanimate "opponents" or the people we are working alongside.

We have found that Boyd's OODA loop gives the greatest agility for rapidly evolving events; far more important, however, is that it is quite easy for the novice to learn and apply. The concept is intuitive. The cycling creates a self-correcting process and aids in information flow by describing information in terms of action-response. Table 6 describes each element; two of the more difficult concepts are the "orient" function and looping back from the "act" function to the "observe" function.

Function	Description
Observe	Observe the situation; after the "act" function, the "observe" function also matches what we predicted with what actually happened; this is not necessarily an in-depth evaluation.
Orient	Process and synthesis of observations using culture, experience, and physiology; a real-world function and does *not* simply orient to the situation.
Decide	Develop the hypothesis to test; decide on a course of action.
Act	Take the action and test the hypothesis; this is the interface between the decision-maker and the environment.
Loop	Note the effect of the action in the "observe" function.

Table 6—OODA loop element functions

The *observe* function is an *attention* function, in which we look for discrepancies, disruptions, and outliers. Initially, these bring us to our initial action and do not require that we have a full analysis of the situation; we will gain knowledge of the situation as we act. We process information by analysis within the *context of the situation*, recognizing that HRO is a high-context system with the environment containing, modifying, and giving meaning to information. The observe function also notices the responses to our just-completed action and whether we received the results we expected. The system can improve, in which case we may continue; the system may deteriorate, in which case our actions generated new information about its structure; or the system may not change. This last option is dangerous, because we might have the wrong dosage, the wrong drug, or the wrong diagnosis.

The *orient* function is probably more confusing to those who are first using the OODA loop, since they may consider this to be orientation to the circumstances. The orientation function is much richer than that, since it includes national, regional, and organizational cultural traditions; genetic heritage; new and updated information; previous experience; and analysis and synthesis from feedback, guidance, and control. In this function we synthesize new information and build support for our decisions; we incorporate our previous experience to guide our decisions and actions as well as our interpretation of events.

As we build experience, we increase our boundaries of safe and effective performance, thereby creating a larger operational envelope. We also build a new and larger repertoire of actions, make use of constrained improvisation (Weick 1998), and exercise "freedom with discipline" (Chesley "Sully" Sullenberger, personal communication).

It is important to note that physiological and psychological influences such as fatigue, dehydration, stress, and fear also impair cognition. These influences exist on a spectrum from "barely perceptible" to "debilitating to self or others." Because judgment is the most sensitive indicator in this case, others will likely notice any incremental changes before the individual can. In high-altitude or cold-weather operations, the first sign of hypothermia or hypoxia (oxygen deficiency, here it would be in brain tissue) is the loss of judgment that fellow operators notice. For this reason, these operators have a duty to watch one another's judgment for subtle decrements that might indicate the onset of hypothermia or hypoxia. This is a model worth emulating in HRO operations.

For HROs, the contribution (or effect) of cultural tradition, either from national or local culture or the organization's culture, is an important consideration. The values and attitudes of a culture are modeled by leaders and internalized by members of the organization. Cultural tradition is more than "walking the walk and talking the talk." It is how one lives in the quiet times when people watch and learn; it is embodied into one's character and beliefs and revealed through behaviors. A final important aspect to mention is one's physiological state. We cannot clearly identify the effects of even mild dehydration or hunger on our own thought processes.

The affective domain of emotion, values, attitudes, and personal evaluation also influence the *decide* function, which is the determination people make for what action to carry out, including what they will do and how they will do it.

The *act* function is the last function; this initiates the *loop action*, which acts in the manner of a control mechanism operating on the environment while changing people's perceptions of the environment. Using the loop action is a method to explore the situation while exploiting any path of least resistance. When we encounter friction as part of the feedback, we can observe whether we should pursue another path that has less friction or identify the friction point as something significant that should remain in focus (Orr 1983, 46). The use of positive feedback through the loop action directs focus and actions toward paths of success, while the use of negative feedback marks practical and safety boundaries that can act as a safety function.

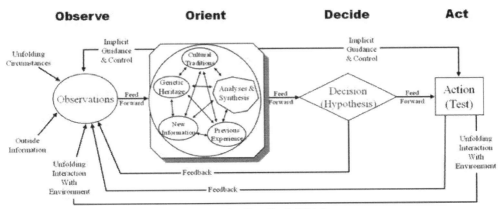

Observe   **Orient**   **Decide**   **Act**

Figure 5—John Boyd's OODA loop

We can think of the OODA loop as the series of capital Os that we were required to write when we were learning cursive, as shown in figure 5. Each finishing loop moves us forward, but only after we have passed through the stages of where we started, where we are now, and where we will be. Each loop back allows us to better ascertain the impact of our actions and contributes substantially to the situational awareness that is imperative for optimal decision-making. There is no border between elements in OODA cycling: everything you do, even your very presence, changes something.

Utility of the OODA Loop

The OODA loop allows for the decentralization of decision-making because of the small increments possible in the decision-action portion. In this way, we find it useful for novices and for more experienced practitioners in novel situations. More significantly, using the OODA loop allows the decision to be made by those who are immersed in the problem, where change is occurring in real time. Information is generated as we learn what works through action while also bringing control to the situation. If necessary, we can probe the structure of a situation to find out where it responds and where it is resistant.

The small steps from OODA cycling contribute to the sensitivity of perception for identifying small, incremental changes. It is this sensitivity to change and resistance that makes OODA cycling an ideal approach for high-risk operations. The OODA loop explains how we evaluate our responses to actions and then compare the results to what we expected; the system is self-correcting and can mitigate confirmation bias and overcome motivated reasoning.

For information and communication purposes, the actions that we take as a result of the OODA loop process through the loop's multiple iterations will create information from uncertainty, give meaning to ambiguity, and increase objective communication. Information, in Shannon's information entropy theory, is uncertainty, because if you know something for certain, then it is not information. Information is learning something. The OODA loop guides interpretation by determining if you have obtained the expected response or if the system is going in a completely unexpected direction. The OODA loop's stimulus-response will convert uncertainty to greater certainty. In the same way, it also gives meaning to ambiguous information. We can also communicate information through the structure of the OODA loop. Rather than saying what you think is happening or stating what you would like to do, you can instead report stimulus-response as action and the response to the action. This contributes to better-quality sensemaking.

By acting, we can probe for remnants of structure or identify hidden structures in what would otherwise appear to be an unstructured system. By moving in a positive direction, we gain control as we learn the system. The OODA loop process, in effect, solves the problem at the same time we are learning what the problem is. The agility of the OODA loop allows us to rapidly change ourselves as circumstances change and helps us adjust the structure of our system in response to a deforming force in the environment. We can exploit opportunities that we could not have planned for. As we learn what works, we then create a new repertoire of skills. OODA cycling decompresses time and inserts operations into chaos. Table 7 shows the benefits of the OODA loop.

Loop portion	Benefit
Observe	Discrepancy, interruption, or outlier
Orient	When rules compete, conflict, or do not apply Decentralization through the ability to integrate other OODA loops Decision migration to those with less experience
Decide	Reduces need for excessive information
Act	Inexperienced individual Novel technique or situation "Black swan event"
Loop	Continuous interaction with the real world Testing your possible worlds

Table 7—Benefits of the OODA loop

OODA Dimensions

Boyd's OODA loop has applications on a number of levels. The first level is one of personal activity, which we can refer to as *OODA in the arena*. The second level, that of looking back at actions we have taken, is more analytical: *OODA analysis.*

OODA in the Arena

The classic example of OODA in the arena is two pilots (one versus one) engaged in aerial combat, as Boyd described it. A simpler aviation example is a single aircraft landing in a gusty crosswind; a parallel example is bicycling along a rock-strewn mountain trail. In either instance, the vehicle must remain under control while navigating constantly changing paths. With every change in the wind (or bump in the trail), the aircraft/ bicycle reacts, the pilot/rider *observes* the change, *orients* to the new situation, *decides* which controls are needed to maintain the desired course, and *acts* to input those controls. This immediately changes the path of the airplane/bike, which produces a new situation requiring another correction—and another OODA loop starts. With each loop taking less than a second and repeating without pause, the person rapidly adjusts the system (plane or bicycle) until the task (landing) is complete. OODA in the arena is a continuous, cycling action. To maintain control of the situation requires full, constant attention.

More complex situations such as tank warfare, mass aerial combat, or triage in a mass-casualty incident benefit from the application of OODA loop actions. Increased numbers of participants and complex situations are greater challenges to individual actors. Observation now includes the OODA loops of nearby participants and OODA loops in various stages due to the local situations or microenvironments. In this stage:

- The *observe* function becomes limited to a finite number of activities, because the number of total activities possible readily exceeds the person's capacity to observe before another action is necessary. When you're going five hundred miles per hour, sometimes you need to do something, *even if it's wrong.* (This phrase was common at the USAF Fighter Weapons School during the 1970s and 1980s, where one of the goals of flight mission debriefings was to discuss "five hundred mph" decisions and how such decisions could contribute to the success or failure of a mission. Actions taken during dynamic, high-stress situations are often based on gut feelings but may be decisive to the success or failure of an undertaking. Many situations require decision-making and action with incomplete information and no time for analysis; that is, there are times when you absolutely must "do something.")

- The *orient* function is constrained to the small part of the overall activity that the person is capable of processing before the next necessary *decision* and *action* functions.
- The *decision* and *action* elements may have just started (and their effect is not assured) by the time the next loop is underway.

OODA Analysis

The time sensitivity and urgency (time compression) of a particular situation limit analysis, which establishes the demand for OODA loop activity. This does not, however, mean that we cannot later analyze a dynamic situation or that we cannot use the OODA process in low-tempo situations.

Boyd's OODA loop can be a valuable tool when analyzing actions that were performed in a time-constrained or crisis situation. These are debriefing or similar analyses, and they become learning situations. The OODA loop model can take the actors back through the crisis situation with a series of questions:

(1).   What did you see or sense? (Observe)
(2).   What were you thinking? What struck you as being most critical at this point? (Orient)
(3).   What did you do and why? (Decide)
(4).   Were you able to execute the way you wanted to? (Act)
(5).   What changed as a result of your action (and, therefore, started a new loop)"
(6).   Return to #1 above.

We must ask, "Did it work every time, only in particular situations, or as a one-off"? Analysis is possible in less urgent situations—those that allow time to consider options without the need for immediate action. In these stable states, the *orient* function increases in importance and becomes a richer source for evaluation.

Culture (national, ethnic, and organizational) has a great influence on orientation in dynamic situations and, in effect, becomes a fixed state. During analysis, we can evaluate the effect of culture on decisions and actions and whether cultural elements support or hinder action (see chapter 14, "Culture").

The results of participants' actions, and their OODA loops, is an easily missed element of the *orientation* function and are commonly absent from analysis. Though an important aspect of interactive group response, this information is fleeting and may not be remembered later. The language of the OODA loop (*action-response*) is one way of capturing this transient experience. Through the *orient* function, the OODA process in a stable situation becomes more like Deming's "plan, do, check, act" model. (Deming 2000) A less urgent situation—one that allows time to consider options without immediate action—more appropriately fits the Deming model.

It is important to note that the use of OODA as an analytical tool is probably more important in assessing crisis situations that have favorable outcomes than those that result in failure. The limits of perception during the event prevent us from knowing the reason for a failure. We do want to publish and promote successful actions and processes to our respective communities; unfortunately, the norm seems to be to focus on events that have resulted in failure.

—Thomas Sokol, Colonel, US Air Force (retired)
Fighter Pilot and Instructor Pilot, Vietnam Veteran

Applied OODA Loops

Learn What Works through Action

The VUCA-T environment, by definition, is not amenable to design or protocols. Even the act of gathering information requires engagement without knowing what information is available, and possibly what information is necessary. We probe for responsiveness and generate information as we act; this reduces the effect of confirmation bias, because the person searches for what will actually achieve a response rather than what will fit the hypothesis. This reduces the effect of motivated reasoning, as people revise their beliefs while engaged in real time.

I entered the patient room in response to an emergency call in the long-term care facility. An infant, dependent on a mechanical ventilator, was in acute respiratory distress. As I walked in, Janet Nichols, the respiratory care practitioner (RCP), was telling the nurse to give the infant a suppository to initiate a bowel movement.

Janet explained that this infant's increased abdominal pressure for bowel movements broke the patient-ventilator synchrony, which caused dangerous acute respiratory distress. Through iterations of the OODA loop, in which she moved toward a calm child by-hand ventilation, she had found that the RCP could calm the infant and facilitate the bowel movement by increasing the "back pressure" in the lungs using positive end-expiratory pressure, or PEEP.

We added this back pressure, or PEEP, to the ventilator settings and had no further bowel-related ventilator crises. Since that time, we have used PEEP for other infants with this problem, previously unidentified in the long-term infant mechanical ventilation literature. The condition is likely caused by the "Valsalva maneuver" for a bowel movement directing abdominal pressure against a weakened diaphragm, thus restraining chest expansion from the ventilator. Calling this procedure "PEEP for poop" has made it easy to teach RCPs and nurses and has made this an important part of patient evaluation during similar crises.

—Daved van Stralen

Titration of Therapy

The use of a linear protocol or algorithm to titrate therapy is more cumbersome and complex than the use of an OODA loop. A linear program risks excessively bulky growth in length if the response is indeterminate, if the amount of titrant is uncertain, or if demands are expected to change after equilibrium is reached. Fluid resuscitation of an infant or child when a physician is not present is one such situation. The amount of fluid necessary to resuscitate a child is not known when the resuscitation starts, adrenaline from pain can mimic the signs of low blood volume, and nonpediatric physicians worry about the volumes used for children. (In a three-year-old child weighing fifteen kg, the initial fluid bolus would be 300 mL of normal saline; in the experience of many physicians, this amount in a frail, elderly woman might cause pulmonary edema.)

Paramedics in the EMS system must follow protocols. The local system wrote a protocol for a 10 mL/kg fluid bolus as indicated by heart rate over two hundred beats per minute and a limb-temperature margin felt on the leg. Vasoconstriction in children is quite sharp, with the margin felt as a band 2 cm wide. The vasoconstriction moves down the leg as blood volume is restored. The pulse is felt in the foot (the dorsalis pedis or posterior tibial): a bounding pulse, or even one that can be palpated (since this is a difficult area in infants), is generally accompanied by warm extremities due to sepsis. Unfelt and prolonged capillary refill, along with the presence of a limb-temperature margin, generally signifies low blood volume. Both conditions are treated with fluids. Liver edge is also felt, because in children, the right ventricle fails before the left ventricle does. (Prolonged capillary refill with a completely cool limb or a temperature gradient along the length of the limb suggests hypothermia, a high risk in infants who are lying unclothed in an air-conditioned room, van Stralen and Kissel 2016.)

The OODA loop is used to guide the administration of the fluid bolus. If the child's heart rate remains high, then the bolus is continued. As the limb temperature warms to the ankle, the paramedic can slow or stop administration. If the liver edge becomes palpable in the abdomen, then fluid administration should also be stopped.

—Daved van Stralen

The drive for protocols written for a specified dose often competes with the logic of the OODA loop when titrating toward a desired response.

A state EMS committee once wrote recommended protocols for paramedics. When it came to administration of a continuous infusion of dopamine, a cardiovascular drug, the experts chose a specific concentration, with several specified rates to reach the desired dosage. Several difficulties lie in the accuracy of weights and the inability to control the rate of infusion. In addition, the committee relied on specified rates as an end-point rather than an outcome measure such as limb perfusion, heart rate, or blood pressure.

The committee was offered another choice: epinephrine, available in a syringe; give half the dose, observe for a response, then continue with a half dose administered when the blood pressure drops. Because no research had been conducted to support this approach, the committee went with the use of dopamine administered at an unknown rate using an inaccurate weight estimate for the child.

—Daved van Stralen

Safety

Negative feedback from actions taken in the OODA loop cycle marks the boundaries of the envelope that someone can safely operate within. On a larger scale, these probes also signal boundaries for system safety and, when developed during interactions with the system, act as an early herald of failure.

The benefit of this approach occurs when the unexpected happens to trigger an event or occurs during actions taken during an event. While we cannot plan for every response or outcome, we can state what we expect to see and ask other participants to be observant for unexpected responses.

Response to Discrepancy, Disruptions, or Outliers

When unwanted or unexpected events occur, some people interpret them as random outliers, far from the routine or expected, or resulting from the convergence of independent, random events, if not independent, random events themselves. Seen this way, such events are unlikely to happen again, so we do not need to make preparations for similar events.

Others see these events as precursors or antecedent events—that is, they are early heralds of a series of cascading events that will lead to catastrophic failure. Viewed this way, it is important to engage the situation while in this covert, compensated state, when interventions are more effective and have fewer complications. When we do not differentiate these events, we risk wasting resources chasing random occurrences, or we miss windows to prevent catastrophes.

The OODA loop describes our interactions with the environment in which we also evaluate the environment's responses to our actions. From this idea we gain a sense of the responsiveness of the environment to our actions. That is, if our actions cause a rapid or large change, then the environment is responsive, while if it resists change, then we should accelerate our OODA loop iterations. We must make a different interpretation if there is no effect from our actions. At some point, we may sense that this failure to respond (combined with the event remaining unaffected or self-resolved) represents a disconnection between our actions and the event. This situation creates clues about whether an event is an independent, random outlier or an antecedent precursor of cascading events.

The field of statistics (the mathematical science of probability—the likelihood of an occurrence—and random, independent events) describes outliers as an observation that is far outside the expected range of measured values in a system. It is far enough out that it lies outside the range of statistical probability. A large number of *independent*, random measured values will produce a Gaussian, or normal, distribution—what is known as the "normal curve." Distance from the average is measured in standard deviations, signified by the Greek letter sigma (as in Six Sigma, the program to achieve error reduction of greater than six standard deviations). Because the normal curve measures independent events, any outlier is independent of preceding or antecedent events and is by definition not predictive of further events. This is cause for the argument that "association does not mean causation."

The Pareto principle essentially describes a system in which, in a series of events, 80 percent of the effects come from 20 percent of the causes. This is a form of power law, where the frequency of some event varies by the power of an attribute of that event. An inverse power law mathematically is a straight line on a log-log plot, representing increasing strength with decreasing frequency. That is, the strongest person in a room is likely a man, as men are generally stronger than women. Among men, the strongest man will have a specific build, so looking for the strongest man among those with a specific build will be more fruitful than looking in a group containing emaciated or obese men. Each observation of the shrinking group increases the chances of finding the strongest man. In another example, to be a moderate city, a city must have started as a small city, and large cities come from moderate-size cities. As a specific attribute becomes more "concentrated," the attribute is found in fewer events because it is built from previous events. In a system described by an inverse power law, events can be antecedent if they develop into larger events. Not all will, but some do.

Comparing the two systems—independent random events described by statistics and precursor antecedent events developing into a larger event—would be like asking the probability of you being the tallest in the room versus there being a tallest person in the room. Another way to see this is that there will be a worst event for the year for your organization: a 100 percent chance of a worst event. But the probability that it will be financial, physical, or social are probability measures between 0 and 1.

After an unwanted or unexpected event occurs, the OODA loop can help differentiate the precursor from the outlier by the behavior of the system—whether the event is influenced by your actions or if the event's responses are random. The difference determines the statistical measure we use, how we evaluate the event, and how we respond.

The Human Environment

We cannot predict how people will respond to a crisis, either people outside our response system or group or within our group. In these situations, if our team (or members of our team) begins to fail then the team becomes our environment.

This failure develops either because of unrecognized fear responses or the instrumental use of fear or threat by someone (see chapter 9, "Threat Responses and Unrecognized Fear"). This failure may also be failure to respond to signs or signals that are undetectable for some reason.

You can use the OODA loop to identify responsiveness in individuals. Your stimulus helps you sort out those who have lost significant cognition from stress, are resistant or oppositional, or have identified new information that drives their action. In the cases of unrecognized fear (the situational cognitive distortions discussed below), people may respond to reframing or identification of new objectives. New information that has created new OODA cycles can be readily incorporated into concurrent OODA cycles.

Purposely disruptive behavior is more difficult. During a crisis, it may be more important to isolate or marginalize the individual in some way. The OODA loop, in this situation, assists in outmaneuvering the disruptor or interfering with the person's own OODA cycles.

> Our teachers watch for early signs of failure. They intervene through observe, orient, decide, act for what works for that student. In five years, the schools' number of suspension hours decreased from seven hundred to four hundred, and the graduation rate increased from 60 percent to 85 percent.
> —Dale Marsden, superintendent, San Bernardino City Unified School District (SBCUSD)

Situational Cognitive Distortions

The orient function of the OODA loop describes a number of influences on decision-making, including fatigue, dehydration, and hunger. The neurochemicals adrenaline and cortisol also influence decision-making in negative ways through interference with critical decision-making.

Critical thinking decision-making has become a desired attribute in those who must rely on judgment. In time-compressed circumstances created by uncertainty or threat, however, such decision-making may lose its effectiveness. Part of the problem is our disregard for the neurophysiology of threat and the cognitive effects of adrenaline and cortisol. It has become trite to say that the fear, or threat, responses are fight and flight—trite because we do not go past fight and flight, nor do we describe them in operational terms. Ask your subordinates what is going on when a superior in authority yells in anger during an emergency, and they will likely respond that they had probably performed inadequately. Ask them to name the fear responses, and they will answer "fight or flight." Ask them how fight is manifested, and they will likely respond with "as anger or yelling." Somehow, we do not put the two together—that the superior was in a fear or a threat response. Performing better will not necessarily make the superior less afraid or stop the superior's fear response.

The amygdala, an almond-shaped organ in the brain, processes perceptions to action with little influence from other parts of the brain. We act without thinking because that is how the brain is constructed—thinking during a live-or-die situation delays attack or escape actions. The amygdala also causes the release of adrenaline and cortisol, two neurochemicals that directly affect cognition and action. Adrenaline "cones" our attention (i.e., extreme focus with loss of attention outside the focus) and accelerates our thinking and movement. Cortisol blocks memory production and recall, freezes the neuromuscular system, and induces a form of passivity. The fear responses of fight, flight, and freeze are directed at self-protection and self-interest.

These neurochemicals distort our cognitive abilities and judgment in the same unrecognized way that hypothermia and environmental hypoxia affect judgment. Because we use our judgment to judge our judgment, we will not see loss of judgment in ourselves, only in others. That is why we watch our buddies in extreme environments and constantly evaluate their judgment. And that is why they listen when we point out their altered judgment.

In time-compressed states of uncertainty or threat, we have similar situations but generally do not necessarily watch our colleagues due to our own needs at the time, or we develop self-awareness of our own cognitive distortions. Because they occur in a tactical situation, we call them *tactical* (or *situational*) *cognitive distortions*: anger, frustration, plausible avoidance, distraction, withdrawal, and freeze.

> After reading James Loehr's book *Stress for Success*, I thought of a terrific example of modulating situational cognitive distortion by watching an accomplished basketball free-throw shooter. By controlling her breath, relaxing her major muscle groups, and focusing her vision on the front of the rim, she can actually reverse the impact in surges in adrenaline and cortisol, which can hijack her brain and body. The modulation allows her to relax and avoid the dreaded "brick" we see when someone is overcome by the stress of the critical shot.
> —Spence Byrum

While in some situations, it will be to our tactical advantage to induce cognitive distortions in our opponents, we will focus on the use of Boyd's OODA loop to develop individual adaptive decision-making. (Adaptive decision-making, or deciding what works, occurs in the anterior cingulate cortex, while binary decision-making, or deciding on right versus wrong, occurs in the prefrontal cortex.)

These distortions are neurochemical and do not reflect the competence of the person; the distortions can resolve themselves as quickly as they appeared. To demonstrate this, have someone recite the months of the year out loud. Then change the protocol to recite the months alphabetically. Few can name as many as six months. You have induced cortisol. (Keep this in mind during incident reconstructions, as cortisol released *during* the event will block memory production; people cannot recall memories they have not made.)

When a situational cognitive distortion occurs, go to an objective that is already reached or easy to perform when in concrete thinking. The use of Boyd's OODA loop takes people out of coned attention by forcing them to observe something simple. They make a decision that was, in effect, already made. They act to do something that will work, which helps move them out of muscle blocks (cortisol) or tension (adrenaline). These simple cycles reduce the effects of the neurochemicals and bring people back to the team.

Giving a concrete objective to people who are demonstrating tactical cognitive distortions with their use of the OODA loop helps move them toward effective participation with the team. When you are dealing with someone who is angry, asking the person *how* you can help forces their thoughts into the prefrontal cortex, as the request requires thinking. Asking "why" or "what" questions can produce a reflex, thus keeping the person in the anger mood.

Steep Authority Gradients

Healthcare has the problem of central authority residing in the physician, while local knowledge of the circumstances lies with the bedside caregiver. While this is not a significant problem for routine situations, it leads to poor medical care in dynamic, time-compressed states or with information that disconfirms the physician's beliefs. Bedside caregivers will commonly resolve this discrepancy by "adjusting" information to be congruent with the physician's views, withholding information that disconfirms the physician's beliefs, or withstanding personal attacks on their abilities. Other work-arounds take place, but none of them will result in the open and aggressive communication necessary for time-compressed and unwanted or unexpected events.

In these circumstances, the OODA loop is not presented in its entirety but as action and response. Presenting *only* one's observation (the observe function) relies on the credibility that the physician places in the caregiver, which is a problem with personal biases going both ways. Presenting *only* one's decision (the decide function) is also problematic, as the physician was trained to view decision-making as a lengthy process of weighing subjective observations, objective data, indications, and contraindications. Instead, by modifying the approach used by fire departments, the caregiver will describe the action taken (act function) and the response observed (looping to a new observe function). This brings focus to the disease process and interventions rather than personal biases and credibility.

> One effective alternative is a Boyd modification of what I learned as a rescue ambulance driver for the Los Angeles City Fire Department. We sometimes received orders from a superior that contradicted previous orders or our personal observations. When this happened, we were to state our orders *and* our observations, then abide by the verbal orders of the officer. John Boyd's OODA loop provides a more effective approach and also increases the responsiveness of medical caregivers to dynamic situations.
> —Daved van Stralen

"Action and response" is an objective way to communicate in uncertainty and high-tempo environments. Limiting this approach is the initiative of people who are blocked or confused about their authority to act. To overcome this problem, we delineate the "command" function; we borrow a military definition that command includes those duties you cannot legally delegate (Mercer, personal communication). For example, a respiratory care practitioner cannot legally delegate the duty of airway control, bag-mask ventilation, or respiratory failure response. That is, a physician or other authority figure cannot order the practitioner to *not* provide these interventions. Once these duties are delineated, practitioners exercise them as indicated but communicate information to their superiors and physicians as the act and observe (looped response) functions of the OODA loop.

> A second way the OODA loop improves communication is through the anticipation of events when suggesting therapies. Mark Rogers, a respiratory care practitioner, suggested to me that we use a helium-oxygen gas mixture to treat a child with severe asthma. We were preparing to use muscle paralytics and mechanical ventilation for treatment. Helium, as a treatment for asthma, had never been used in our medical center, though it was somewhat common as an asthma treatment before World War II. (It became unavailable for medical treatment when helium became a strategic war material for barrage balloons.)

He knew and routinely used the OODA loop and presented the information as the benefits we might observe. He then followed his suggestion with the observations that would demonstrate if the treatment had made the child's condition worse and the length of time he would treat the child before deciding the treatment would not work at all.

The child responded to therapy in a matter of minutes. After more experience, we published our use of helium-oxygen mixtures for asthma in a medical journal, and its use became routine in our medical center. We now teach caregivers to make their suggestions with this "anticipatory" OODA loop of action (the act function) and possible results (the observe function). This demonstrates that people understand how to identify if their therapy is making things worse and how to adjust treatment if it is helping.

—Daved van Stralen

The use of the act and observe loop functions to communicate in the presence of steep authority gradients encourages engagement, facilitates communication during events, and is an effective means of suggesting courses of actions.

When Rules Compete, Conflict, or Don't Apply

Principles, rules, and protocols create a discrete spectrum of actions one can take, yet environmental challenges occur over a continuous spectrum. To solve any dilemma of action, people have a tendency to fit the situation into a protocol and create what James Reason calls "the strong but wrong rule." To avoid this problem, we work with staff members to identify when the rule does *not* apply. Describing how the rule *did not* apply is far more difficult than it at first appears. We must know the indications and triggers for the rule, then document and describe their absence at that time. This creates a void between the rules, however. John Boyd's OODA loop provides guidance for action in this void between the rules.

During routine discussions, the team develops an objective for each problem (what could be considered "commander's intent"), then decomposes the objective to a series of smaller objectives that novices can more easily reach. We can then discuss actions they can take, develop multiple actions for each objective, and discuss how the decision to act is a criterion for action and not a demand to act in a specific way. All actions are described in terms of the responses we want or do not want, which makes it easier to discuss how to maneuver when a patient's pathology evolves while the patient's physiology is simultaneously responding to treatment.

Operationally, this teaches staff members to observe (perception versus collecting all available data), orient (acquiring support from superiors, learning what the strategy is, knowing what tactics to use, and determining what the response tells the person, among other things), decide (a decomposed objective), and act (in a reversible way). Observing the response to action generates new information, which then guides the next iteration and avoids taking the deterministic approach of algorithmic protocols.

Decomposing objectives in our discussions has two advantages: staff members learn the process and importance of decomposing objectives, and they learn how to amalgamate a sequence of objectives for smoother operations as they gain experience. During a resuscitation, for example, they will encounter events that do not respond to treatment. Rather than viewing this as a failure on their part to select the correct treatment (or that they have the wrong diagnosis), they learn to decompose the objective and try again. They now have a rapid way to learn the problem's structure and can determine if the failure is due to overreaching rather than having incorrect diagnoses or treatments.

People commonly believe that they will achieve speed and agility by increasing the rapidity in which they think, decide, and act. By decomposing the problem, they focus on circumstances and become more aware of how the situation unfolds. With experience, they spontaneously fold two actions together into one step. Within a short time, they have amalgamated a series of actions to one, thus increasing their speed and agility. Speed and agility come from becoming fluent and smooth in one's actions.

The civilian novice team now has a common objective for the team as a whole, which helps to develop shared sensemaking or situational awareness. They can also work the problem with their own decomposed objectives in a manner that will not interfere with others. The end result is a team that can move smoothly from individual circumstances to a common objective through cohesive team actions—all in a group of civilians who are not accustomed to such coordination.

One unintended benefit occurs when people encounter a convergent "helper" who joins the team and begins to use an algorithm or begins to take command. In one resuscitation I can recall, a senior resident physician began shouting orders that were inconsistent with the team's actions. Besh Barcega, the lead physician already in command (but junior to the interloper), would allow certain orders to pass through as long as they did not interfere with her objectives. Talking to the people later, the interloping physician believed he was in charge and that things had gone smoothly, while the nurses had followed the original resident physician in command.

—Daved van Stralen

Identifying when the rule does not apply avoids Reason's "strong but wrong rule," gives the team freedom to respond to the circumstances (thus pushing them to develop shared objectives that they can decompose), and directs them toward response to therapy as a guide to further actions. John Boyd's OODA loop replaces algorithms, increases responsiveness to situations, and brings the team to a common focus.

Other Decision-Cycle Systems

Boyd developed his OODA loop as a means for the fighter pilot to get inside the decision cycle of his adversary and outmaneuver his opponent. We have modified its purpose for agile responses in rapidly changing environments. The loop has other uses that we will discuss later in the chapter.

The structure of the OODA loop is similar to the PDCA cycle (plan, do, check, and act also called PDSA cycle for plan, do, study, and act) used by Deming for continuous quality improvement and learning. (This is also called the Shewhart Cycle developed by Deming's mentor, Walter A. Shewhart, for statistical analysis to follow improvements, Deming 2000.) The OODA loop differs, in that it is not a prospective plan and does not include long-term predictions of results. Rather than reducing the "do" function to multiple small steps to gain control, the OODA loop decomposes its loops to shorter and quicker complete loops, including the shortest possible time frame a human being can process information into action. Deming's "plan" or "planning" function requires prediction (Deming 2000). The "check" or "study" functions would take too long in a rapidly changing crisis. The "act" function, for Deming, is directed at standardizing or improving the process, while for Boyd the "act" function is directed toward creating change in the environment. Looping for Deming is a change in the program, an internal process that makes the organization better or more standardized. Looping, for Boyd, is an external process directed toward survival in a hostile environment. While two systems appear to be structurally similar, they are not interchangeable.

Boyd's looping design processes information as fast as neurologically possible to change a rapidly changing environment; Deming's looping design identifies and captures system deficiencies to improve the organization.

"We can reach Deming's plan-do-check-act through
the orient function of the OODA loop."
—Patricia E. Sokol, RN, JD
Analyst, health policy and point of care

These uses of cycles or the OODA loop will engineer new approaches but will not necessarily test hypotheses in real time.

Conclusions

(1). The VUCA-T environment interferes with protocols, algorithms, and open-tree decision-making methods.

(2). The Boyd OODA loop utilizes rapid, short feedback loop for decision-making that adapts to rapidly changing situations.

(3). The orient function, sometimes mistakenly considered orientation to the situation, is the most complex function, including culture, personal attributes, mental state, stress and fear, and the physiological condition of someone's body.

(4). The OODA loop finds utility to ensure safety, engages threats, identifies and responds to discrepancies and disruptions, and supports novices and beginners.

(5). Fear and threats can disrupt thinking and create situational cognitive distortions; the OODA loop assists people in navigating these situations.

(6). Steep authority gradients impede the flow of information, particularly with subordinates who are unsure of the situation; the OODA loop facilitates the flow of information upward, against the steep gradient.

(7). The OODA loop assists people in making decisions when rules compete or conflict.

CHAPTER 7

DECISION-MAKING IN HEALTHCARE

The engagement of any situation in the VUCA-T environment—volatile, uncertain, complex, ambiguous, and threatening—means that we make time-compressed decisions with limited or imperfect information. Threat too easily acts as a strongly negative stressor if we lack the ability to regulate our emotional state, thus impairing cognition and our cognitive functions. At worst, threat and fear reactions cause us to pursue self-preservation at the expense of the common good.

Conventional	Emergency
Biases	Situational cognitive distortions
Bounded rationality Practical rationality	Disrupted rationality
Uncertainty	Limited, imperfect information
Time-dependence	Time compression
	Threat or stress
	Contextual

Table 8—Impairments of decision-making

The situation itself is in flux. Embedded in the environment, information becomes contextual and dependent on hidden environmental variables. Nonlinear interactions create unpredictable trajectories and outcomes, from which emerge novel, unexpected properties.

Common approaches to medical decision-making cannot rise to these situations. There is a risk of identifying a standard or correct approach, thus creating normative decision-making at the expense of adaptive decision-making. Medical decision-making developed as clinical reasoning from physiology and pathophysiology for diagnoses, tests, and treatments. The cognitive sciences have contributed the identification of cognitive errors (such as biases and heuristics) and decision methods for uncertainty and time-dependence. Evidence-based medicine and epidemiology have refined the use of statistics to evaluate experience with probability to better understand the future.

HROs are involved with the VUCA-T environment in an uncertain, time-compressed, threat state. The affective domain comes into play by placing value on attitudes and information and modulating emotion. Rather than uncertainty and time-dependence alone, we must also work with time compression and threat or stress impairment of cognitive functions. The ease of occurrence (possibility) may take precedence over the likelihood of occurrence (probability).

Medical Decision-Making	Emergency Decision-Making
Action and problem solving	Enact a preferred end-state
Diagnosis and treatment	Control system energy
Cognitive	Cognitive and affective
Biases	Situational cognitive distortions
Evidence-based	Experience-based
Uncertainty, time-dependence	Uncertainty, time-compression, threat
Normal distribution	Power distribution
Likelihood of occurrence (probability)	Ease of occurrence (possibility)
Outlier more easily disregarded	Outlier is threat or early herald of threat

Table 9—Medical and emergency decision-making

The use of probability functions may be of less use in the VUCA-T environment. The outlier, or distance from the norm in a normal distribution curve, can more easily be disregarded. We should bear the following in mind:

- If our concern is frequently occurring events, then we focus on the central portion of the probability curve: the hoof beats come from horses. (See the discussion of zebras and horses in the "Possibility" section of chapter 3, "The Logic of Practice and the Logic of Operations.")
- If our concern is reliability and operations for rare events, then we focus on the distribution tails (i.e., the hoof beats come from zebras).
- If our data is additive (that is, random and independent), then we use the normal distribution to calculate statistics and probabilities.
- If our data is multiplicative, then we use the lognormal distribution, as in trauma or critical-care scoring systems.

- If the process is a power function, then we find the best fit of the power distributions, such as the Pareto distribution (Bob Bea, Professor of Civil Engineering, University of California, Berkeley, personal communication).

Connecticut Paramedics

Two paramedics arrived on scene to find a woman in her late sixties lying face down in the street. It was summer in the late evening with a light rain, and the street was wet. They rolled her over and saw that she was nonresponsive and pale. Her skin felt damp, more so than just from the rain, and she had oxygen saturation in the low eighties with a very slow, weak heartbeat in the forties. On the EKG, they identified a normal electrical pattern except for extra beats coming from the ventricle (premature ventricular contractions, or PVCs). The first thought was that she'd had a cardiac event, so they began to consider cardiac protocols. The two paramedics were not sure which protocol to use, but each paramedic had 15 years of experience and could see that she was dying. They began to feel helpless to stop her death.

While accomplishing this evaluation, they had also made a rapid visual respiratory exam and observed very shallow breathing; they identified lower airway obstruction from the prolonged expiratory phase. This indicated treatment with a bronchodilator drug, something they would not have considered without the rapid visual exam. They were not sure, however, if they should treat what could be a second disease, if the bronchodilator would work, or if the bronchodilator might stimulate the heart and cause the extra beats to fibrillate, creating cardiac arrest.

They decided to administer the drug and observe the response, which is something they would not have considered without the use of Boyd's OODA loop decision-making. After the bronchodilator treatment, the woman's chest expansion increased, the expiratory phase shortened, her oxygen saturation increased above 90 percent without supplemental oxygen, and she became more alert. Most critical, her heart rate increased, and the extra beats (premature ventricular contractions) resolved.

Approximately four months earlier, the senior paramedic had learned the rapid visual respiratory exam and OODA loop decision-making. The OODA loop is a rapid decision-making pattern that employs immediate feedback to guide the next decision. He had not used either the exam or the OODA loop before this. This woman's life was saved by treatment the paramedics would not have considered without the concepts of a rapid visual respiratory examination and Boyd's OODA loop decision cycle.

—Daved van Stralen

First, Do No Harm

As we stated previously, "First, do no harm" has become a maxim to help ensure safety by not commencing an action that we cannot reverse. The maxim encourages reflection to identify the best and safest treatment. In the above vignette, however, the patient is dying, and the paramedics do not have sufficient information to confidently administer a drug—they initially see cardiac disease as the greatest danger, then they observe respiratory signs, but they do not connect respiratory disease to the heart rhythm and fear that treating the respiratory disease may make the heart disease worse.

With these conflicting thoughts while faced with a worsening condition and limited time, they treated the respiratory disease. It was the response to therapy that told them that a severe asthma attack had lowered the blood oxygen level low enough to create the heart problem.

Their fear in treating the airway disease came from the effect the bronchodilator might have had by stimulating a weakened heart. Treating airway disease might make the heart disease worse and possibly cause death. Doing nothing while we collect more information and think of the right course of action does not stop the progression of heart disease and could cause death.

"First, do no harm," improperly interpreted, can force reflective thought over investigative action and delay treatment. The paramedics' initial assessment, coupled with an overreliance on the concern to "do no harm," temporarily incapacitated their processes associated with continuing to seek additional information.

It is the purpose of this chapter to identify methods for decision-making that will support investigation during treatment while minimizing the possibility of harm from our actions: in other words, "interactive, real-time risk assessment and management" (Bob Bea, Professor of Civil Engineering, University of California, Berkeley, personal communication). The interactive approach of crisis management focuses on the support of both people and systems (Bea 2008).

Dual-Process Thinking: Thinking Fast and Slow

In the situation described in this chapter's initial vignette, the paramedics struggled between using controlled thinking to analyze the situation and automatically responding to the immediate problem. Each option may seem reasonable, and we do not naturally synchronize our thinking with those around us when these events happen. Depending on your point of view, the paramedics may have jumped the gun and should have looked before they leaped, while others believe the paramedics avoided "paralysis by analysis."

Dual-process theory is an explanation of these two processes of conscious thought and immediate actions, described as the difference between performance and introspection. The two processes are not distinct in time; we shift between responding and thinking about the various bits of information in rapid continuous feedback to help interpret what we see, to process relevant information, and to identify irrelevant information (Wason and Evans 1974).

Contextualization

Stanovich (1999) described overlearned response patterns as decontextualized cognitive styles. That is, the response occurs without regard to the context and can be considered a skill that enables the operation of reasoning processes independent of what he calls "interfering context." While decontextualizing, as a domain generality, is an important component for critical thinking, doing so poses a problem when context provides important information or gives meaning to existing information (Stanovich 1999, 172).

Contextual cognitive styles, which are more commonly studied in developmental psychology, emphasize specificity. The expert level of skill performance is a measure of the ability to use knowledge specific to the area of expertise: a higher level of performance described by the Dreyfus brothers' work on expert performance (Dreyfus and Dreyfus 1980) and Rasmussen's description of the knowledge-based domain for interacting with technology (Rasmussen 1983).

Highly contextualized reasoning tends to be associative, interactive, and experiential and makes use of heuristics to process information. Decontextualized reasoning, in contrast, tends to be rule based, analytical, and rational and to make use of analytic processing for information. Stanovich (1999) calls this system 1 and system 2, respectively, with system 1 being quick and inflexible; at times it needs the flexibility and intellect of system 2 to override it. In the best cases, metacognition will influence which system is used.

Patricia Benner: Skill Acquisition and High Reliability in Nursing Practice

Patricia Benner made a significant contribution to nursing professionalism in the 1980s with her adaptation of the Dreyfus model of skill acquisition (Benner 1984; Dreyfus and Dreyfus 1980) to nursing practice. She demonstrated the advancement of skills, from novice to expert, as the nurse develops from classroom principles and theory to what Dreyfus and Dreyfus call context-dependent judgments and skills that only can be acquired in real situations.

The Dreyfus progression is most commonly described as advancement from rigid adherence to rules to an intuitive model of reasoning based on tacit knowledge (i.e., that which is understood but not spoken). Brothers Stuart and Hubert Dreyfus developed their model at the UC Berkeley Operations Research Center for the US Air Force Office of Scientific Research.

In Benner's book *From Novice to Expert*, she describes the novice as being rule based, having little or no contextual experience, and having very little situational awareness. At this level of skill, the student nurse is supervised closely. Generally, the nurse begins clinical practice at the "competent" level of nursing, in which the nurse is able to standardize and routinize procedures and see actions as long-term goals. At the competent level, the ability to achieve most tasks using the nurse's own judgment allows the autonomy necessary to work independently. The "expert" nurse has acquired the highest level of skill and no longer relies solely on analytical principles to understand situations and initiate appropriate actions. Rather, the expert nurse has a high level of situational awareness, is highly intuitive, and has a vision of what is possible.

HRO principles correlate with Benner's adaptation of the Dreyfus model. Benner provides the milestones of the journey that is HRO (i.e., nursing decision-making), context to nursing encounters, and the development of a repertoire of experiences for the nurse to interpret and analyze in new situations. Benner clearly states that the Dreyfus model, as it applies to nursing, measures skill and not the person. In addition, Benner stresses that her adaptation of the Dreyfus model does not necessarily associate time with proficiency. Like the Dreyfus brothers, Benner bases someone's level of proficiency on attributes and characteristics that are a necessary foundation for situational awareness, analysis, contextual adaptation, deference to expertise, resilience, and sustainability.

—Patricia E. Sokol, RN, JD

Intuition and Reasoning

Stanovich and West (2000) later focused on these neutral terms as system 1 for automatic, unconscious reasoning (action) and system 2 for analytical conscious reasoning (thought).

The Nobel laureate Daniel Kahneman (2003) distinguished dual-process thinking between intuition and reasoning. Intuition is fast, instinctive, and emotional (system 1), while reasoning is the slower, more deliberative and logical approach (system 2). A long list of cognitive biases and heuristics are associated with each system. Kahneman (2011) elaborated on this concept in his book *Thinking, Fast and Slow*. system 1 is fast, automatic, frequent, emotional, stereotypic, and subconscious, while system 2 is slow, effortful, infrequent, logical, calculating, and conscious.

These models academically describe what happens in these situations and can help us understand and interpret outcomes and actions taken. They may be of less use for conditioning in decision-making or teaching us how to make decisions. We seek an approach that is of immediate use, much like that used by the paramedics in the opening vignette of this chapter. The approach must be pragmatic and based in daily practice. While VUCA is a useful description, we must remember that it goes along with very real and immediate physical danger (the "threatening" of the T in VUCA-T). It is this time-sensitive threat that impairs cognition, essentially blocking efforts to use system 2 analysis and deliberation in an emergency.

Our approach must incorporate the effect that threat and the associated fear response has on thinking and decision-making (thus creating immediately applicable practical decision-making skills that are in fact immediately applicable) rather than engage in scientific discussions of how the decisions are made.

Conflicted Decision-Making

Irving Janis and Leon Mann (1977) studied stress from unexpected threats when we face time pressure, have no good choices, and face the restriction of activity, sensory deprivation, and lack of contact with supportive people. Their work, which is not commonly referred to today, is significant in the study of large-scale, high-risk decision-making events such as the Cuban missile crisis. The authors identified five patterns, but we have found two to be useful in teaching decision-making. Their five patterns are unconflicted adherence, unconflicted change, defensive avoidance, hypervigilance, and vigilance; we discuss hypervigilance and vigilance.

In the hypervigilant state, we do a nonselective search for information and a rapid, cursory evaluation of data. People only consider limited alternatives and do not review the decisions they make. Thought processes are simplistic and easily disrupted. If an action is not fruitful, then we develop a new action plan; we continue this cycle in response to local successes and failures.

Vigilance is mediated by awareness of serious risks for *no* protective action taken but also for the risks when protective actions *are* taken. This is significant to keep in mind, as risk-benefit discussions often focus on action: what is the risk of acting, and what is the benefit of acting. In vigilance, we compare the risk of acting and the risk of doing nothing. Part of this risk discussion identifies limits to new actions; if the action is not fruitful, then we stop and revert to our original plan.

With vigilance, we hope that a search for information will lead to a better solution and believe that we will have sufficient time to search and deliberate. Vigilance is characterized by a systematic, organized information search, where we reexamine and review data before making a decision. We thoroughly consider all available alternatives and devote sufficient time to adequately evaluating each alternative.

The response to actions is perhaps the clearest way to compare vigilance and hypervigilance. Vigilant operators will try a new approach for a limited time; if not productive, then they will return to the previous course, which serves as an anchor during the process. In hypervigilance, operators try a new approach and change approaches when one does not work. They do not revert to an anchor process. The risk of this strategy is becoming lost in orientation, while the benefit is potentially uncovering a desired response.

Looking at hypervigilance and vigilance as two separate entities, we might prefer the vigilant state, where we take sufficient time and energy to evaluate information and prospective decisions. Compare this thoughtful deliberation to hypervigilance, where we begin a rapid action cycle, change course every time something happens, and don't conduct reviews of when to start over.

But if we take hypervigilance and vigilance as extremes on a spectrum, then the value of integrating the two (depending on the particular situation) becomes apparent. In our earlier discussion, we remarked on the significance for HROs of the situational evaluation of information for particular circumstances. We can seek balance between vigilance and hypervigilance, for example by proportionally using reevaluation and starting over while at the same time rapidly taking action following a cursory evaluation of the situation.

Decision Interference
Many sources of interference and distraction can happen during a crisis. That is obvious. But maybe it is only obvious in retrospect, because we do not know if that distraction is actually an early herald of further deterioration or a separate

problem that is developing. For example, a team member who is responding to fear through avoidance may need redirection. Some people may have an immediate emotional response to abrupt failure.

> As the attending physician for the pediatric ICU, I responded to a code blue on the pediatric ward. Among the flurry of activity around a small child, I heard a rhythmic "I have the A, I am doing the B, do your C. I have the A, I am doing the B, do your C." Richard Spencer, the respiratory care practitioner, was hand-ventilating the child and saying this mantra in a soft, soothing voice.
>
> The day before, the surgeons had placed an intravenous catheter into a large central vein inside the child's chest. Some of the staff members wanted to use that line for the fluids, while others wanted to give medications to sedate and paralyze the child for endotracheal intubation. Richard responded with, "I have the A, I am doing the B, do your C. I have the A, I am doing the B, do your C."
>
> The team established an intravenous line and gave a fluid bolus for a heart rate of over two hundred. Cool extremities and a high heart rate indicated low blood volume. A chest x-ray revealed that the surgically placed line had migrated into the chest wall. Overnight, all the intravenous fluids had moved to the chest and were pushing the mediastinum to the other side. (In infants and small children, the mediastinum is very pliable. It does not take very much pressure on one side to cause tension on the other; this can also lead to rapid cardiac arrest.)
>
> Had the team given the fluids through the central line, the most likely result would have been loss of both lungs and cardiac arrest. Had the team given a sedation medication, the blood vessels would have dilated; with insufficient blood volume, the blood blister would have plummeted, and the most likely result would have been cardiac arrest.
>
> It was Richard's soft mantra to keep to the plan: he had the airway (A), he was doing the breathing (B), and he asked the team to take care of the circulation (C).
>
> —Daved van Stralen

Leaders during crises have the responsibility of maintaining their own focus in order to support others in maintaining their focus as a team. But then we have the problem of determining whether this is proper focused attention for effective operations or if have we focused our attention on some piece of minutia.

The commercial and military aviation fields now have stringent rules regarding the distribution of responsibilities and the maintenance of focus during in-flight emergencies. These rules provide a very clear, spoken delineation between which crew member will fly the aircraft and which will focus on the emergency. This situation came about after a number of fully avoidable fatal accidents occurred in which the pilot flying (PF) developing such channelized attention that he focused so much on resolution of the emergency (in several cases a relatively minor issue like an indicator light that was not properly functioning) that he failed to maintain separation with the ground, water, or other aircraft.

Because this phenomenon has happened many times, a significant amount of simulator time is now also dedicated to flight crews encountering numerous simulated emergencies that are closely monitored and debriefed by experienced instructors. The potential impacts of interference and distraction have been significantly mitigated, and the incidence of avoidable accidents attributed to those factors has been greatly reduced.

—Spence Byrum

Biases and Heuristics

The difficulty with biases, heuristics, and cognitive distortions is our ability to identify these things in others but not in ourselves. Because we use our judgment to judge our judgment, we are unlikely to judge our judgment as lacking. In these situations, we find it difficult to see where we have gone wrong. In this section, we will discuss the material that is most pertinent for your use, since we realize this is a large topic with many experts and numerous favorite positions. This limitation creates a situation called confirmation bias, which essentially means that we sort through a plethora of information, grasping only that which supports our initial judgment. It is contrary to objective decision-making and unquestionably not in the best interest of the patient. We need to discuss tools that can overcome confirmation bias and be used the same day we learn them. Our most basic bias is that we use our judgment to judge our judgment.

During one emergency I recall, members of the team offered to help and gave me a few ideas. They felt their ideas were compelling and important, because in a similar situation, the ideas had worked. But this was not that situation, and it had only a cursory similarity to their past experience.

Feeling frustrated, I told them, "You can remember your successes. I have to remember my failures."
—Daved van Stralen

Of the many biases and heuristics, we find that four cause most of the interference in effective decision-making: availability, representativeness, confirmation bias, and over conservative revision. A fifth core bias, motivated reasoning, prevents the acceptance of information that contradicts a strongly held belief and is a form of confirmation bias.

Bias or heuristic	Effect
Availability	What you think of first is most important
Representativeness	What you see represents events
Confirmation bias	Search for supporting information
Motivated reasoning (a form of confirmation bias)	Over-scrutiny of information disconfirming strongly held belief
Over-conservative revision	Require more information to stop action than to start

Table 10—Bias and effect

Availability, also called frequency bias, leads us to accept our first impression. You may more easily see this in others who come up and tell you what to do, giving you unsolicited and poorly thought-out advice. Availability bias also occurs when redundant variables influence our perceptions. These are variables where we measure the same thing, but we do so in several ways, unconsciously placing more weight on variables with multiple ways of being measured, despite the fact that they measure the same thing. We put more weight on what we first see. Availability will bias us toward precision and the use of numbers (also called quantitative information, but it seems the number itself is what makes it important) over qualitative values.

The strength of availability bias can easily be demonstrated in several ways. We can ask our students what cows drink (the common answer is milk, because we think of milk when we think of cows). But more effective in a group is to ask someone to spell the word "folk." Then ask, "What is the white of an egg called?" The student will generally answer what you made more available to his or her brain: "yolk." Your other students will attempt to correct, though some may side with the student and a few will become argumentative.

Representativeness, closely tied in with complexity and "refusal to simplify," is a bias that leads us to regard partial information as if it were complete information. In other words, what you see represents what is happening. This is a difficult one to break, because we must use partial information when we begin to engage. If we recognize this as a bias, however, then we will more likely continue to reevaluate our situation to obtain and refine new information.

Confirmation bias derives from cognitive dissonance, the discomfort of holding conflicting beliefs. To avoid the dissonance of having conflicting beliefs, we tend to search for information that will confirm our current belief. We look for evidence that will support our conclusions while ignoring disconfirming, discrepant data.

These biases often combine to distract from or confuse the facts we believe we are faced with. A subtle availability bias we might face is the preference for what worked last time. When this combines with representativeness bias, we may first look for familiar information (likely connected to our last experience) and assume that what is happening now represents what happened last time. Next comes confirmation bias as we seek information to support our new conclusion, which starts a cascade of failure based on only a few unrecognized biases. Confirmation and availability bias are insidiously dangerous, because they cause us to stop considering other alternatives when we encounter situations that require additional analysis.

Overconservative revision leads us to continue treatments long past the point when we would not have treated the patient had the patient not been sick. In other words, once we started with treatment, we find it hard to stop, even when the reason to treat is gone. We require more information to stop action than we initially required to start.

I came on service with a patient who was in dire straits; all members of the treating and consulting teams supported the withdrawal of support from the patient. One night we had lost vascular access, so we tried an uncommon approach to placing the vascular catheter. Review of the chest x-ray showed that it lined up in the superior vena cava. The child went into abrupt respiratory distress during the early-morning hours. A chest x-ray revealed a large amount of fluid in the chest on the side with the catheter. Further studies revealed that the catheter was alongside, rather than inside, the vein. All the required fluids and medications were entering the chest cavity rather than the bloodstream. Oddly, the child had improved.

Working on the assumption that the medications were not necessary, I stopped them. The child continued to improve. It seemed we were treating our treatments. We gave medications for the heart to be stronger, but those caused the child's blood vessels to constrict and the kidneys to fail. We then gave medication to dilate the blood vessels that had been constricted because of the heart medicine. We also gave diuretics to maintain kidney function and fluid balance. Other medications also became involved to help maintain physiological balance.

I would like to say the child survived, but the baby died a week later because of mechanical ventilator interactions with the lung and airway.

It is easier to identify the symptoms of "treating the treatment" in others rather than in your own care. Consultants and second opinions play an important role in high-risk environments, since they bring new points of view.

—Daved van Stralen

Motivated reasoning is the ugly sibling of confirmation bias, in that it causes over scrutiny of *disconfirming* information, while confirmation bias leads to under scrutiny of *confirming* information. Disconfirming information is a marker for safety in an HRO. It is a sign that we are approaching the edge of our safe operational envelope, that a discrepancy has developed, or that a disruption has commenced. Ignoring this sign is tantamount to looking only one way at a four-way intersection.

In a world where facts are few and unreliable, we routinely work with beliefs and interpretations. When these beliefs become too strong, they interfere with the incorporation of new information and our thought processes. People who have not experienced severe failure will too easily develop motivated reasoning. Some leaders can develop motivated reasoning if they attribute their rise in the organization solely to their own effort and not to the larger network of people around them or to supportive mentors, leaders, and subordinates.

Situational Cognitive Distortions

Fear can become normalized in high-risk environments, which makes its influence subtle and often unrecognized. The normalization of fear can be worn as a badge of honor, which can preclude any consideration of less dangerous or drastic alternatives to the situation. Such normalization has a greater effect on decision-making than cognitive biases and heuristics or system 1/system 2, fast and slow thinking.

As discussed in chapter 9, "Threat Responses and Unrecognized Fear," the fear responses of fight, flight, or freeze are manifested cognitively. The overall fear response limits perception and cones our attention to a singular focus. We become inattentive to new information and voices. We lose our peripheral perception.

> The FAA's Federal Aviation Regulations (FAR) require the copilot to take over flying of the airplane if the pilot does not respond when asked the same question twice. This rather dramatic change to protocol, called the two-challenge rule, came about out of necessity. The two-challenge rule was developed after research and accident analysis showed that an unacceptable percentage of copilots would allow a captain to continue flying the aircraft in an unacceptable manner as long as that incapacitation was not obvious. The incapacitation was found to not only constitute physical incapacitation but also cognitive incapacitation due to stress, distraction, or fear. The rule states that the copilot or pilot not flying (PNF) would assume control of the airplane if the captain or pilot flying (PF) did not respond appropriately after two callouts. The belief is that functional loss of hearing and cognition results from something that is stressing the pilot, who then becomes focused on a specific problem at the expense of flying the airplane.
> —Spence Byrum

Fight responses include anger and frustration. When you sense yourself becoming angry or frustrated, it is important to pause and differentiate between expectations and demands. Focus on demands (and your ability to meet those demands) and think of which resources are immediately around you that could help. Using physical activity, particularly your hands, also helps to solve problems.

When you see anger in another person, ask "*How* can I help you?" Asking *what* you can do or *why* the person is angry seems to increase the fear (anger) response. Speaking slowly and comfortably while employing a softer voice may also help. Do not become carried away with the slow, soft voice, as doing so can come across as condescending if you do not do it in a subtle manner. Giving the person a physical task to perform may also help.

The flight response often presents as avoiding tasks, responding to distractions, or addressing easily accomplished tasks to the detriment of essential efforts. In such cases, solving a problem at hand can also help to bring people back to the team.

The freeze response, which can manifest as confusion or as an actual cognitive or physical freezing up, can often be resolved through physical activity.

This can take the form of reevaluation of a previously resolved problem by visual inspection or manipulation or by physically accomplishing a new procedure.

Fear responses are manifested by anger, frustration, avoidance, confusion, and/or physical or cognitive freeze. Other effects of decision-making in the VUCA-T environment include the need to value information and objectives. Decontextualizing, as in system 2 decision-making, is fraught with peril. For example, an automated car, while attempting to avoid an obstacle, may drive on the sidewalk and hit people in order to avoid hitting a tree.

> A critical care fellow came up and told the story of why he had come to accept concrete thinking during emergencies. During a resuscitation, he said to the staff, "I want to give a twenty-five percent albumin infusion." The nurse gathered the material and handed it to him. "What is this for?" he asked.
>
> "You said you wanted to give albumin," she answered. She had thought the physician wanted to personally install the intravenous infusion apparatus and start the albumin infusion. What he wanted was for the albumin to be infused into to the patient, but his wording was taken concretely by the nurse. The nurse wasted time and distracted the physician from managing a critical event.
>
> A few days later, I told this story on rounds, anonymously, to emphasize the presence and effect of concrete thinking in an emergency. We should always assume that everyone thinks concretely (even us); in effect, we should *always* speak concretely. After my patient-care rounds, the nurse came up to me and said, "That was me. The reason I gave him the albumin was because he said he wanted to give it." Even that next day, without pressure, this excellent, experienced nurse continued to think in concrete terms.
>
> Abstract thought is not reliable when we are giving and taking orders during an emergency.
>
> —Daved van Stralen

The most significant, and unrecognized, consideration is that stress not only impairs cognitive function, but severe stress, and particularly fear, also reduces abstract cognition. Someone who is under threat tends to think in concrete terms.

Error Recognition and Self-Correction

Can there be error in uncertain or ambiguous situations? In the dynamic state, we have little time for evaluation and reevaluation and even less time to suffer the consequences of an error. Every action is an evaluation for the border of safety; we constantly search for the envelope we operate within. Self-correction includes this type of feedback and also includes articulation of the problem and accuracy over precision.

> When hiking a trail at night above the timberline, you walk by the feel of the trail. A foot that lands too closely to the vertical rock on the mountainside can cause you to stumble; a foot that lands too closely to the edge can lead to a dangerous fall. You feel for the hard-packed center of the trail, and you also feel for the edge of the trail, which has a looser surface. The only wrong step is the one that hurts you, so you constantly feel for the looser surface. That is what attracts your attention. In a sense, you are feeling for the early herald, that of leaving the center of the trail. This gives you the envelope you can walk within.
> —Daved van Stralen

In a rapidly evolving state, we must identify error early and correct it. To achieve early error identification and correction requires each member to be observant of any undesired results and to communicate these observations to the person who is making the decision and the person in charge. A steep authority gradient impedes information flow and can have deadly consequences. Later in this discussion we will describe outcomes as good, bad, or no change; it is important that all members of the team know what to look out for.

> "If you can articulate the problem, then you have half the answer," a US marshal told a group of training recruits. This was his answer when the recruits asked him about probable cause, a legal term regarding the belief that a person has committed a crime. If you can articulate in an objective manner that someone is out of place in a manner that is not normally expected, then you're halfway to answering the question of probable cause. For example, an adult in business dress driving through an industrial zone at two in the morning would give you little probable cause to search the person. The person may be an executive of one of the companies. On the other hand, an adolescent in the industrial zone at two in the morning is more serious, as the adolescent likely has no business being there; this establishes probable cause for a search.
> —US marshal

Other organizations have taken delineation of these responsibilities further.

Aviation has overcome much of the ambiguity associated with individual views of the same situation overlaid with the need to have a designated leader. Federal rules now require members of the flight crew to speak up when they identify a situation that might have an impact on flight safety or mission accomplishment while still acknowledging that the pilot in command (PIC) retains the ultimate decision-making responsibility. Responsibility, coupled with timely team inputs, has dramatically decreased accidents.

—Spence Byrum

The Decision Frame

A common fear derived from "First, do no harm" is making a wrong decision. We have found it helpful to work with the operator to create a frame for decisions that are found along a scale of "too soon" versus "too late" and "too much" versus "too little." This is similar to what Tversky and Kahneman (1981) described as a *decision frame*, a representation of the decision problem that contains acts, outcomes, and contingencies with different alternatives.

Is the decision reversible? Often, we find the novice decision-maker worrying over an action that can readily be reversed. For example, we can reverse the effect of a diuretic with the administration of fluid. We can reverse the administration of too much fluid by corrective action with a diuretic. This problem arises when we titrate fluids for dehydration or blood volume and, though we can calculate ideal weight and expected blood volume, we still do not know exactly how much fluid would benefit our patient.

> "Doctor, do you want to give this patient fluids?" the licensed vocational nurse (LVN) asked. She wanted an order for fluids to treat thick pulmonary secretions; the fluids would be given through the gastrostomy tube. We then had two discussions, one for treating the secretions and one regarding the fluid.
>
> I asked her, "What would happen if we didn't treat the secretions, or if we treated them and didn't need to? And what would happen if we gave too much or not enough fluid?"
>
> She answered that treating the secretions too early would cause excess fluids and increased urine output. Waiting to treat the secretions could lead to the formation of thick mucus plugs, an obstructed airway, and cardiac arrest. For the fluids problem, she said that giving too much fluid would increase the urine output, while giving insufficient amounts of fluid would delay response and increase the threat of thick secretions, which could lead to cardiac arrest.

In balance, she had answered her own question. The client faced two risks: increased urine output versus cardiac arrest. The LVN became vigilant for secretions and had a better understanding of what we were treating, how we treated it, and why we make the decisions we do.
—Daved van Stralen

Another important factor in the decision frame is the outcome, whether it is good, bad, or there is no change. If it is good, then we continue doing it. If it is bad, then we do not express it as a poor decision but as new and important information. Like the footsteps on the mountain trail, a bad or unwanted result identifies the boundary of our envelope for operational purposes and helps us identify structure within what initially appears to be an unstructured situation.

The most dangerous outcome is "no change." In the medical field, we may have the wrong dose, wrong drug, or wrong diagnosis. "No change" increases our uncertainty and supports more vigorous attempts to characterize the structure of our problem.

As part of the evening check out before I left the Pediatric Intensive Care Unit, I reviewed a patient's treatment plan with the resident in some detail. She asked when to call me, and I told her to call if the patient did not respond to her care. Typically, during night call a resident will collect data, labs, vital signs, and the like then develop a working diagnosis before calling the attending physician. Collecting this information or confusion about the diagnosis delays immediate and necessary medical care. Knowing this may happen, I reiterated that she should call me if the patient was not responding. Early in the morning, I received that call with a simple, yet effective, statement: "The nonresponder is not responding." With that, and without what others consider requisite information, we could begin an intelligent, informative conversation and start treatment much earlier in the deterioration than otherwise would have occurred.
—Daved van Stralen

You'll recall from our earlier discussions that "decisions not made" can be exceptionally harmful if all the elements of the decision were present yet not acted on. This is a culpability of inaction that no one in an HRO would accept or tolerate. Within our decision frame is the decision "not to act." Please note that "not acting" is a decision and not a passive move or something you don't do because you don't know what to do. If you do not act, then look for any changes and discrepancies or developments that will help you understand or lessen the worry. The most important thing is to watch for points where you can intervene.

Many would say that they "don't have time" to conduct even a cursory review and say that the healthcare environment is too dynamic for such an approach. We maintain that, to the contrary, if you don't take the time to review, then you won't capture the things that went well to "lock them in." In that case, you most certainly are going to repeat the things that did not go well. Our response when people say that they "don't have time to do that in medicine" is that "you don't have time *not* to do it."
— Spence Byrum

Boyd's OODA loop (see chapter 6) can help overcome the fear of causing more harm than good in these situations. The OODA loop provides the ability to sense events through short feedback loops, better reading of the situation, and improved agility to act effectively and meaningfully. The use of the loop builds a decision frame within which we can use the OODA loop to navigate toward resolution of the problem or control of the situation when protocols cannot help.

Having the knowledge of what it means not to act can give us confidence to intervene and to use greater effort when a situation deteriorates. The OODA loop's focus on response to actions (therapy in this case) supports action more quickly and forcefully. The only other part we need to discuss is the question, "Is this reversible?" Nonreversible interventions are more serious and require greater thought before we act, although this is part of the decision framework within which these interventions freely work.

Utility of the Decision Frame

The decision frame described here refers to a frame within which any decision or action can safely work. Any decisions made outside the frame results are not predictable and may result in loss of control. This is similar to hiking a trail at night. Identify your boundaries of safety: too much or too little, or too soon or too late.

To teach safe driving, the officer-instructors at the Los Angeles Police Department "skid school" had students drive in a tight circle until the rear of the car began to swing outward, making the car drive in a circle but sideways. The purpose was not to teach the students how to perform trick driving but to let them know how it feels when the back tires break loose, or lose friction, from the road. It is at that point when the driver is in the most danger of losing control of the vehicle. The instructors wanted the students to know how it feels as the car begins to go out of control so that they could recognize the feeling during real-life high-speed driving maneuvers.
— Daved van Stralen

The next step in the decision is to determine whether the person can reverse the decision. Irreversible decisions, no matter how minor, can begin a series of events that can cascade out of control. If the person can readily reverse a decision, then he or she can make it with greater safety while under less supervision.

As a medical student in the 1980s, I studied a trauma-scoring system paramedics performed to see if it predicted the need for ICU care. If the patient transferred out of the ICU the day after admission, then I classified them as not needing trauma care (this was a false positive).

Dr. Martin Eisner, the trauma surgeon, disagreed with my interpretation. "Trauma surgeons at a trauma center might not operate on a patient that other surgeons working at a nontrauma center might. This is because the trauma center nurses are better educated and experienced at observing physiological changes, early signs of infection, or shock, which allows the surgeon not to operate. Instead, the surgeon can observe and rely on the skilled nursing staff." Trauma centers prevent the performing of operations because of these critical nursing skills.

—Daved van Stralen

The most critical decision is the decision "not to act." This "nonacting" can signal to others that no action is necessary or that the problem is not severe. Observation, the key to "not acting," may be passed over. The leader must reiterate that "the decision not to act *is* a decision."

We had recently passed a policy that the respiratory care practitioner could cancel a breathing treatment order if the patient did not respond after two consecutive treatments. A physician on the ward approached me, angry that our policy stopped a very necessary treatment. His anger had shifted discussion away from any logic, and the ward physician angrily announced, "OK, if you won't authorize the breathing treatment, then you take the patient on your service." The patient was evaluated on my service with flexible bronchoscopy and found to have bronchomalacia—a weakening of the cartilage in the airways that causes collapse during breathing. This disease does not respond to bronchodilators; it needs a different treatment.

—Daved van Stralen

We monitor our decisions for success or failure: Did the patient improve from treatment, or did a complication from treatment arise? What is left out of this analysis is the patient who does not respond. Too commonly, the team does not pursue the failure to respond to treatment. Failure to respond can represent a deteriorating condition, a new and more severe disease that needs different therapy. Failure to respond can also be due to administration of the wrong drug, wrong dose, or wrong disease.

This is distinct from enactment failure *from not acting*, which may be a response to social knowledge that action is dangerous. By not acting, we do not learn what caused the failure (or even if there will be failure). For example, as noted earlier, it was once taught that administering adrenaline by aerosol to an infant with croup would lead to "rebound croup." From this developed a belief that administering adrenaline by aerosol could actually make an infant's condition worse. In reality, if the child deteriorated later, it was due to progression of the disease, not the treatment. This situation is similar to ibuprofen wearing off followed by a return of the headache pain. We do not call this "rebound headache." Action creates information.

Use of the Decision Frame

The child had had severe asthma for over a week in the PICU and was gradually deteriorating. We would need to use paralytic drugs, place a breathing tube in the airway, and then use a mechanical ventilator, possibly for several weeks. These children are difficult to hand-ventilate, which makes this a high-risk procedure. Mark Rogers, the respiratory care practitioner, suggested a helium-oxygen mixture. The right ratio would slow the oxygen in the airway, shifting it from turbulent flow—resistance from flow velocity—to laminar flow, or resistance by airway diameter. (Helium has low density with high viscosity; like Silly Putty breaking when pulled quickly by becoming "stiffer," this helium-oxygen gas mixture becomes "thicker" with higher gas flows, slowing the gas and reducing the resistance.) We had not used helium-oxygen mixtures in our medical center.

I asked for his plan. Mark said, "We'll start the helium-oxygen mixture. If his oxygen saturation drops, then we switch back to our original plan. If he gets better, we continue. If he doesn't improve after two hours, we go back to the original plan." He had included signs for improvement, deterioration, and no response in one brief statement.

—Daved van Stralen

Decision-Making

The Boyd OODA loop is not a replacement for conventional decision-making approaches. It is of great utility when conventional methods do not apply or do not work, and it can augment conventional methods. The first decision methods we learned were linear—we collect the information we need, arrive at a conclusion, and then act. For more advanced problems, we may follow a protocol that guides thinking to ensure we are complete in our actions. The algorithm decomposes a larger problem into a series of smaller problems that we can more easily solve; in the algorithm, we complete one action before moving on to the next. Academics developed the decision tree to help identify alternatives and guide decisions when the decision is made today but the information will come tomorrow. In the 1960s, John Boyd developed a rapid feedback loop for decision-making that is nimble and increases accuracy (J. F. Magee 1964a, 1964b).

The Boyd loop creates a decision architecture for decision structures that meet the needs of various purposes. When we must solve problems in a stepwise fashion, with the solution to one problem becoming input for the next step, we will use an algorithm. If we have a straightforward problem that needs minor decisions to be made in a series, then we would use the protocol, an early example of which (from 1839) is the Jacquard loom for mechanically selecting yarn colors to create patterns in cloth. Mathematicians developed decision trees in the late 1950s; this structure found use in business initially for capital-investment guidance in the mid-1960s. The utility of decisions trees, which draw on outcome probabilities, benefitted numerous fields. Boyd, as discussed earlier, developed the concept of OODA loop decision-making to explain the unexpected kill ratio in aerial combat during the Korean conflict and World War II tank battles. He used the loop for the purpose of outmaneuvering enemy pilots by thinking in rapid cycles. We will evaluate each of these for use in particular situations that lack predictability.

Linearity

We too easily fall back into deterministic, or predictive, thought processes and think of a situation as a series of linear events to be dealt with sequentially, one after the other, and that we should stay "within the lines." Linearity is strongly supported by universal principles and generalizations. Our situations have severe local effects that can expand to affect the larger community. We have limited resources, so we must evaluate where to place them and when. These situations are not amenable to the linear approach.

Protocols

The ability to control a sequence of operations in weaving allowed for the production of numerous patterns in cloth. The aforementioned Jacquard loom was the first system to use punch cards to control this sequence—an important event in the history of computing that also corresponds to medical care as a clinical protocol. Protocols, like lists, reduce variance in procedures while permitting a higher level of function than is normally achievable when relying solely on reasoning and recall memory. Protocols are tremendously useful when applied as the tool that they are. Dynamic events lack the predictability necessary for the linearity of a protocol.

Protocols must be specific, both for indication and procedure, which leaves gaps between the protocols where the person must choose which adjacent protocol to use (Weick 2011). See the spectral-analysis figure below for an example.

Life and our perceptions are a full and continuous experience, represented by the continuous light spectrum below. Protocols and rules are discrete, the clear boundaries necessary for clarity of when to apply the protocol or rule. Concepts are similar but may have somewhat fuzzy boundaries or wider spectral bars. They are represented by the bright lines in the emission spectra below. The different bars might represent the experience of different organizations leading to a concentration of rules and protocols in one area of the continuous spectrum that is black in the other organization. This would be the difference between experiences and events or the opinion of an administrator or executive.

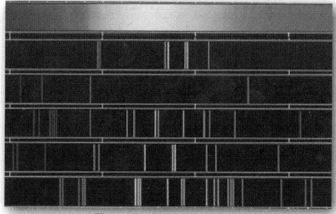

Figure 6—Spectral analysis

One thing to ask yourself is: Are your protocols a concrete wall that keeps reality out, or a picket fence that lets reality in?

Algorithm

An algorithm is a set of rules in a finite number of steps that is used for problem-solving. The computations are carried out in discrete stepwise fashion, not as continuous methods or processes. The history of the algorithm started in ancient Greece as a method to decompose the solving of a larger problem into a *series* of smaller problems. An algorithm follows a sequence in which the solution of a subproblem is used in the next subproblem of the sequence; it generally follows a defined sequence, such as in the procedure for endotracheal intubation:

- open airway
- clear airway of secretions
- visualize airway
- place endotracheal tube

Each of the four subproblems can be further decomposed to smaller subproblems, each of which must be completed before moving to the next in the series.

The Decision Tree

In the late 1950s, the decision tree emerged along several lines of thought, then was applied to business in 1964 through J. F. Magee's two articles published in the *Harvard Business Review* (Magee 1964a, 1964b). Decision trees identify alternatives and guide decisions that must be made when only incomplete information is available.

The phrase "decision tree" first appears to have been used by Herbert A. Simon (1957) as a tree of subproblems that correspond to proofs, each node of which represents a subproblem from a branch descending from the original problem above. He developed the system by combining algorithms in a larger flow chart to reach a final answer. Decision trees help in identifying alternatives when you do not have perfect information. Martin Shubik (1962) used a "game tree," where each branch represents an alternative choice, for processes where you do not have perfect information or do not know the rules. J. F. Magee (1964a, 1964b) also used a decision tree to represent alternatives, with the addition of outcome probabilities at each alternative he designated as a node. In this case, the leader must decide on what happens *after* the decision is made; that is, "today's" decision depends on information we will learn tomorrow. In the "tree of decisions," Magee used a node to represent change, each node representing a chance event that has a payoff with a known probability. This decision tree combines *actions* with *results*.

The decision tree we use today appears closest to Magee's model. It is important to recognize that the original decision nodes had a *known* probability. Today's trees often have alternatives listed in a tree of algorithms, which is functionally closer to Simon's tree of subproblems. The uncertainty and ambiguity inherent to complex, dynamic events limit the utility of decision trees.

Naturalistic Decision-Making
Naturalistic decision-making (NDM) describes how people use their personal experiences to make decisions when faced with uncertainty and complexity under time pressure. Rather than reducing decision-making to elements amenable for lab study, NDM researchers work in the field or closely to realistic settings. They focus on the expertise one develops over years of experience and emphasize environmental context in decision-making. Essentially, NDM studies examine how people use their knowledge and experience to make decisions in complex and uncertain conditions (Zsambok 2014).

The four themes of NDM include (1) a complex and dynamic stochastic environment, (2) experienced decision-makers, (3) situational awareness and diagnosis, and (4) research directed toward strategies that are actually used rather than what is prescribed by procedures that ought to be used. The concept of environment is expansive and includes tasks, poorly structured problems, and shifting, ill-defined, or competing goals. Individuals are included in the concept of setting. People are faced with feedback loops, time pressure, high stakes, other participants, and the need to meet organizational goals and work within organizational norms. Researchers are generally interested in plan generation rather than a focus on the moment of choice (Zsambok 2014).

The experienced decision-maker is the standard for performance in NDM, which allows researchers to build on the strategies experts use. Researchers tend to focus on decisions with high personal stakes of the type a novice or inexperienced operator would not encounter. Such studies also place a greater emphasis on situational awareness, a form of context-dependent information that they find to be more critical then deliberating over other courses of action. Further context-dependent characteristics include cues, information, decision requirements of context-specific judgments, and decisions and specific tasks. Contextual sensemaking, the manner in which one rapidly evaluates a situation, is a more critical driver for effective decision-making than the manner in which one decides (Klein 1993; Zsambok 2014).

Decision skills for NDM must be learned within the operational-context setting for which they will be used. Five types of NDM skills have been identified: (1) situational awareness, pattern matching, and cue learning; (2) typical cases and anomalies; (3) mental models; (4) the time horizon; and (5) managing uncertainty and time pressure (Klein 2014). The goal is to make a good-quality decision—that is, a decision with as few serious deficiencies as possible.

Yates (2001) describes five varieties of deficiencies: (1) failure to reach an explicitly formulated aim, (2) failure to meet the actual need in the situation, (3) failure in which the aggregate outcome of decisions leaves the person worse off than an effective reference, (4) failure in which the aggregate outcome of decisions is inferior to a competing alternative, and (5) failure where the cost of arriving at the decision is inordinately high. Simon (1957) coined the term "satisfice" from *satisfy* and *suffice* as a decision-making step where an acceptable threshold has been met, which applies to situations where an optimal decision is not possible due to the limits of bounded rationality (see chapter 3, "The Logic of Practice and the Logic of Operations").

NDM focuses on the cognitive functions of decision-making, sensemaking, situational awareness, and planning. The study of these cognitive functions in natural settings differentiates NDM from other models of decision-making that attempt to describe decision-making from laboratory studies or compare decision-making to a normative standard. NDM is an effort to categorize the complexity of time-dependent decision-making with imperfect information within the environment where the decision is made.

Recognition-Primed Decision-Making

Recognition-primed decision-making (RPD) describes how people use experience to solve problems with uncertain information and under time-significant pressure. Their experience rapidly creates mental models of the encounter that also suggest solutions. Rather than conducting analyses by decomposing the situation to its basic elements, experienced people limit their choices and quickly make a decision. The experienced decision-maker rapidly makes a situation assessment and option evaluation. The dynamics of the situation have a greater influence on decision choice than the second component of RPD, option evaluation (Klein 1993).

The RPD model arose from studies of firefighters' cognitive-task analyses to better understand how experienced fire ground commanders deal with time pressure and uncertainty. An RPD identifies patterns in the new situation that people have learned from previous experience. These patterns are picked up by relevant cues. This is a system of matching the situation to learn patterns. It may seem paradoxical, but the rapid decisions made from RPD are more effective than decisions made after careful analysis (Klein et al. 1989).

A note on cognitive engineering: cognitive engineering applies cognitive psychology to the design and operation of human-machine systems. Congruent with cognitive psychology, human factors, and ergonomics, this kind of engineering goes beyond human factors to study the worker in the work context and the controlled environment. It is a growing field in decision-making and may, at some time, enter the medical field and healthcare. The field of cognitive engineering examines decision-making from a normative standard, or how people *ought* to make decisions. The principles and constraints for the right decision come from rational choice theory, which is built from formal mathematical systems, deductive logic, Bayesian probability theory, and decision theory. Human intellectual and computational capacity limits the achievement of the ideal normative decision. Cognitive engineering attempts to bridge this gap between the desired normative decision model and how decisions are actually made; this is known as descriptive decision research (Lipshitz and Cohen 2005). Behavioral decision research identifies targets for intervention. Cognitive engineering would then identify if the prescribed decision training, decision analytic consulting, or decision aiding were successful in aiding people to more nearly satisfy the normative ideal, which is measured by the reduction in departures from formal normative standards.

We have discussed naturalistic decision-making, recognition-primed decision-making, and cognitive engineering in some detail, because their derivation from engineering principles makes them attractive for implementation. They are structured, have clear categories, and are able to measure outcomes. They rely on cognitive function but without the acknowledgment that stress will impair the prefrontal cortex and its higher cognitive functions at the moment when this part of the brain is most needed. These models do not account for novice or expert decision-making in completely novel situations, however, nor do they describe methods to modulate the fear response or ways in which one can assign value to information that changes.

The Limits of Naturalistic and Recognition-Primed Decision-Making
Naturalistic decision-making, recognition-primed decision-making, and cognitive engineering rely solely on cognitive capacities. The researchers who developed

the theories of NDM and RPD relied on highly experienced decision-makers and focused on high-risk decisions in dynamic, uncertain environments where the decision-maker is also under time pressure. All three systems define error as a deficiency of some type or failure to reach the desired level.

We do not take issue with their approach or these models. The situation we have in an HRO is quite different, though overlapping does occur. What distinguishes HRO from these models and organizational management strategies is a need for people to place value on information and their objective, keeping in mind that new information is constantly acquired, and previously acquired information needs constant updating. The attainability of objectives may change, and people will have multiple objectives. People must constantly change the value of their information and objectives.

> The director of an emergency department at a nearby medical center called to transfer an infant who was undergoing cardiac arrest. Through medication, he could gain a heartbeat, but it was quickly lost. We could not place a child this fragile in an ambulance with only three caregivers: a physician, a nurse, and a respiratory care practitioner. I asked the director if he could stabilize the child's heart long enough for the transport. He called back over an hour later and told me he had been unable to stabilize the heart for any length of time. We discussed whether this met the criteria for futile care and if would be more ethical to stop the resuscitation. Their medical staff bylaws stated that a physician could not pronounce death if a heartbeat could be obtained through treatment. I advised him that we would send our team.
>
> Because I was busy with some very sick children, I sent a second-year pediatric resident who was in her second week of her PICU rotation. Her goal was to be a general pediatrician without subspecialty training. Not too long after she left, she returned with the child, who was now stable on medication.
>
> After we completed the admission-stabilization process, she approached me to talk about the incident. She said, "They did what you said they would do—they walked away when I came in. That was the fear response, wasn't it? Avoidance."
>
> "Yes," I replied. Then I asked her if they had helped her with the resuscitation.
>
> "No, they did not." She added, "And I felt that freeze response in myself that you did to me last week." As part of my decision-making program, I have the residents recite the months of the year in order, from

January to December. Then I tell them, just like in real life, the proto-col has changed: recite the months in alphabetical order, out loud, without any help from your colleagues. Many people can reach six months, though they almost always mention only one month beginning with A. One combat veteran reached seven months, and one nurse reached eight.

I asked her what had happened, and she told me that she'd checked the endotracheal tube. Confused, I wondered why she suspected the endo-tracheal tube if it was working. She told me, "That's why I checked it— because it was working." She then elaborated that, by physically checking something that was working well, she was able to bring herself out of the freeze response and could then resuscitate the infant. She achieved stabil-ity of the heart sufficient for transport after twenty minutes of treatment.

Was the earlier failure to achieve heart stability because of a lack of knowledge or from the influence of the stress neurochemicals on the brain? An experienced emergency physician working with an experi-enced healthcare team responded to the stress of an infant undergoing cardiac arrest. Their response was neurochemical, which caused situa-tional cognitive distortions.

That is what I have taught: when you feel these reactions coming on, they are not a sign of weakness, inexperience, or lack of knowledge. They are a neurochemical reaction that can go away as quickly as they came.

—Daved van Stralen

Time pressure in the HRO is not about multiple tasks but about the time one has before the threat causes damage or irreparable harm. This situation does not refer to game theory but to how we manage to secure the environments we enter. The threat is not failure or harm to others. HROs developed with the threat imperiling those who were making the decisions.

I asked the officers in my training classes if they had ever been in *the fight*. "Yes," they answered, "we've been in fights before." I said, "There's a dif-ference between a fight to escape and *the fight*, where a suspect is able to escape but stays to try to kill you." This is the first time most officers have faced a threat like this. Many of the police officers I train have no expe-rience with people who are comfortable with extreme violence. Once they've been in *the fight*—and survive—they report that they now see and experience violence much differently than before.

—George Williams, international police force and tactics trainer

NDM, RPD, and cognitive engineering are similar to all cognitive models of decision-making in that they do not acknowledge that stress impairs the prefrontal cortex. Not only do people lose their higher cognitive functions, but they also will not recognize this loss. The role of the amygdala in the fear response is often discussed, but the notion that the loss of rational thought is part of the fear response is not. That is the importance of modulating the fear response to enable function during a crisis. Growing evidence shows that the anterior cingulate cortex plays a role in this scenario. The cingulate cortex can suppress the amygdala. It also is involved in error identification, and decision-making in this cortex is adaptive to reaching answers that work, rather than the binary yes/no or good/bad answers of the prefrontal cortex.

Error is also viewed differently in the HRO. How can you be wrong if you do not know what to do? "Can you commit an error once you discover it's an error? Was it an error before you discovered it?" These are two questions Karl Weick has posed (personal communication).

Error also calibrates our sensemaking and gives us a sense of our edges. If we only experience successful decision-making, then we may encounter serious problems. In an environment of uncertainty and threat, error gives us the negative feedback we need to identify the boundaries of safety. If you have not made an error in this case, then you do not know where safety lies or whether you can sense what is about you.

> "Remember: when making decisions, the threat has a vote."
> —JAMES P. DENNEY, LOS ANGELES FIRE DEPARTMENT BATTALION CHIEF

One of our two vignettes describes how a novice can successfully operate in a situation and environment novel to her and yet familiar to the experienced team that had been unable to succeed in the same situation. The other vignette describes how a very experienced professional can still encounter a novel and extremely life-threatening situation. We can see in both the same response, both neurologically and behaviorally. Rasmussen's skill-rule-knowledge framework is not objective and does not hold an experienced decision-maker as a standard for performance. An experienced professional may know the rules for routine experience and can operate almost without thinking. When encountering something completely novel, the experienced professional will be in the knowledge framework. A novice who is working in this routine situation may not know or recall the rules and will then also work in the knowledge-based framework. This is a way of thinking that can be taught.

A sensed absence of error does not mean that error is not present. I characterize the potential for error as being omnipresent in threatening situations, and it is our ability to employ calibrated sensemaking to root out small errors that can grow to catastrophic errors if not recognized and acted upon in a timely manner.

—Spence Byrum

Finally, we must acknowledge that people with limited experience (in their teens and early twenties) have performed exceptionally well in crises. They did not have the experience necessary for naturalistic or recognition-primed decision-making. They were also under threat, yet they were able to operate despite having impaired cognitive performance.

Affective Decision-Making and Cognitive Decision-Making

We most commonly study, learn, and use the cognitive domain in decision-making. In this chapter, we hope we have demonstrated that the affective domain of decision-making becomes a greater priority in a crisis. This is not to diminish the importance of cognition in decision-making but to recognize that the fear response will impair cognition, although not necessarily to the point that all is lost. HRO is built on affective decision-making in threat environments, and it is in the affective domain where the impact of impaired cognition is mitigated.

One part of affective decision-making assigns value to information, which means more than weighing the reliability or validity of information; instead, this refers to the relevance or importance of the information in that moment when the value of information changes in the flux of time. What helps us one moment can hurt us the next. Information must also be weighed for the degree in which it helps us reach the end-state. A more difficult concept is that information and multiple objectives must be weighed when they conflict or compete.

For the management of mechanical ventilators in a pediatric long-term care facility, we used the lowest possible breathing rate (below twenty breaths per minute) in case the child unintentionally disconnected from the ventilator. One cause of these disconnections is patient agitation. If a child became agitated, the respiratory care practitioner (RCP) would ventilate by hand with a ventilator bag and find a pattern that would calm the child. Then the RCP would adjust the ventilator to the new setting, thus freeing the RCP to call and discuss the situation with the physician. I generally accepted these new ventilator setting.

These new settings, however, tended to be 22–28 breaths per minute, and it might take several weeks to wean the rate to a safe rate. I became frustrated with the RCPs for not using the lower rates. One day, I became angry with them. Peggy Clements, a bedside RCP, became equally angry with me. She said, "You say we're supposed to hand-ventilate to calm the child. We do that, and you're mad." Now that we had the central problem identified, we could talk. (Probably not a method I recommend.)

I wanted a rate below twenty breaths per minute for safety, in case the child disconnected from the ventilator. The RCPs found that rates averaging twenty-five reduced agitation and *prevented* disconnection from the ventilator. We decided to allow the higher rates to stand, which prevented the emergency I was trying to treat.

Shortly afterward, all rates were higher than normally used in the PICU. But we noticed that most of the children were smiling; some laughed, and some cried. Some of the parents came to us and told us they hadn't seen their children smile for years. The higher breathing rates allowed the children to feel. They could now express their emotions.

Our new end-point for setting ventilator states was to "make the child smile." Our new end-state for the mechanical ventilator changed from maintaining life to *enhancing* life.

—Daved van Stralen

Deductive Reasoning, Inductive Reasoning, and Critical Thinking

We know of deductive and inductive reasoning as the universal to the specific and the specific to the universal. This is a somewhat confusing description and of little practical use. Of more practical use, we can think of deductive reasoning as "the facts *guarantee* our hypothesis," while in inductive reasoning, "evidence *supports* our conclusion." Though we find great comfort in deductive reasoning, it is of little use with uncertainty and ambiguity. In the HRO setting, we do not have facts; if we do, we do not have sufficient facts to prove a deductive hypothesis.

Inductive reasoning is close to how we work in an HRO. We seek evidence and strengthen the evidence we have. Stronger evidence convinces us to keep our conclusion. When we find that our evidence has become weaker, we adjust our conclusion to this new, evolving reality. This approach is shown quite well in the television show *House, MD*, where Dr. House will learn something or obtain new evidence and suddenly change his diagnosis, or where he looks for more information.

The ability to modulate the decision-making process is difficult for many clinicians. Because a fairly rigid, scientific, rules-based approach is taught in medical school, many clinicians find it difficult to "step away" from their initial diagnosis when presented with new evidence. Rather, they spend a disproportionate amount of time trying to conform the evidence to support their first impression rather than seeking additional information that is outside of their initial diagnosis.
    —Spence Byrum

The Bayes estimation theory for decision-making is also a major component in our reasoning. While the theory can be described in mathematical terms, we will use it in its more general form, where we adjust the probability of an event based on current experience. Imagine that you are deciding to bring an umbrella to work. You hear that it's cloudy outside, so you choose not to bring the umbrella. It rains. Were you wrong? In some parts of the world, clouds do not predict rain. Rather, the season or the time of day is a better predictor. Your subjective prediction comes from past experience and may not serve you well when you move to different parts of the world. What we accept as real in the complex, dynamic environment is less what we perceive or observe and more what we sense through interaction with the environment.
    The following are a few comparisons of reasoning strategies.

Reasoning	Deductive
Speed	Slow
Linearity	Linear
Basis	Facts; identify facts; data and facts are reliable
Process	Accumulative; facts guarantee hypothesis
Methodology	Classical logic
Objective	Precision

Reasoning	Inductive
Speed	Rapid
Linearity	Nonlinear
Basis	Evidence, strengthen evidence, discard weak evidence; data and evidence are not reliable
Process	Adjust conclusion from evidence; multiple iterations
Methodology	Modal logics; awareness of biases and heuristics
Objective	Accuracy

Reasoning	Critical thinking
Speed	Deliberate
Linearity	Linear
Basis	Facts; evidence; evaluate facts and evidence; data, evidence, and reasoning are not reliable
Process	Hypothesis derives from reasoning; multiple iterations
Methodology	Classical logic; awareness of fallacies and sham arguments
Objective	Best result

Conclusions

(1). Prevailing methods such as "First, do no harm" and dual-process thinking can inhibit adaptive decision-making and delay necessary care.

(2). Ambivalence or conflicted decision-making arise from unexpected threats with time pressure, restricted information, and not having a good choice readily available.

(3). A synthesis of vigilance and hypervigilance in decision-making may be the most prudent approach in situations with conflicted decision-making, while interferences with decision-making arise from stress impairment, biases, heuristics, and unrecognized fear.

(4). Only a few biases and heuristics interfere with decision-making.

(5). Unrecognized fear distorts cognition to create the fear responses of anger and avoidance and the freeze response.

(6). Early error identification/correction enables people to maneuver in dynamic and uncertain states.

(7). While deductive reasoning and critical thinking have a place in decision-making, inductive reasoning, for us, provides greater utility in uncertain or ambiguous situations.

CHAPTER 8

PROBLEM-SOLVING AND END-STATES

We make decisions for action; we solve problems for solutions. In both cases, because of time compression and uncertainty, we look for what works at that moment rather than the best action or solution. Time continually branches throughout the event and can take new turns unexpectedly; therefore, what action or solution works for us now may not suffice in the very near future. Numerous scientific studies and many discussions have discussed the difference between decision-making and problem-solving; we will make the division between decision-making and problem-solving as actions (decision-making) and solutions (problem-solving).

We have borrowed the concept of the "end-state" from the military to describe the course of action when we encounter an undefined or poorly defined event and we cannot make out what the problem is. The military defines "end-state" as "the set of required conditions that defines achievement of the commander's objectives" (Gortney 2016). In military science, the concept of end-states may be more useful in a crisis than deciding on an action or solving a problem. In a crisis, the problem may be undefined or so poorly defined that we cannot find a solution. We then may seek resolution of the events that will lead to a more preferable end-state.

In fact, the end-state may be the best method for the intuitive or undefined problem. In this situation, you are trying to reduce the amount of energy and resources that are drawn into the failing system. Our objective is to gain functional operational control, followed by collecting information and creating a solution.

It is the nature of the high-context VUCA-T environment—volatile, uncertain, complex, ambiguous, and threatening—that we cannot clearly define a problem. (See "The Environment" in chapter 2, "What Problem Does HRO Solve?") Different people might identify different problems, we might face multiple interacting problems, or we might have to deal with an active, threatening environment in addition to the initial problem. In these situations, we do not solve problems as much as bring resolution to the situation. We work toward a favorable end-state, then reevaluate.

Problem-Solving versus End-State Resolution

Problem-solving is a mental activity that combines the cognitive and affective domains of the mind. *End-state resolution* is organizational and includes command, leadership, and team formation. Both approaches share the same practical logic and logic of operations, but end-state describes a more ordered approach to the situation.

Problem-solving relies more on thinking, reasoning, logic, and decision-making. For our purposes, problems can be characterized in four classes: (1) intuitional, (2) undefined or ill defined, (3) defined, and (4) trivial. For decision-making we can generally correct our decisions more quickly; to correct a solution is more difficult because of the longer feedback loops necessary to differentiate successful from failed solutions. This delay can effectively mask any confirmation bias we may have. "Motivated reasoning" describes holding onto a strongly held belief despite disconfirming evidence (the cognitive dissonance complement of confirmation bias). Motivated reasoning can increase internal friction among participants and make solutions more difficult to identify or achieve.

We can plan for problems, particularly those that are defined or trivial in nature. The activities directed toward a solution commonly following the following approach: (1) define the problem; (2) generate alternatives; (3) evaluate and select alternatives; (4) implement solutions.

End-state resolution is an organizational approach that is used to engage an emergent crisis situation; it is directed toward the resolution of complex situations (versus problems) in VUCA-T environments. We approach this resolution with both safety and operations in mind. In this form of resolution, we: (1) ensure safety through operations, and operations through safety; (2) contain the problem and redirect the trajectory; (3) implement interactive, real-time risk assessment and management (per Bob Bea, Professor of Civil Engineering, University of California, Berkeley, personal communication); (4) control the energy and resources that enter the problem space.

If we cannot develop a way to reach our objective, then we decompose it into smaller steps that we can reach sequentially. This is an effective means of teaching problem-solving: the student decomposes the problem, often a procedure, into multiple steps. The student then amalgamates the steps as psychomotor skills and improves decision-making capabilities. We must emphasize that speed comes from smoothness, not quickness. In this manner, we decompose problems to make them more accessible and solutions to be more achievable.

Directing our actions toward an end-state may be more profitable by pursuing avenues with the least friction while also obstructing events that pose the greatest danger. We also work simultaneously to *increase our chance of success while decreasing the risk of failure.*

Reframing the problem or event is critical for both approaches. People bring their own frames to the problem (as well as the frames' importance), what solutions or outcomes they desire and will accept, any information necessary for a solution, the actions they are free to take, and their perceived abilities. When they encounter difficulty, they are unlikely to change any of these problem attributes; it is here that a more experienced person can reframe the problem by choosing select attributes to change and then observe changes in the other person's problem-solving actions.

The environment and problem both change over time, thus making communication with others critical not only for the events but also for whether reframing should or did occur. Reframing will change the problem-set or frame and our operational approach.

Problem-Solving

Problem-solving is goal directed; this differentiates it from decision-making, which is action directed. We seek a solution to a problem and don't simply decide on an action. In complex, dynamic situations, multiple solutions to the problem and even multiple objectives may be found. For example, we can solve the problem of fever and possible infection with any one of three approaches: (1) physical examination and expectant management, in which we do not treat but observe for changes; (2) laboratory evaluation; or (3) the empirical administration of antibiotics. Dieterly (1980) proposed a model of problem-solving that we find useful in our situations; it is based on whether or not we know the situation, the intervention, or the objective/result.

The new nursing home administrator met with the CEO, who wanted a specific problem solved. This had been a low-trust organization. The administrator met with the management team, stated the situation, and asked them for a solution. A week later, they presented their solution but were unsure if it met the CEO's criteria. They thought this assignment was a trick to make them look bad. He took a solution they had provided and used it, unchanged—much to their astonishment and further suspicion. Their solution needed revising, which they earlier would have interpreted as an error. When they were finally successful, they recognized that it had all been their work.

The CEO continued with this approach for problem-solving and distributed decision-making. The management team's sense of duty increased, and they began to work toward the greater good of the program. Sixteen months after the CEO arrived, the nursing home was in the top twenty-five nursing homes in the country and was listed in *US News and World Report* out of roughly seventeen thousand facilities. This happened three years in a row, with the only change being the use of distributed problem-solving.

— Jeff F. Lewis, LVN. NHA, MA, Sr. Vice President / Administrator

In Duncan Dieterly's model (1980), as shown in figure 7, to know all three elements (situation, intervention, and objective) makes the problem trivial—not trivial in the sense of not important, but trivial in the sense of being somewhat straightforward to answer. This may be compared with complex situations, where answers have different degrees of usefulness or safety. The defined problem is a well-defined situation, but we do not know what intervention will work or if we can reach our objective. These two problem conditions, the trivial and defined problems, are examples of where we can make the best use of protocols, algorithms, and clinical pathways. This is also a situation where the use of lists will have the greatest influence in reducing complications, errors, and other undesired outcomes.

I sent a ladder truck company to the rear of a factory to effect entry. After some time, the captain contacted me with an apology. He had attempted entry through a number of doors that he couldn't open, and he was sorry he'd wasted time on those doors. I told him, "You didn't waste time on those doors; you identified doors we can't open. That's important information."

—Joe Martin, retired fire department battalion chief

The danger of trivial or defined problems is the focus on knowing what the situation is and what rule to apply. We may disagree on the situation or rule, which can create friction between people that derives from their different sensemaking. Internally, we may fear that we have made the wrong choice and will be heavily criticized, so we focus on supporting our decisions, which is easy to do through confirmation bias. Doing so disengages us from the environment, and we no longer search for the discrepancy or disruption that may signal a serious problem down the line. Our focus, instead, is on the organization's rules, which make the problem conform to our biased sense of well-being.

Problem Type	Strategy
Trivial problem	Protocol
Defined problem	Identify what works
Undefined problem	Choose an objective
Intuitive problem	Engage

Table 11—Problem type and strategy (Dieterly 1980)

The most dangerous situation is strongly held belief, described above as motivated reasoning. This type of reasoning derives from cognitive dissonance, much like its twin, confirmation bias. In this case, belief carries more weight than evidence, which leads us to over scrutinize evidence that conflicts with our strongly held beliefs. When a threat is not personal, we may more easily develop motivated reasoning. This type of reasoning is more common than we may realize. Motivated reasoning is uncommon in people who have become conditioned to operate in dangerous environments with the live-or-die situation of their own physical vulnerability. People in these situations have likely seen the outcomes from those who strongly hold on to their beliefs as failure engulfs them. This is the reason we look to those historic HROs for decision-making and problem-solving approaches.

In an HRO, we are concerned with the unknown situation, as this drives the structure of Dieterly's undefined or intuitive problem. In this problem, we do not know our situation or the structure of the environment, yet we must act. Decisions can be made with a bias toward action for containment, control, or to generate information. Because the OODA loop, as we use it, is an information generator, this way of thinking has no errors. What we commonly would consider error becomes a marker of boundaries, the envelope within which we work. Negative feedback serves to ensure safety when we have recognized the error early and can change operations, and it becomes a sign of what path not to pursue, thus making our progress more efficient.

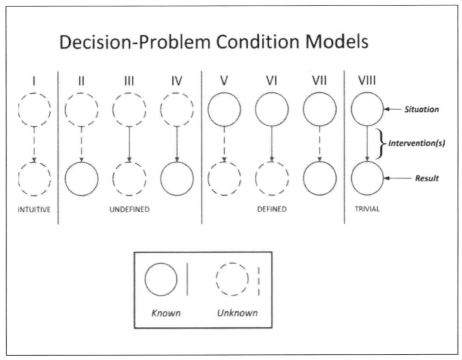

Figure 7—Decision-problem condition models (Dieterly 1980)

Decomposing the Problem and Amalgamation

If we cannot identify or reach an objective, then we can decompose it to smaller, achievable objectives. As mentioned earlier, the ABCs of resuscitation have been decomposed as resuscitation to airway, breathing, and circulation. We can decompose the airway factor further to manually acquiring the airway, identifying any obstruction in the mouth, identifying any obstruction in the upper or lower airway, and then protecting the airway.

When teaching complex procedures, we do the same by teaching multiple steps. For example, in the well-known ABCs for resuscitation, we open the airway, which in simple situations is quite straightforward. If we cannot open the airway easily with the head tilt, then we thrust the jaw forward and look for obstruction in the mouth. We teach this to a novice as several steps, but to an experienced rescue worker it is one step. We allow students to amalgamate the steps in the order of their preference and by what makes sense to them.

It is common in an emergency to have two simultaneous objectives. We strive for the desired objective while simultaneously striving for a less-desired, though more easily achieved objective. In a sense, we hedge our bets. This can confound the novice who is looking for economy of action—why do something you don't need to do?

In high-risk situations, we work to achieve success while also avoiding failure; this is a critical operational approach that is represented by the HRO principle "preoccupation with failure." As you observe people in an emergency, you will note that they are working for success. Observe closely to see if they are also avoiding failure. This is less common. Avoiding failure is more than redundancy; it means being vigilant for things that can go wrong and what people are missing. We work to increase our chance of success while simultaneously decreasing our chance of failure.

In teams with shared objectives, you may find that you cannot reach your objective. In that case, you have a subordinate or parallel objective, or you assist others in reaching their objectives and work to increase their chance of success. A French fighter pilot once described this to us: "If I can't accomplish my mission, I continue on and support the other pilot; I work to increase the chance of success for his mission."

The Undefined Problem

Trivial and defined problems are straightforward—we know the objective and, for the most part, know what will work. Top down approaches make use of cognitive processes, knowledge of the object and general principles (Gregory 1970) making top down methods useful in planning and situations where effectiveness and efficiency are paramount. Top-down processing uses contextual information to recognize patterns which one interprets from knowledge and past experience. The individual can then construct categories for the selection of plans and protocols. This direction of processing and problem structure is more amenable to planning and a straightforward, generalizable approach to problem solving. Cognitive processes predominate in top down processing.

Cognitive processes are neocortical, computational, intentional, with actions controlled by perception (Cromwell and Panksepp 2011). This is where we find the greatest use for skills and rules from Rasmussen's skill-rule-knowledge framework (Rasmussen 1983). James Reason (1990) built his error work from this approach. The advanced beginner and competence levels of the Dreyfus (1980; 2004) performance model of problem-solving use lists, rules, protocols, and algorithms which work quite well.

Undefined and intuitive problems, as described by Dieterly, present far greater difficulty because in these cases, you must engage in problem-solving without knowing your situation; you may not even have an objective you can identify from the circumstances. Bottom-up processing has greater utility in novel circumstances as it relies less on learning (Gibson 1966). Furthermore, because perceptions have greater influence on interpretation than previous knowledge and concepts, bottom up processing represents greater fidelity to the "real world." Neural process limits misunderstanding of the real world (Gibson 1972).

The individual will perceive useful stimuli despite the paucity of detectable, relevant, or salient information. The mind's ability to censor perceptions that do not make sense (Gregory 2015) poses a significant risk, but suspension of disbelief and reliance on *analog* data or signal processing reduces ambiguity. Analog processing refers to continuous values that change by time or situation. Affective mental processes give the ability to process analog data through use of analog processing to accept or reject by degree information based on the value at that time and in that situation (Cromwell and Panksepp 2011).

Use of analytical principles such as rules, guides, and maxims do not help the individual grasp the particular situation, necessitating the intuition of the expert level of skill performance (Dreyfus and Dreyfus 1980). Rules for control are no longer available moving the individual to the higher conceptual level where performance is goal-controlled and knowledge-based (Rasmussen 1983). Problem-solving must move beyond top-down cognitive processes and classical logic.

The subjective and emotional component of affect leads some to diminish its relevance even though judgment is an affective process. But it is the affective processes we use for uncertainty and threat: motivation, variable value on information, regulating fear responses, and modulating threat reflexes.

The undefined problem utilizes both affective and cognitive processes and from both a bottom up and top down approach. It is in such cases where we advocate having an objective of some type: always have an objective when going into any such situation. In some ways, the ABCs of resuscitation are objectives we have available to us when we see a patient undergoing respiratory or cardiac arrest.

When developing a free-standing pediatric long-term ventilator unit, we discussed methods to manage the ventilator without the need for blood-gas analysis, routine chest radiographs, medications for sedation, and an off-site physician. For the most part, we planned to transfer the patient to the nearby medical center with a pediatric intensive care unit. This worked fine until a severe respiratory disease season occurred, and the PICU could not admit patients. I discussed the predicament with the respiratory manager, Racquel Calderon. Along with the patients' baseline vital signs and the staff's familiarity with the patients, we decided that a calm, awake patient with good oxygen saturation would most likely have good blood-gas values. We gave this objective to the respiratory care practitioners (RCPs); if they could not reach that level of calm, then we would arrange for transfer to a higher level of care.

We felt comfortable with this situation because, for several years, we had calmed long-term pediatric ventilator patients using a faster inspiration and larger tidal volume (due to the use of pressure control ventilation) than that routinely used in the ICU, which is a technique I learned when I managed home mechanical ventilation for a young child with a complete upper neck spinal cord transection. She began to experience the sensation of suffocation despite having normal oxygen and carbon dioxide levels and despite having no sensation in her body. An increased rate for inspiration and a larger tidal volume relieved her feeling of suffocation. Upon checking her blood gas, we found identical values—there had been no change! (Since then I have learned that this is likely a lung sensation transmitted by the vagus nerve which bypasses the injured site of the spinal cord.)

With the objective of a calm patient, we managed nearly every patient who had developed pneumonia, severe reactive airway disease, or status asthmaticus while on a ventilator and initiated mechanical ventilation for dozens of patients in acute respiratory failure over the years. Later we learned to give faster ventilator rates to calm agitated children, which resulted in smiling children, even those with profound intellectual disabilities. Some of these children began to laugh, while some performed somersaults or learned to walk while attached to the ventilator. With this single objective, the RCPs adjusted the ventilator settings for the individual child rather than a standard or rule-based approach.

After experiences described elsewhere in this book, our objective in ventilator management advanced from a calm patient to a smiling patient. This objective created a discrepancy for ventilator settings between the intensive care physicians and us. Forced to explain this to our ICU colleagues, with the assumption that both groups were right, we studied the different goals, procedures, and physiology. In the ICU a patient is acutely ill, with either a damaged respiratory system or the need to control oxygenation or ventilation. The settings are a response to arterial blood gas analysis guided by minimizing damage to the lungs from mechanical ventilation. Long-term ventilation has a different situation, where there is chronic lung disease, use of a tracheostomy tube without a cuff to allow leakage of air, and an awake patient. One goal is to control arterial blood gases (i.e., maintain oxygenation and ventilation), and the other is to calm a patient (i.e., influence sensation).

With different circumstances and objectives, we use the same tool but in a different manner. The difference is in managing mechanical ventilation for oxygen and carbon dioxide (oxygenation and ventilation, respectively) or sensation (stretching of the chest wall). After years of success, the science caught up to us: this was likely stretch receptor sensation from the vagus nerve. We have taught our approach to hand ventilation of a breathing patient to EMTs, paramedics, and military combat medics.

—Daved van Stralen, MD, FAAP, and Racquel Calderon, MA, RRT, RCP, HACP

Approaches to Engagement

The following approaches allow those encountering an emergent situation to engage it, thereby changing the response from reactive to interactive, then becoming "enactive." The approaches vary, but the need to respond is particularly critical in time-compressed emergency situations.

Situational Awareness

Situational awareness (SA), sometimes called situation awareness, is often described as the intersection of what has happened, what is happening now, and what might happen in the future. Spending too much time in any one area can lead to a situation where we miss pertinent facts. Further, humans are poor judges of SA in others unless they are properly trained. We make the assumption that others are "seeing" what we see; as a result, people who are looking at exactly the same set of factors may make totally different assessments of the situation.

Situational awareness is an important attribute of an HRO and of the people who constitute the emergency response portion of the entity. Mica Endsley (1995a) defined SA as being comprised of three levels, defined by (1) perception (including recognition) of the elements within the environment within a volume of time and space, (2) comprehension of those elements' meaning, and (3) the projection of the elements' status in the near future. This concept is also often depicted as three *levels* of SA: level 1 (what has happened), level 2 (what is happening now), and level 3 (what might happen in the future). The system can be depicted as three spheres, the intersection of which represents SA.

The emergency responder, in cases of high stress and an urgent need for action, must make decisions predicated on the *balance* of the three levels of SA, as spending an inordinate amount of time in consideration of any one of the particular levels risks further loss of situation as the dynamic nature continues.

Spending insufficient time at any level has the potential to exclude information relevant to the decision to be made. Devoting inordinate time at any level leads to *channelized attention,* which may subsequently preclude the individual or team from recognizing new developments. It should be noted that both the team and each individual have SA; a degradation of either or both puts the decisions of the team at risk.

In his summation of Endsley's 1995 articles on situational awareness theory and management, Christopher Wickens (2008) points out that (1) "SA is not an action or performance, meaning that the understanding of a situation is quite distinct from the manual or vocal action taken in response to a situation"; (2) "SA is not the same as long-term memory knowledge, meaning that *static* knowledge is less relevant to SA than *dynamic* knowledge"; and (3) "The product of SA is not the same as the process of updating SA," meaning that it is possible to make the clear distinction between the learned (over a long period of time) properties and rules embodied in the mental model and its more dynamic outputs, thus reflecting the changing environment (the SA product).

What all this means in healthcare is that SA, both of the individual and of the team, is critical for the resolution of significant problems in time-compressed situations that affect patient outcomes, yet virtually no formal training associated with SA takes place in care delivery. Practitioners who are "good" in pressure situations do many of the things that are generally recognized to contribute to enhanced levels of SA, yet their knowledge has no formal means of being conveyed to the many other practitioners who would significantly benefit from their knowledge. It is incumbent upon all of us who are knowledgeable of SA to press for aspects of HRO training to be included in the curriculums of training for physicians, nurses, respiratory therapists, administrators, and all other professionals who deliver patient care.

Framing and Sensemaking

Framing brings the discussion toward what you saw, thought, and made sense of. Framing and sensemaking will more strongly support your decisions and actions to those who are not present, particularly those who review from a distance. Framing directs the discussion toward learning for yourself, for the system, and for the organization, which all develop from how you make sense of the situation and how you transmit your sensemaking to others.

One of the best wildland firefighters in the world is Paul Gleason. His stature comes in part from his work in over 500 serious fires as Crew

Chief leading a 19-person Interagency Hotshot Crew (the ZigZag crew). Gleason said that when fighting fires, he prefers to view his leadership efforts as sensemaking rather than decision making. In his words, "If I make a decision it is a possession, I take pride in it, I tend to defend it and not listen to those who question it. If I make sense, then this is more dynamic and I listen and I can change it. A decision is something you polish. Sensemaking is a direction for the next period."

When Gleason perceives his work as decision-making, he feels that he postpones action so he can get the decision "right" and that after he makes the decision, he finds himself defending it rather than revising it to suit changing circumstances. Polishing and defending eat up valuable time, preclude learning and encourage blind spots. If, instead, Gleason treats an unfolding fire as a problem in sense-making, then he gives his crew a direction for some indefinite period, a direction which by definition is dynamic, open to revision at any time, self-correcting, responsive and with more of its rationale being transparent.

—Karl Weick (2002, S10)

People act in a way that makes sense to them at the moment; no system or leader can prevent this. While this is a chapter on decision-making, we have found that, regardless of what people are taught or what the science of decision-making supports, *how people make sense out of situations drives their decisions.* After the crisis has passed, however, they often describe their actions in a different manner, most likely to justify the decisions they made or the actions they took.

For this reason, we work with novices to frame situations in a way that will help them make sense out of them. But even for the expert, as noted above with Paul Gleason, we may want to focus on how we make sense of the situation and frame our decisions and actions inside the frame of sensemaking.

Decision-making builds on sensemaking—we do what makes sense to us at that moment. Influencing sensemaking and reframing the situation or problem are effective methods to influence decisions when you, as the leader or expert, are not immediately present.

Police academy recruits are trained and tested in a variety of scenarios, including crimes in progress, robbery calls, building searches, domestic violence situations, ambush response, car stops, and dead body calls, among others.

The typical protocol for developing the recruit's skills for handling these scenarios is to provide a checklist of appropriate and exacting action and response steps which, when tested, are in essence a "pass/fail" evaluative measure. In other words, the evaluator will either check the box for "accomplished," "not accomplished," or "not applicable," depending on the recruit's performance within the scenario test.

When queried about learning how to perform in these scenarios, the recruits admit, when they are up front and honest, that they are memorizing the checklist rather than deciding to concentrate on "working the problem." In other words, their focus is on "getting it right" rather than "doing it right." This mind-set is often reinforced by well-meaning instructors, who take the initiative to write long narratives for the recruits to memorize that incorporate each step of the response process.

Added to this procedural memorization is the testing stress recruits find themselves under. These scenarios can be career ending when recruits fail; when asked what they're thinking as they process the scenario, the honest recruits respond, "I'm trying to remember what step 2.1.3 is on that testing form in the evaluator's hand."

It's been my experience that, given the opportunity, recruits welcome a dramatic modification to the training regime. I've had the occasion to tear up an evaluation form or instructor-provided narrative and tell a recruit that we're going to work on "sensemaking," "cue recognition and tactical prioritization," "problem-solving and decision-making," and "teamwork and shared goals." That is when their interest, excitement, and motivation to work and learn dramatically increase. They understand that the procedural checklist does not allow for a "problem-solving" mind-set, nor does it provide training that in any way tells them "how it's really done" in the open and ambiguous real world.

—Steve "Pappy" Papenfuhs, Retired Police Sergeant, Instructor Law Enforcement Constitutional Use of Force

Affect

How we feel about something is not objective; the value we give something is not objective; the attitudes and values we use to judge things are not objective. Feelings, valuation, attitudes, and values are subjective and personal judgments.

Psychologists call these things emotion-based sensations, or, more academically, "affect." Scientists and academics often discuss this affective element of sensemaking and the affective influences on decision-making. These definitions have insufficient clarity and utility, but we use these concepts for someone who makes decisions under stress. Stress may arise from the circumstances, or they may be caused by the "tacit" social environment of the organization.

When we discuss affect, it is common to think of emotion and the subjective as the polar opposites of objective. This is not a negative thing, as we may not objectively say why we like, or don't like, a specific food or a type of weather. This placing of value on things is affect. Affect also describes our attitudes and values.

The affective domain has a significant, though somewhat misunderstood, influence on our sensemaking and decision-making. In this discussion, we do not depreciate the importance of the cognitive sciences and the role of rationality in making decisions. Instead, we want to focus on the influence of attitudes, values, local valuation of information, and regulation of emotion/fear during these events. Not only is this difficult to measure, but it is unlikely to be observed by those who have not, themselves, experienced a live-or-die situation.

The denial of affect becomes a problem in decision-making. Some people participate in risky, thrill-seeking sports, or they participate in high-risk operations or actions without realizing they are being protected by experienced operators and do not, themselves, perceive the risk of death. They tend to openly denigrate the idea that "it could happen to me." The denial of affect also includes people who believe that they've "seen it all." This notion melds into a belief that they know how to work in extreme situations where their survival is in doubt. We provide an example below as an illustration. In this situation, police officers with experience in hands-on fighting with suspects often come to believe that they can handle a life-threatening fight—*until they are in one*. (The sidebar is also included in the "The Limits of Naturalistic and Recognition-Primed Decision-Making" section of chapter 7, "Decision-Making in Healthcare.")

The Fight

George Williams, international police force and tactics trainer and expert in the police use of force, describes "the fight." In training, Williams asks who has been in "the fight." Police officers tell him that they've been in fights with suspects before. He points out that this fight is from someone who is trying to escape from the officer. What Williams means by "the fight" is an assault where the suspect injures the officer sufficiently to attempt to escape but, instead, remains with the intent to seriously harm or murder the officer. Williams has observed different attitudes and different decision-making among officers who have had "the fight." Before that, these officers had a tendency to discount procedures, vigilance, and specific decision-making methods.

There are three types of hands-on fights police face where the suspect is not apparently armed with a weapon: the scuffle, the determined escape, and "the fight." While every cop will gain experience in going "hands-on" with resisting subjects, it is not a given that an officer will experience the most severe form of suspect resistance in his or her career.

An arrest goes sideways, and the officer's response assumes the typical methods of controlling the scuffle—until that unexpected flash of white light and pain of being struck, surprise, and loss of grip creates the space the offender needs to flee. Except this time, he doesn't run. He not only stays but closes the gap, renewing his assault with ferocity. The suspect isn't just attempting to injure the officer; the officer's murder is the goal.

Almost universally in this first experience of "the fight" is a feeling of shock. The officer is surprised by the suspect's fierce, ongoing attack. The officer has no context with which to orient to the suspect's intentions. From his or her middle-class background and prior police experience, the officer may academically have believed it might be possible, yet "What's going on?" and "Why isn't he running?" are questions that often cycle over and over again in confusion at the onset of this focused attack. Confusion increases the perceived urgency to solve the problem, but the officer cannot yet recognize what the problem is. An underlying panic may take hold, robbing the officer of problem-solving capabilities and resulting in ineffectual efforts to counter the suspect's actions. Often these increasingly futile attempts are a response to something the suspect did seconds earlier and will have no positive effect on the present necessary tasks. At some point, the officer may be too far behind, and any hope of survival ends.

Nearly unanimously, officers who have survived "the fight" report perceptual distortions, especially involving perceived time, saying that "it felt like it took forever" for them to realize these suspects' existential threat to their lives. They also report that they felt like they were "moving in slow motion and unable to catch up." In real time, this contextualization of the evolved threat likely required less than two to five seconds.

Time lost in a fight or on a battlefield is often time lost forever. The officer in this looping cycle of uncertainty and indecision is now in a severe tactical deficit, having given the suspect more than sufficient time to draw the officer's handgun from the officer's holster or produce his or her own handgun or knife or strike the officer several heavy blows or take the officer down in a chokehold. The essential tactical element of surprise saps the officer of the ability to act, while the suspect takes full advantage of the officer's hesitation. Injuries accumulate, creating a greater time deficit and deeper confusion and hopelessness. It is this gap in orienting to the violent context of the suspect's intent that is likely causational in a significant percentage of officer murders and a larger percentage of serious injuries.

—George Williams, international police force and tactics trainer

Doubt and Uncertainty as Strengths

HRO is a system of decision-making in uncertainty in which error and success cannot be differentiated until final resolution. The goal is to move the system from the indeterminate toward the deterministic, where decisions are fewer and more predictable. This occurs on the individual level and in organizations that permit such individual actions.

This model is focused on the difficulties in HRO implementation: rigid, vertical hierarchy to ensure communication; resistance to decision-making; and blindness to weak signals and error.

Judging Judgment

Judgment means as many things as there are people. The manner in which you think, or "how your think" invariably matters more than "what you think" when it comes to accurately assessing a critical situation.

How You Think Matters More Than What You Think

> "The fox knows many things, the hedgehog one great thing."
> —ARCHILOCHUS, GREEK POET

Philip E. Tetlock (2005) studied the success rates of forecasters in politics, intelligence, and journalist commentary. He found the worst success rate from those with the greatest certitude and higher rates from those who entertained the most doubt. To explain this finding, he looked to Isaiah Berlin's essay *The Hedgehog and the Fox.*

Hedgehogs, or the confident poor predictors, know one thing, and they know it well. They will extend their one theory to many domains with great confidence. Following Occam's razor, they believe that their parsimony of having one

theory overrides the numerous theories other people use. Their occasional correct predictions sustain them, thus strengthening their confidence. What makes
them most intransigent is to be right with an extreme prediction. But the cost
from their large number of false predictions is high. They did not entertain the
idea that other views may be correct. When they are wrong, they argue about the
implications of the event and focus on justifying their decision.

Foxes, the "superforecasters," know many things but to a far lesser degree.
They are shy about forecasting, adjusting predictions with new information. They
readily admit to being wrong. Foxes are self-critical and use a point-counterpoint
style of thinking that sustains doubt while reducing excessive enthusiasm. Foxes
understand that opposing and contradictory forces yield stability, a feature that
confounds prediction.

Superforecasters are diligent in pursuing information, updating their information, and revising their conclusions as more information becomes available.
They have a greater tolerance of operating under uncertainty, easily learn from
their mistakes, and improve over time.

Tetlock identified several quandaries of superforecasting and criticisms
against the methods that fox superforecasters use to reach their conclusions, this
despite the fox superforecaster's success rate:

1. The line between logical rationality and subjective rationality will often
   be blurry.
2. Failing to learn everything is not the same as learning nothing."
3. "Prediction and explanation are not as tightly coupled as once supposed"
   (Tetlock 2005, 14).
   a. *Explanation is possible without prediction*—we do not know if the ante-
      cedent conditions are present or if chaotic oscillations interfere with
      outcomes.
   b. *Prediction is possible without explanation*—for centuries, humanity has
      made predictions without knowing scientific cause and effect; in the
      complexity of the HRO universe, we rarely have explanations.
4. We must make our predictions clear and articulate. A falsifiable prediction cannot be made using hedging expressions such as "remote chance"
   or "maybe" or vague words such as "likely."
5. Ambiguity exists in the events and in the implication of actions:
   a. Ambiguity supports numerous predictions that depend on interpreta-
      tion and the meaning given to information.
6. We do not always learn from our mistakes:

    a.   Though everyone agrees we should change our minds when we make mistakes, in practice it is not clear what caused the failed prediction and which evidence is actually disconfirming.

How you think matters, and it *is* predictive.

Planning and the Puzzle versus the Mystery

In Chapter 3 "The Logic of Practice and the Logic of Operations" (Disrupted rationality) we described Adrian Wolfberg's (2006) mystery-solving as the application of full spectrum analysis to problem-solving. We find this level of analysis, *mystery solving*, is more productive in uncertainty and ambiguity than puzzle-solving. In dealing with uncertainty and complexity, it is difficult for us to separate information into various categories, and it is also unreasonable to follow a linear progression of actions. Instead, we consider information as a continuous spectrum for use simultaneously in a process where the situation is constantly developing. An example of this is the patient with respiratory findings developing into respiratory distress, respiratory failure, and, finally, respiratory arrest. Rather than using a cutoff value of oxygen saturation or level of CO_2, we want you to see this as a progression where the rate of change is more important than an actual number.

> We persuaded ourselves that we had conceived of virtually all possible scenarios and, by having observed a wide range of the pieces of the scenario, that we could effectively extrapolate a behavior that was underway or being planned. This was the puzzle approach we used in an attempt to understand the cold war world. What kept us from seeing clearly was a lack of healthy respect for the principle of uncertainty. Taking uncertainty into account—*approaching a problem as a mystery and not as a puzzle*—is at the heart of full-spectrum analysis.
> —Adrian Wolfberg (2006, 39); emphasis from the authors

We experience our perceptions in a continuous spectrum, while we make our classifications and categories in discrete divisions (Weick 2011). How people align their perceptions to a category leads to differences in sensemaking. Recognizing the presence of a full spectrum and using mystery-solving can reduce friction and miscommunication, particularly when the members of the team are kept apprised if the situation or the plan changes appreciably.

When we see the problem as a puzzle, we believe that data will fit in specific positions; with enough data, we will solve the puzzle. This thinking also contributes to the belief that digital data sources are perfectly reliable. When we see the problem as a mystery, we perceive it as being multifaceted and on a continuous spectrum rather than in terms of the binary either/or. We then move toward adaptive decisions and away from a preference for viewing decisions as binary or right versus wrong. We begin to collect information and constantly evaluate its position in context of the situation and the environment.

> "Insanity is doing the same thing over and over
> again and expecting different results."

Solving a problem in a complex, dynamic environment as a puzzle will mislead us in our solution and will make us believe the problem is over while it continues to fester. Solving problems as a mystery will keep us engaged and close to the situation. We do not know what pieces we need, where they fit, or how they function. We continue to work the problem or situation until it fully resolves.

Conclusions

(1). Decision-making is for action, problem-solving is for finding a solution, and we enact the desired end-state.

(2). When the situation is undefined or poorly defined, our best approach is to start with a clearly defined objective.

(3). If we cannot reach our objective, HRO supports decomposing the problem into subproblems and developing multiple interventions.

(4). Safety and operations are intertwined. Remember: "Safety through operations, and operations to safety."

(5). Doubt and uncertainty are strengths that protect us from making premature diagnoses and rigidly following an erroneous pathway.

(6). Rather than a puzzle, viewing the problem as a mystery and using full-spectrum analysis both provide a more robust problem-solving approach.

CHAPTER 9

THREAT RESPONSES AND UNRECOGNIZED FEAR

Failure *is* an option. Organizations react to stimuli from inside or outside the organization. Arousal is the sudden increase in alertness and ability to respond. Both good and bad stimuli cause arousal. Arousal from good stimuli can lead to complacency or decreasing defenses, but this chapter will focus on arousal as a challenge. The acceptance of arousal as a challenge gives us the insight of athletes who engage challenges to improve their performance and increase their strength. The final goal is to maintain system homeostasis through resilience.

Fear is the feeling of perceived danger that we observe in the classic fight-or-flight response. Threat describes something that can bring harm. We differentiate the fear and threat responses to reflect the physiological responses of fear from the threatening object that causes the fear. We have no control over what triggers our fear response, but we may have some control over the fear response itself—a dichotomy between adaptive or maladaptive responses. The threat response describes how we engage the threat in an adaptive way.

The Los Angeles Fire Department (LAFD) trained all rescue ambulance recruits in a specific "Rescue Ambulance Driver Drill Tower." (The "Drill Tower" is the LAFD training program for fire recruits that includes fire drills to learn procedures for firefighting.) To learn emergency vehicle driving skills we attended the Los Angeles Police Department's "Pursuit Driving School." Our final exam was a one-mile course for time, taken twice. Our first attempt was to drive as quickly as we could, and then we repeated the drive with the siren turned on. We all passed, but they did not tell us our times. We wanted to know what the passing time was and if we had beaten the cops. They told us, "If you drove faster with the siren than without, then you failed. We don't want you if adrenaline makes you drive faster." In fact, they did not want us if adrenaline affected us in any way.

—Daved van Stralen

Neuroscience has begun to distinguish fear from threat, which brings the field's views closer in congruence to those who work in hazardous environments. Science has used "fear" as both conscious feelings and as the behavioral and physiological responses (LeDoux 2013). Joseph LeDoux (2014, 2876) now recommends restricting the term "fear" to what happens "when the sentient brain is aware that its personal well-being (physical, mental, social, cultural, existential) is challenged or may be at some point." This brain mechanism operates through the prefrontal cortex and is felt as the emotion of fear. The mechanism for "threat-induced defensive reactions" occurs through the amygdala to create behaviors (LeDoux 2013, 155). These two classes of threat responses make intuitive sense— one of feeling afraid and one of physical reactions to threat. As described by Joseph LeDoux and Daniel Pines (2016, 1083), the two mechanisms are "(1) behavioral responses and accompanying physiological changes in the brain and body and (2) conscious feeling states reflected in self-reports of fear and anxiety."

This chapter begins with our reasoning for using live-or-die circumstances as our exemplar and foundation for HRO. The human body achieves homeostasis through a balance between maintenance and growth systems (the parasympathetic nervous system, or PNS) and the emergency system (the sympathetic nervous system, or SNS). This interaction produces unexpected results, such as gastric distress with difficult decisions.

This balance between two systems is also represented in the brain, though with several orthogonal systems; that is, they have separate axes yet interact. (Orthogonality is the relation of two axes perpendicular to each other.) Paul MacLean (1990) has described a popular model of a "triune brain" (i.e., in three parts) built in several layers upon the reptilian brain. We will incorporate his model into our discussion of orthogonal axes. The two axes are (1) between lateral hemispheres of the cortex and (2) between the prefrontal cortex and the amygdala.

Perceptions enter our brain through the left or right hemisphere, which is a laterality that differentiates novelty (the right hemisphere) from the familiar (the left hemisphere). A separate axis is found between the prefrontal cortex responsible for cognition and the executive functions and quickly impaired by the amygdala's fear reactions. The cingulate cortex appears to have a modulating influence in this impairment, which is possibly the source of the conditioning needed for military and public-safety operations. The two axes of perception and thought include:

- the *lateral cortical hemispheres*—the novel (right) and the familiar (left); with age, they meld to produce wisdom;
- the *cortex-amygdala*—cognition and rationality (the prefrontal cortex) and behavioral threat responses (the amygdala), moderated by the cingulate cortex.

Two more specific locations, rather than axes, are the pleasure center of solving problems and the calming effects of socialization. Because these things are neurochemically mediated, we will also discuss the neurochemicals that help us and those that hurt us. We close this chapter with the physiological causes of fear, why we do not recognize them, and the effect they have on performance and operations.

The Origin of High Reliability: Live-or-Die Situations

We use the live-or-die situation as the standard for operations in this book, because all of us use and have the same brain structures and the same brain responses, whether we're working on a dangerous fire line, facing a dangerous suspect, or making a mistake on the first day at a new job. We do not trivialize near-death situations but use them to more clearly identify the array of brain responses and to avoid superficiality—that is, those responses that work well for large but less dangerous affairs but will fail us in severe situations.

Live-or-die situations create a threshold, or liminality, marking an existence between realms of the survivor and day-to-day society (Morris 2015, 19). Within an HRO, the resultant behaviors and beliefs become normalized, and the individual is not set apart. This normalization is as much a part of the source of HRO operations as engagement in a particular event. The use of conventional management methods across this liminal threshold can result in catastrophic failure (Tempest et al. 2007). These threshold events can cause significant cognitive disruption to people's personal narratives; as their narratives normalize and *become comprehensible*, they become manageable (Calhoun and Tedeschi 2014). The social support and shared stories and anecdotes of the HRO facilitate comprehension toward congruence in a now-shared culture, thus preparing people for subsequent demands and increasing individual and organizational resilience.

This liminality, which marks the threshold between structured environments with a recognized internal logic and unstructured environments with unrecognizable or absent internal logic, is difficult to categorize and find words to describe. Historically, this information was shared through stories, yet stories are often derisively dismissed as "anecdotes" in the culture of healthcare. Within an HRO, stories carry vital, life-saving information as well as social knowledge. The stories HRO operators tell carry meaning and demonstrate a principle or truth, which is a process that teaches the expectations of how to behave, prepares the novice for these events, and transmits the social norms of HRO operations. After novices engage an emergency, these stories contribute to their new self-narrative, thus contributing to their resilience (Neimeyer 2014).

The literature on post-traumatic growth (PTG, discussed in chapter 10, "Sensemaking of Noise") shows parallels with the culture and operations of high reliability operations. Highly stressful events require a restructuring of our world view. While this restructuring can take a negative form, we will discuss the positive growth elements. After such an event, elements similar to HRO characteristics develop, including strength from the recognition of vulnerability, the acceptance of the novel, a feeling of greater connection to others, and the giving of personal values to priorities (Calhoun and Tedeschi 2014). Many high-tempo groups ensure the development of relationships between peers and between peers and superiors, thereby reducing authority gradients during emergencies. (Note that this situation does not mean "having your best friend at work," as described to one of the authors by a hospital's safety and reliability administrator as being similar to an FBI SWAT team: you want your best friend behind you. The program the administrator referred to exhorted managers to have their staff develop friendships. They missed the point that intimacy and openness are necessary for high-tempo operations. The "best friend" concept is not a matter of socialization but of the intimacy between colleagues that is necessary to openly discuss fears, concerns, and errors without fear of judgment or criticism.) These organizations do not allow individual people to become isolated from the organization or groups. They redefine their priorities *during* an event.

> "Always redefine your priorities."
> —WILLIAM J. CORR, CAPTAIN, LOS ANGELES FIRE DEPARTMENT

PTG creates wisdom and knowledge of the fundamental pragmatics of life and gives people the insight necessary to balance reflection and action, weigh uncertainty and ambiguity, and accept paradox (Tedeschi and Calhoun 2004). In the dynamic and complex events of an HRO, we continually encounter situations where the favor or disfavor of events rapidly changes, and the value of interventions can change not only with the situation but with time. Performed well, this creates a "dynamic nonevent."

Studies have found that even thinking about one's own death, without having experienced severe trauma, elicits reduced greed and selfishness, heightened spirituality, and enhanced gratitude (Cozzolino 2006; Burke, Martens, and Faucher 2010). Thinking of abstract, global concepts of mortality does not have the same effects as the specific personalization of one's own death. People with lower levels of death denial or fear of death have an enhanced sense of (self-reported) self (Cozzolino et al. 2014). Terror management theory (TMT) holds that the realization of the inevitability of death can lead to different responses—one bad and one good. The bad is the severe enforcement of rules and norms and intergroup conflict, while the good is open-mindedness and treating those outside the group with respect (Greenberg and Arndt 2011). (See "Sensemaking and the Post-Trauma Experience" in chapter 10, "Sensemaking of Noise.")

> In a class of forty police officers, it is not uncommon to have fewer than four officers who have created a last will. Very often, only officers with prior military experience have "death letters": letters for loved ones that often begin, "If you're reading this, it means that I've died, and I don't want to go out of this world without telling you..." Those in law enforcement often have a great sense of denial of death and of personal vulnerability.
> —George Williams, international police force and tactics trainer

PTG also contributes to resilience, which can be resilience on three dimensions: reaching the outcome, dynamic interactions between risk and protective factors, or reconfiguring one's life (LePorte and Revenson 2014). What is important to someone after experiencing trauma often differs from what was important before the trauma. What is important before the trauma is commonly theoretical or conceptual, while what is important after trauma is perceptual and functional. The aftereffects result from perceptions during the event, interpretations modeled by others after the event, and functional anticipations before the next event.

Someone who has limited or no experience in traumatic situations is more likely to make ineffective performance or operational recommendations for high-risk operations, while those with experience may not have the language to describe their experience or know the science that supports their recommendations. This is the quandary of following someone who knows the science but lacks experience versus someone who has the experience but lacks the words needed. This scenario underscores the importance of the self-correcting approach to accommodate both the lack of scientific knowledge and the use of imperfect, unreliable "street" knowledge: real-time interactive risk assessment and management (Bob Bea, Professor of Civil Engineering, University of California, Berkeley, personal communication).

The asymmetry of HRO is that the concepts and models that are developed, evaluated, and used in an environment sufficiently safe for the researcher may not work in a dangerous situation. On the other hand, what can work in dangerous situations can also work in routine times if we modulate some of the more severe responses. We act in a certain manner because we *choose* to, not because we *have* to. Unfortunately, emergency responders may not have the language necessary to translate to low-tempo environments, and researchers who observe high-tempo, dangerous environments may focus more on their own safety than on their evaluation of the operations currently underway.

HRO is both social knowledge and common knowledge; that is, all members are aware of this same knowledge that others have, thus creating a functional relationship between participants. In a crisis, we take actions because we *choose* to, not because we *have* to. To help with this idea, we will look at how brain structure and function help *exploit* the environment for growth and development while also *exploring* new areas and protecting the organism from environmental threats and predators.

The mammalian brain has evolved beyond the reptilian brain with the development of the PNS as a monitor of the organism's internal environment and the SNS as a monitor of the external environment. The brain contains various regions that bring these two systems together. This integration allows the organism to respond to internal threats such as hunger and thirst by acting on the external environment. Threats from the external environment galvanize an effective response from within the body. The vagus nerve, sensing thirst, hunger, pleasure, and suffocation, among other sensations, is a primary internal monitor for the internal environment. In extreme situations, these states of arousal are threat responses. When people interpret these states of arousal as the emotion "fear," these states become incredibly powerful motivators. Unfortunately, people have learned how to use fear responses to artificially or gratuitously motivate others. Fear can also become pervasive within the social environment to the detriment of individual people and the organization.

Homeostasis: Growth-Development and Threat-Emergency

We all have an alarm and response system to maintain homeostasis and operate against adversity. In human physiology, we see this in the autonomic nervous system, with its divisions into the PNS and the SNS. These systems run automatically, without the need of our awareness. The PNS is responsible for growth, while the SNS is responsible for alarm and protection.

Events in the environment can unexpectedly disrupt the organization's homeostatic mechanisms of self-regulation. The purpose of HRO is to use knowledge gained across the liminal threshold to prevent these consequential disruptions.

Many proposals have been put forth to prevent these disruptions, but few *prescribe* methods for *preventing* system failure that can also *respond* to system failure. HRO responds in this way through error identification, error correction, and interaction with failure. The limiting factor of other models is how (or if) they prescribe interaction with failure. The great majority of approaches rely on cognitive models, sensemaking, decision-making, and problem-solving but seldom discuss error management or failure recovery.

We will show in this chapter the limitations of cognition and offer insights into brain functions that support the interaction with uncertainty, time *compression* (versus time *dependence*), and threat.

> "There are no secrets to success. It is the result of
> preparation, hard work, and learning from failure."
> —GENERAL COLIN POWELL, US ARMY (RETIRED)

Remember, failure is an option. Thinking that failure is not an option contributes to aversive behaviors, dismissive language, withdrawal, and failure from *not* acting. Without interaction, the organization does not learn, does not become strong, and institutionalizes into its culture the belief that we cannot act.

The threat response to emergencies is not as simple as the SNS responses of fight or flight; the response also includes the PNS responses (1) the parasympathetic freeze response; (2) a parasympathetic nausea response; and, for our purposes, (3) the choke response. The fight-or-flight response is mediated by the SNS and adrenaline, processed through the amygdala. The PNS mediates the freeze response with cortisol and the nausea response through the vagus nerve.

Parasympathetic Fear Responses

It seems odd to include the PNS—a system for growth—as a fear response. This part of the nervous system supports feeding and lowering metabolism to reduce energy expenditure. Calling upon this system in the first stage of an emergency makes sense if the animal must stop moving to not be seen or to appear as though it were dead (many predators will not eat a dead animal because of the risk of putrescence). Another tactic is to become unpalatable through the evacuation of body fluids or waste (Natterson-Horowitz and Bowers 2013).

The Vagus Nerve

We tend to think of the vagus nerve as the nerve that slows the heart rate. In this capacity, it acts in a similar manner to a motor nerve by carrying commands from the brain to the organs. The vagus is also a sensory nerve that tells the brain about the body's internal state. The vagus is not only active in homeostasis but also in the body's emergency-response system.

Vagal response to fear. The initial fear response is actually a parasympathetic response to the vagus nerve. The freeze response protects a prey species from being seen by the predator. The animal must reach complete stillness, which is assisted by the vagus nerve causing, bradycardia (slow heart rate, usually accepted as less than 60 beats per minute).

Vasovagal syncope. When the heart slows down into bradycardia, the condition can induce fainting or vasovagal syncope. The medical term for this is "fear-induced, vagally mediated bradycardia." The same response in animals is called "alarm bradycardia" (although animals faint less often than humans).

Nausea and vomiting. Stimulation of the vagus nerve also causes loss of sphincter tone for some body functions to induce vomiting, defecation, or urination. Research suggests that this may serve a protective function by making the prey animal unpalatable. People experiencing extreme fear, such as from combat or rape, may vomit, defecate, or urinate. Victims of motor vehicle collisions may do the same thing; it is not uncommon to see small spots of urine in the crotch, evidence of mild urinary incontinence at the time of the collision. We are more likely to observe this response as nausea or an upset stomach when confronted with an unexpected event or having to make a decision. The response contributes to the commonly occurring aversion that prevents decision-making or impairs engagement of the situation. Of these responses, the nausea encountered in high-consequence decision-making, particularly someone's first solo public decision, is the single greatest block to bringing people to a High Reliability approach.

Air Hunger

Shallow breathing alarms the brain and gives a sense of "air hunger" or suffocation. The sensation of shallow breathing feels worse than breathing against resistance (Banzett, et al. 2008) and is caused by the state of the stretch receptors within the lung. For example, shallow rapid breathing is fairly comfortable, but holding the chest completely expanded during shallow rapid breathing soon induces a feeling of air hunger, despite no change in blood-gas levels *and* respiratory minute volume (the volume of gas inhaled in one minute, a produce of respiratory rate X tidal volume or volume of one breath). We observe this situation in novices when they have shallow, rapid, and sometimes irregular breathing while concentrating on a task. This kind of breathing increases their sense of distress, which can be relieved when you tell them to take a deep breath (taking a deep breath provides a generalized pleasant sensation).

The Freeze Response

The freeze response as loss of muscle tone. When we experience the sensation of severe threat, our muscles may not seem to move. This is actually a survival mechanism found in prey species that freeze or play dead, a process called "tonic immobility." The response is based in the cerebellum, specifically the cerebellar pyramis (Koutsikou et al. 2014).

The freeze response as mental freeze—cortisol and working memory. Under even modest pressure, such as when questioned by a superior, the brain seems to freeze and we cannot answer straightforward questions or solve even the simplest problems. This situation is neurochemical and not a deficit in our intellect. Acute stress releases cortisol, which appears to interfere with our working memory in the prefrontal cortex. When unrecognized, this gives us a feeling of anxiety at being placed in such an uncomfortable situation (LeDoux 2000; Dickerson and Kemeny 2004; Duncko et al. 2009; Elzinga and Roelofs 2005; Lupien et al. 1999). Unfortunately, some supervisors may have learned how to use this response on their subordinates as a means of control or abuse. Putting people into situations where they must answer questions under stress can induce this freeze. The unscrupulous leader or teacher will then continue the pressure and increase the freeze, thus decreasing people's performance, neutralizing their self-efficacy, and driving good people out of the program under the guise of removing incompetence (albeit artificially induced incompetence).

Chronic fear, stress, and memory impairment. Long-term exposure to cortisol, for example in chronic stress, damages cells in the hippocampus and impairs learning. This is important to understand for those people who believe that putting people under stress improves performance, since doing so actually prevents learning (McAuley et al. 2009) and can be responsible for a significant physical decline if allowed to persist. Poverty is one factor independent of stress that measurably diminishes cognitive performance (Mani et al. 2013). While this factor is not a problem within the healthcare field, it does have a pronounced effect on some of our patients by decreasing their health literacy, independent of educational opportunities.

Fight-and-Flight Responses

The fight response. The fight response is any offensive or defensive method that is used for protection. In animals, the response includes biting and clawing; for humans, we could add hitting, punching, and kicking. These are all physical manifestations of fight. Both the animal and human fight responses include intimidation and threat displays. Fight, in human behavior, is manifested by anger, frustration, posturing, intimidation by countenance, raising of the voice, and any other anger response.

The flight response. The flight response is obvious in animals but far less obvious in the professional workplace. Nobody wants to appear afraid; therefore, the flight response must appear plausible. We often observe avoidance, distraction, preoccupation with other duties, following other priorities, and various other "acceptable" excuses that plausibly allow the person to disengage.

Passiveness. Passiveness in these situations is not uncommon. We include it here because passiveness has multiple causes and reasons. It is easiest to think of passiveness as passive-aggressive behavior, a personality disorder with specific findings or a term laypeople use to describe their frustration when encountering passive people. Passivity can arise from the immediate fear responses of fight, flight, and freeze; function as a coping strategy to avoid stress; or a means to control when disagreeing with others: in effect, saying "yes" but doing "no." The leader or coworker will use different approaches based on the situation, the person, and the history of this behavior. Awareness of these different causes can reduce frustration while better targeting interventions such as the use of better decision-making methods and better education, the identification of purposes and goals, or the separation of the individual from these situations.

Choking. Choking, which refers to performance decrements that happen under pressure circumstances, differs from poor or freeze performances. We learn new complex motor skills in the cerebral cortex. With experience, the skills are transferred to the cerebellum. Because we cannot consciously control the cerebellum, any efforts to check our progress slow the normally fast cerebellar sequences. Though we discuss choking in this section about fear, choking is not a fear response but occurs from interference with routine. While we are performing a task, we experience an increase in demand to process too much information during the process or procedure. Even slowing down to take one's time can increase the chance of choking. Worrying about things one cannot control or becoming self-aware during an automatic process can cause over-analysis. Distraction that draws attention away from the task can cause choking. This is one reason that in Olympic gymnastics, no one but the coach can approach the gymnast during the fifteen minutes before the competitor performs. Contributing factors to choking include fear of a negative evaluation, the conscious awareness of an audience, and (oddly) overconfidence. These factors help us understand why the instructions we give people to help them during procedures actually may increase their risk of failure. The use of complex instructions increases our efforts for conscious control, which in turn increases choking. The use of single-word instructions is actually more helpful.

The Triune Brain versus the Reptilian Brain

We often hear of the reptilian brain as a cause of survival through self-interest in a crisis. This refers to the understanding that the brain efficiently keeps older structures and behaviors while adding on new structures and behaviors in layers. Paul MacLean (1990) proposed an influential theory of the brain as three interconnected units, known as the "triune brain":

- The reptilian brain (archipallium), as the oldest brain, includes the brain stem and cerebellum. This is where automatic behaviors are controlled. The reptilian brain serves for self-preservation and aggression (survival).
- The paleomammalian brain (limbic system) corresponds to the brain found in most mammals. It is concerned with the emotions and instincts, including the fight-or-flight responses and sexual behavior.
- The neocortex (neopallium or neomammalian) brain is found in the primates and is where higher cognitive functions occur. This is the rational brain, which is used for intellectual tasks.

This model of the brain is no longer well accepted when used to explain behaviors such as the "reptilian brain" or the "limbic system." We prefer the updated concepts found in neurophysiology.

Brain Laterality, Cognition, and Fear

Perception enters the brain and is related to novelty and familiarity. This information is not fixed, i.e. the novel can become familiar, as in the process of learning. (Handedness and its laterality are separate from the brain laterality of this discussion.) Cognition occurs in the prefrontal cortex and is easily impaired when threat perceptions initiate the fear responses through the amygdala. Mounting evidence shows that the cingulate cortex, particularly the anterior cingulate cortex, modulates this impairment. We cannot presume that this modulation will occur, just as we must not presume that cognitive functions will operate without decrements during the HRO event.

Brain laterality, or simply laterality, describes the specific functions or biases between the left and right cortical hemispheres (laterality, again, in this context does not refer to right or left-handedness). Asymmetry between brain and behavior is found in most vertebrates and has also been found in invertebrate animals (Frasnelli 2013). This asymmetry does not refer to left or right-handedness but to the processing of perception and motor activity. Whether the asymmetry is homologous or analogous is not clear. For example, foraging and prey-capture behaviors tend to have rightward-directed responses, which arise from specialization of the left hemisphere (Rogers 2002). Lateralization may have survival value by allowing animals to search for food while monitoring for prey (Vallortigara and Rogers 2005). Lateralization can come about because the right hemisphere has rapid, diffuse responses with global analysis, while the left hemisphere has focused attention with considered responses. In fact, some vertebrates use the left eye/right brain to explore novelty. This side bias can be seen in the response to prey on the right side and "agonistic" responses to individuals of the same species occurring on the left side (Rogers 2002).

The right hemisphere is adapted to respond to the unexpected or to identify novelty and support avoidance; it assesses multiple properties of objects and their context, noticing small differences between stimuli. It can maintain high levels of arousal and supports a negative, intense affect. The right hemisphere provides attention to spatial information and has diffuse attention, rapid response, and parallel processing. Right-hemisphere behaviors include the survival behaviors of avoidance, fear responses, predator escape, and aggressive responses (Rogers 2002). The right hemisphere also has a bias toward social interactions with bonding and affiliation, including facial recognition and reading facial expressions, gaze directions, and intonation (Cozolino 2006, 70).

The left hemisphere is adapted to identifying the familiar and supporting the approach to food and animals in the same species. It provides considered, sequential responses, which include inhibition of the right hemisphere and inhibition of responses while deciding between alternatives. The left hemisphere also focuses attention and is involved in feeding and prey capture (Rogers 2002). The left hemisphere is more developed for cognition, semantics, and abstract abilities. Socially, the left hemisphere has social emotions, awareness of other beings, and a general positive affect (Cozolino 2006, 70).

Across vertebrates, the left hemisphere is specialized for routine and established patterns of behavior in familiar circumstances, focused attention to specific targets, sustained response without distraction, differentiation between objects and categories, the attention to "landmark" usage, top-down processes guided by learning instructions, and sequential processing.

The perception and expression of emotion is asymmetric, with the right hemisphere superior for emotion processing compared to the left hemisphere. We also see this situation with asymmetry in expression, though we are rarely conscious of it. Emotions tend to show stronger on the left side of the face, which is also found in subhuman primates.

The basic difference, then, is that the right brain is global, with rapid responses and species-specific behaviors, while the left brain is specific and focused, with considered responses following decision-making. These behaviors are not fixed in a hemisphere but can transfer from one side to the other. For example, the right hemisphere responds to novelty, whether it is a threat or anything new, but with experience, the left hemisphere will process behaviors from novelty or threats. This shift creates an integration between the two hemispheres to produce a more balanced response. Learning also takes place in this manner.

Laterality is also visible in storytelling. Young adults tend to tell stories about their immediate personal experiences, while older adults often integrate both inner and outer realities, a process that produces understanding and is a central component of wisdom (Cozolino 2006, 46). Narratives are well-crafted anecdotes that describe the experience and the underlying principle, which are ordered sequentially but must be understood as a whole. Narratives integrate the neural systems and socialize us into a culture, because they require the participation of various structures in the brain, including conscious memory, knowledge, sensations, feelings, and behaviors (Cozolino 2006, 303–4).

Brain laterality is an underrecognized part of HRO. It can contribute to modulation of the fear response through a shift in the processing of perception and consequent change in location of sensemaking from the left hemisphere to the right hemisphere.

Because it processes language, the left brain has the dominant function in communication. It tends to recognize the familiar, name items, and categorize, all of which are necessary functions for communication. Vague boundaries and overlapping characteristics are accepted in our natural communication, particularly when the context is known between the parties. Discrete boundaries must separate categories for the purposes of academic studies, rule-making, and protocol formation. An HRO is *reluctant* to simplify because boundaries, borders, and categories are simplifications. It is in this creation of borders and the action of categorization where we lose information (or, paradoxically, we corrupt our communication).

The right brain dominates in novel situations where we do not have clear or shared definitions for communication. Members of a cultural group may have developed group-specific categorizations that, when shared out of the group, will lose their qualitative values. People have several nonverbal ways of communicating, such as with changes in tone, word selection, or body language.

We can see the effect of categorization when we draw a picture of something or someone right-side up and right-side down. Because we cannot categorize when we use the upside-down approach, we often find that this kind of drawing produces a more accurate representation (Edwards 1999). To the spatial side of the brain, drawing something upside down represents a shift from the verbal side of the brain to the spatial side of the brain.

We can also see the effect of *negative space* on comprehension by drawing a picture of our hand and then drawing a separate picture of what appears between our fingers and around our hand. Drawing what appears around our hand gives a more accurate likeness (Edwards 1999). Negative space is the space in a painting that is left empty in order to bring attention to the subject of the drawing. In sculpture, negative space is the stone that is carved away from the subject to focus attention on the subject. We find the use of negative space to be useful in describing and understanding situations. For example, if we look between the positive space—the part that attracts our attention—we see things we would have missed. This does not refer to seeing the forest for the trees; it is seeing *between* the trees. Negative space forces a shift from the verbal side of brain to the spatial side of brain.

In situational awareness, we must note that the situation (environment) can communicate to the brain (right side), or the brain (left side) can communicate to the situation (environment). This is the difference between searching for meaning in the situation (right side) versus giving meaning to the situation (left side).

The right hemisphere specializes in responding to novel and threatening stimuli (such as predators), control-escape responses, and the expression of intense emotions. The left hemisphere categorizes stimuli and controls established behavior with focused attention.

The Cognition-Fear Axis

Cognition is a broad term describing how we learn, understand, and make decisions. As noted earlier, the executive functions describe how the brain synthesizes information for the control of behavior. The prefrontal cortex (PFC), at the center of this activity, is well connected to other parts of the brain. The PFC also has some ability to modulate the amygdala, although for the most part, the amygdala impairs PFC function during stress.

The amygdala is the emotion center of the brain; it processes fear and pleasure responses and involves *emotional memory*, a memory that does not get extinguished with time. The amygdala monitors the external world as the alarm center critical for survival of the organism. Like the cerebral hemispheres, it demonstrates lateral differences. The anterior cingulate cortex (ACC) regulates behavioral flexibility, signals error events, is active in reward processing and performance monitoring, and informs the value of decisions (Kolling et al. 2016b; Shenhav et al. 2013). The ACC can also modulate the amygdala.

It is the interactions of the PFC, amygdala, and ACC in response to threats that create an adaptive threat response through the ACC or a maladaptive fear response through the amygdala.

The Prefrontal Cortex and the Executive Functions

Executive functions or tasks describe the activities of the cortex to orchestrate higher-level cognitive functions for complex thoughts and behaviors. While these functions are associated with the frontal lobe, they may occur elsewhere in the brain. They do not become fully developed and mature until people are about twenty-five years of age. These tasks may be categorized in various ways. We will look at basic functions such as forming goals and objectives, working memory, cognitive flexibility, fluid intelligence, decision-making, and problem-solving.

The prefrontal cortex plays the central role in *forming goals and objectives* and then in devising the plans of action required to attain those goals. This is forward looking and proactive rather than reactive, since it requires one to conjure internal representations of the future.

Working memory, both verbal and nonverbal, involves holding information in mind and mentally working with it. This type of memory is critical for making sense of anything that unfolds over time, because we must hold in our mind what happened earlier and relate that to what comes later. This situation differs from short-term memory, which refers to simply holding information in mind without manipulating the information. The two systems are linked to different neural subsystems, with working memory relying on the dorsolateral prefrontal cortex.

Cognitive flexibility refers to having the ability to change perspectives spatially or interpersonally; the term also refers to being flexible enough to adjust to altered demands or priorities, to admit you were wrong, and to take advantage of sudden or unexpected opportunities. Inhibitory control involves being able to control one's attention, behavior, thoughts, and/or emotions to override a strong internal predisposition or external stimulus and instead to do what is needed.

Fluid intelligence is the ability to reason, problem-solve, and see patterns or relations among items. This form of intelligence includes both inductive and deductive logical reasoning and involves being able to figure out the abstract relations that underlie analogies.

Decision-making can be deterministic or ambiguous. Deterministic decision-making is a single correct solution intrinsic in the situation. This system is called "veridical" (i.e., truthful) decision-making because it is directed toward a truth that can be known and is often accomplished algorithmically. "Ambiguous" decision-making does not have an intrinsically correct solution; it has value. Ambiguous decision-making is a form of adaptive decision-making, such as choosing what is good at the time, what is practical in a given situation, or prioritization.

Related functions include self-regulation, which refers to processes that enable us to maintain optimal levels of emotional, motivational, and cognitive arousal. The term refers primarily to the control and regulation of one's emotions and overlaps substantially with inhibitory control.

The Amygdala

The amygdala plays a key role in processing emotions and is linked to both fear responses and pleasure; it also contributes to our feeling of safety. The brain learns what is dangerous when fear pathways are activated and what is safe when its pleasure-reward circuits fire. The amygdala is involved with both. The amygdala has more projections into the prefrontal cortex than the other way around. Thus, when activated, the amygdala impairs cognitive thinking, which is the function of the prefrontal cortex. This is a critical fault of many sensemaking and decision-making models, since stress impairs cognitive thought.

The optic nerve takes stimuli into the brain and the amygdala. Some of these actions are hardwired, such as the sinusoidal form (represented in snakes) that alarms primates. The amygdala can also identify a threatening or frowning face in a crowd of faces. Some of these behaviors are present from birth, and some are learned through emotional memory (as noted earlier, the only memory that does not get extinguished with time).

The olfactory nerve (the first cranial nerve) is one of two cranial nerves (the other is the optic nerve) to go directly to the brain, bypassing the brainstem. A smell can rapidly increase psychological (emotional) and physiological states (Zald and Pardo 1997). For example, smells are associated with nostalgia, which evokes a pleasant yearning for the past. Smells are also alarm signals; some smells will immediately induce vomiting. Our sense of smell warns us of spoiled food, a danger to those with anosmia or for elderly people whose sense of smell has faded. This sudden alarm response will also fade rapidly, and we soon become unaware of the smells around us.

Emotional memory. The amygdala also links emotion and memory. Through classical fear conditioning, the animal associates fear with a stimulus. Later, any related stimuli will elicit the same fear response. This system is the neurophysiology behind post-traumatic stress.

The identification of subtle danger is adaptive. Someone who consistently works in a high-risk environment may develop sensitivity to the environment for these cues. A benign but similar cue may elicit a response to a past danger. That is, *the trigger is from the past, but the response is in the present.*

We can see some evidence of emotional memory in ourselves when something, innocuous or otherwise, not only catches our attention but also begins a drive to action. Likely, that innocuous trigger was an early herald to a previous emotional experience. Old-timers may respond out of proportion to the event, which is likely linked to a stressful moment in their past. This may be linked to a stressful on-the-job event or an event from another experience. We must also realize that the trigger may be from an experience from the family in which they grew up, "family of origin" in psychology.

A colleague once called for assistance in treating a child with severe upper airway obstruction. Afraid of complete airway blockage, the physician asked me for treatment advice. After I heard the child crying in the background, I knew the child was in far less danger than the team surmised. Rapidly covering the elements of a specific respiratory exam the physician had used for the child, the physician acknowledged that the previously administered therapy was having the desired effect.

I drove to the hospital and helped the team complete the care for the child and start management. The physician then took me into a private room, angry that I had not come immediately but instead had "just talked on the phone." I tried to explain, but he was too angry. His anger built to a crescendo, then the physician rapidly told me of a personal experience he'd had in the military at a medical care facility with a critically ill or injured sailor. The corpsmen were worried the sailor would die. The physician had called for helicopter transport, but the commanding physician at the main hospital had refused: he said the sailor could be cared for at the facility, and there was too much fog. The physician told me that helicopters had flown in worse fog, and he didn't know why the commanding physician had refused the transfer; he would only talk on the phone.

The trigger for his anger was my action on the phone. His response was to that commanding medical officer.

—Daved van Stralen

People with post-traumatic stress show exaggerated amygdala responses, deficient PFC function (particularly in the ventromedial PFC, closely linked to the ACC), and the ACC. Van Wingen et al. (2011) studied soldiers deployed to combat and found a change in amygdala reactivity in soldiers following combat stress in the absence of self-reported post-traumatic stress symptoms. This finding suggests that these changes are an adaptive response to stress: the people who *perceived* little threat showed an enhanced ability of the ACC to suppress the amygdala. This idea supports the view that it is the cognitive appraisal of threat that determines the response to stress, rather than the actual threat exposure itself.

The locus coeruleus mediates many of the sympathetic effects during stress and plays a factor in stress and panic.

The Anterior Cingulate Cortex

The anterior cingulate cortex (ACC) lies between the thinking, cognitive prefrontal cortex and the feeling, emotional amygdala. Through its connections with the two systems, it plays a significant role in affect regulation to control any emotions that may interfere with thought processes during a dangerous situation. The ACC is the cortical area where error perception and identification occurs; it is also where regulatory and executive processes interact.

Self-regulation. The ACC regulates the perception of physical and social pain, processes reward information, monitors conflict, and detects error (Posner et al. 2007). This regulation contributes to controlling incoming information and providing orientation to avoid conflicting responses in behavior.

Conflict resolution. The rostral anterior cingulate cortex is associated with the resolution of emotional-conflict activity. Activation of this area during high-conflict resolution trials is accompanied by a concomitant reduction of activity in the amygdala. The degree of reduction, as well as the reduction in autonomic responsivity, is related to subjects' behavioral success at emotional-conflict resolution, which increases with experience.

Conflict monitoring. When two competing choices must be made in a difficult task, the ACC interprets the conflict between choices in the task difficulty. Doing so requires the ACC to place subjective value on choices.

Updating of information and beliefs. The existence of multiple signals to the ACC allows it to update information, beliefs, and internal models of the environment. This updating contributes to commitment to a course of action, evaluation of associated costs, and exploration of alternative courses of action (Kolling et al. 2016a).

Adaptive decision-making. Decisions involving evaluation of the outcome of choices, positive or negative, show as brain activity in the anterior cingulate cortex. In contrast, decisions that attend to explicit consequences show activity in the orbitofrontal cortex.

Top-down regulation of the amygdala. In the beginning of this chapter, we discussed post-traumatic growth. We now see that the amygdala plays a part in this growth. It can both suppress growth and create incapacitating emotional memories. The PFC and the ACC can suppress a portion of the amygdala's response, thus contributing to suppression of the fear response.

Reappraisal. We can modulate the processing of an emotional stimulus through deliberate and conscious use of top-down executive control over the amygdala through reappraisal (Etkin et al. 2011). Reappraisal is a cognitive technique used to modify the appraisal of a stimulus to change its ability to initiate an emotional response. We do this by creating an additional positive appraisal that competes with the initial negative emotional appraisal we had made. This activity occurs in both the ACC and a portion of the PFC. Reappraisal, distraction, and distancing are associated with decreased amygdala activity, while PFC activity is increased (Stevens et al. 2011). Suppression increases amygdala activity. Cognitive-reappraisal strategies appear to suppress the amygdala through a specific region of the PFC and by a separate network containing the ACC and the insular cortex (Diekhof 2011).

Regulation of emotional conflict. We want any signal of potential danger to interfere with our attention or task at hand, but not to the degree that we cannot think; nor does every threat require our attention. The amygdala (and a part of the PFC) tracks the amount of emotional conflict from an environmental signal, while the ACC resolves the conflict (Etkin et al. 2006). In high-conflict situations, the ACC appears to reduce the activity of the amygdala.

Fear conditioning. Fear conditioning is the regulation of fear responses (rather than the inhibition of the fear response) and is combined between the ACC and the PFC (Etkin et al. 2011). A specific region of the PFC may be a general controller of the perceived fear and aversion that modulate the amygdala (Diekhof 2011).

Neurofeedback. By using positive autobiographical memories and neurofeedback, people can self-regulate the amygdala (Zotev et al. 2011).

Reward System, Social Rewards, and Neurochemicals

The brain's reward system includes the neurotransmitter dopamine, probably the most important reward system in the brain. The ventral tegmental area (VTA), a principal dopamine-producing area, connects to the nucleus accumbens through one pathway and to the cerebral cortex through a second pathway. Dopamine mediates the rewarding effects of an activity such as problem-solving, though it may have gained more attention for its role in addiction. Dopamine release during problem-solving explains why people will solve crossword puzzles or engage in other mental exercises. Dopamine creates pleasurable feelings when it is released. This general arousal, and the single focus it generates, are important in creative thinking and problem-solving. This may be the driver for change to HRO methods.

The amygdala helps establish a relation between environmental stimuli and whether an experience was rewarding or aversive. Dopamine and reward or reinforcement are our sources of motivation and incentive drive.

The SNS, when activated, releases adrenaline and cortisol. Adrenaline is responsible for the increased metabolic activity in the fight-or-flight response. The cardiovascular effects of this release include increased heart rate and blood pressure, while the respiratory effects include an increase in respiratory rate and tidal volume of the lungs as well as opening of the airways through bronchodilation. Other metabolic effects include the release of glucose. The central nervous system's effects include increased attention and dilation of the pupils.

Cortisol, as a stress hormone, prepares the body for fight or flight by increasing glucose release from glycogen in inhibiting insulin production. Cortisol narrows the arteries and also releases proteins that can cause inflammation. As a short-term release, cortisol helps with stress. In contrast, chronic release of cortisol is damaging to the body.

The neural chemicals—oxytocin, dopamine, and serotonin—are not only present in the absence of stress, but they also mitigate stress. Oxytocin is a neural peptide hormone originally identified to cause postpartum uterine contraction and the "letdown" reflex for breast-feeding. It has since been identified as a behavioral and prosocial hormone released through touch. Oxytocin has been shown to increase bonding, trust, facial recognition, and empathy while reducing fear and anxiety. Dopamine stimulates the pleasure and motivation circuits in the brain and is released with problem-solving. Testosterone decreases talking and interest in socializing. Serotonin provides calm, but it is not clear if this can be manipulated for our benefit.

While events, the system, or the culture can propagate the fear that triggers the release of the stress hormones of adrenaline and cortisol, these factors can also propagate the hormones of oxytocin and dopamine. The latter hormones also increase motivation and mood.

Stress

The following discussion of stress and fear is drawn from the model of Richard Lazarus (2006) and Raymond Novaco (1979). Demands and expectations come from the environment. Demands are external to us and are a part of the problem frame. Expectations are social and subjective; they develop from our own mind or from those around us (either from our team or the public). Demands must be met; expectations do not. Yet it is often expectations that act as the greater drivers, rather than demands for our actions; expectations are also how we judge success.

As leaders, we must work with our staffs to clarify whether it is an expectation or a demand that must be met. If we receive an expectation, then we must identify if the expectation comes from outside the organization; from peers, subordinates, or superiors; or from one's own, internal, expectations. In the final analysis, this must be weighed and valued by the individual.

Attributes and resources are found within the organization and the individual. Attributes are what people bring to the situation and include knowledge, attitudes, and abilities in decision-making and capabilities in problem-solving. Resources are external to the person and are what people can call upon. "If you don't have it with you, then it doesn't exist" is a common fire department saying. Time is a separate element in resource management, and resources must be available *when* they are needed.

Resources describe the ability to draw upon support, not simply having access to the support. One author wrote a chapter for a book on patient safety and included the phrase, "Call me if you need me, but remember, calling is a sign of weakness." The editor removed the paragraph because the statement could not be verified by an academic article (though, oddly, the editor had heard this phrase during his residency training). Nonverbal communication methods can limit or block in private the support people publicly offer.

Resources contribute to someone's strength long before a crisis. During routine or extramural interactions, someone who acts as a resource may confer knowledge or skills. This background resource material is not recognized but is made significantly different by the status of the person. For example, an administrator may have a friend who is a lawyer or physician. If the administrator has a legal or medical question, then an informal phone call is a learning experience that could prove useful in a later emergency. This informal resource experience will not be nearly as available to someone with lower social status or experience. An unrecognized source of strength in more senior people that reflects "common knowledge" is not necessarily common.

As leaders, we help staff increase their attributes, internal strengths, and abilities by modeling, teaching what is salient, framing the problem, showing how to make decisions pre-event, and interpreting the details after the event. The organization is a resource, and people's job is to call, and call early, for those resources.

Stress occurs when demands and expectations exceed attributes and resources. Stress, in this model, leads to coping behaviors. Maladaptive coping behaviors include all the unrecognized fear responses (see figure 8). Adaptive behaviors include reevaluating demands, evaluating expectations, turning to resources, and reframing the problem, among other things. In this model:

- Stress occurs when demands and expectations are greater than resources and attributes.
- Coping can be negative or positive.
- Positive coping leads to reevaluation of demands and expectations.
- Long-term coping increases people's knowledge and skills.

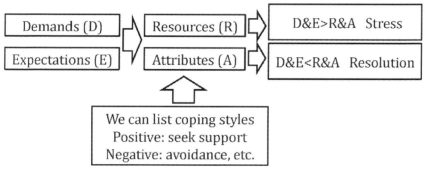

Figure 8—Stress schematic

People have an easier time approaching a problem when they can differentiate expectations from demands, feel supported, and are free of meeting expectations if necessary. Also, more often than organizational leadership will freely admit, staff members are not always fully aware of the support and resources available to them. Waiting for the staff to ask for assistance may instill confidence in leaders that they are a resource, but in truth the staff needed assistance but did not want to bother their superiors. This model also supports lessons learned that are specific to particular experiences as a means of increasing people's attributes and identifying where the organization's resources can be improved.

Unrecognized Fear Responses

We tend to think of a fear response as something physical, such as the fight-or-flight response. Most people do not recognize anger or avoidance as fear responses. We also tend to see confusion and fear as weakness or failure. These are all fear responses mediated by neurochemicals. They can come on with incredible speed and can be interrupted almost as quickly when we accept them as simple neurochemical effects in the brain eliciting an emotional response.

Calling fear "fight or flight" leads people to consider fear as belligerence or patently running away. We characterize these unrecognized fear responses as unrecognized because, in a more civil environment, we do not hit people or run away in response to fear.

> When I ask people about the meaning to them, personally, when their superiors angrily and publicly criticized them or complained about their actions, people generally respond by saying that they probably didn't do the right thing, and they would then actively work to improve their performance.
>
> I then describe the fight response as reactive anger that is often directed at someone and is actually a fear-driven response. They quickly understand this sublimation, or redirection, of fear to be the emotion of anger. They just as readily appreciate that nothing they can personally do and no amount of improvement in their performance will resolve that person's anger, because it is a fear response to something else in the environment.
>
> We then return to the first response: anger in a superior was a signal that the subordinate's performance was inadequate. They now accept their previous misunderstanding of anger as being caused by their performance and accept anger as a fear response within their superiors in reaction to something independent of them, the subordinates.
>
> —Daved van Stralen

Adrenaline mediates fight and flight; cortisol mediates freeze. Fear is a neuro-chemical event that is triggered from the environment through the amygdala but operates within the prefrontal cortex. Once triggered, self-awareness can lead to reappraisal. In the unconditioned person, however, this is unlikely to happen. Unfortunately, the fear behaviors manifesting in aggression and anger have become common and accepted in today's culture through social learning and through movie and television representations. Character-driven movies with introspective lead actors (such as *Shane*) have been replaced with action, retribution, and vengeance movies. Sadly, the effects of these fear responses on those who are subjected to this behavior, as well as the results within the organization, generally go unrecognized.

HRO is a functional approach—how the fear response affects high-risk operations. The effect of the fear response is a continuous spectrum ranging from mild to debilitating, experienced to surmised, and witnessed to assumed. We are interested in academic categorizations and mechanisms to the degree that we can better understand the sources of fear responses and their mitigation. In fact, this categorization has been the only way we have been able to connect neuroscience, fear, anger, aversion/avoidance, emotion, and leadership to the unrecognized, almost gratuitous, causes of performance deficits. The fear responses are real and damaging to both personnel and the organization.

The academic separation of anger from fear may clarify academic discussions and research, but this separation comes at a cost to understanding human performance and operations in adverse or hostile environments. Anger and fear both arise from high-arousal states reliant on context and past experience. Fear is an aversive state that causes protection and withdrawal, while anger is an approach system (resource acquisition) that occurs when our goals are blocked. Blocking withdrawal can shift the defensive system into defensive aggression, and the fight response can then ensue. Blocking the fight response—since doing so leaves belligerents without an escape or route for withdrawal—increases the severity of their anger. This is a reason to never publicly corner people into situations they cannot escape—physically, emotionally, or verbally—since this affects their public image.

Because fear is such a strong motivator, some people intentionally use fear as a tool for motivation. Unfortunately, over the long term, this use leads to docility, the loss of initiative, aversion/avoidance, submissive behaviors, and avoidance of making decisions. Self-protective behaviors include the careful use of words, phrases, and clichés that put a distance between people and their statements or decisions. Talking to people with an ear for this "self-protective talk" is one method of identifying the presence of unrecognized fear and the use of instrumental anger in a program.

The unrecognized *fight* responses include anger and frustration, which manifest in aversion, plausible avoidance, distraction, delay, and denial behaviors. Unrecognized *freeze* responses include freezing, confusion, an unsettled feeling in the stomach, and possibly nausea. Nausea is commonly associated with the first critical decision people make or the first time someone provides information that is not verified and will be used for an action. If people cannot get through the nausea and make the decision, they may then become averse to making decisions. This situation also contributes to being averse to uncertainty and ambiguity, thus preventing engagement in unexpected or evolving situations. In our experience, this is a major impediment when introducing HRO or when developing people who will engage a discrepancy or disruption in the VUCA-T environment. People who do not move past this feeling of nausea often move upward in the hierarchy. One hallmark of this type of person is the avoidance of engaging difficult situations. We will leave this for another discussion, but studying a problem for an effective solution is different than avoiding the problem, delaying conclusions, or "kicking the can down the road."

Anger in Our Patients and Families

Anger among patients is caused by a variety of factors. We present two examples of anger as the expression of an underlying emotion. These two cases come from chronic illness and critical illness.

(1). People who have a chronic illness, or the parents of a child who has a chronic illness, may feel cheated of their health. They cannot publicly acknowledge or discuss this emotion, however, because they believe "we must play the hand we've been dealt." That is, accept their circumstances. The limits of this belief arise when circumstances overwhelm a chronically stressed person or family. Outside their system, we are unaware if a small demand will overwhelm a weakened person; sadly, some treat these unfortunate people as being overly demanding. The patients or their families, over time, come to believe that they only receive help when they express anger, or that their frustration leads to this anger, which elicits their desired response.

This situation may be similar to Kahneman's finding among fighter-pilot instructors (see chapter 4, "HRO and the Environment") when students improved after criticism and deteriorated after praise: regression to the mean. With the same dynamic, family members may remember improvement in the condition of their loved one after they express anger at healthcare staff and remember any apparent deterioration in level of care after they give praise to healthcare staff. It also may be that anger is the patient's remaining means to impress on staff the seriousness of the situation or the patient's only means of gaining the necessary medical attention. Operant conditioning (i.e., the environment operates on the unaware person), in a taxed healthcare environment, then creates these behaviors and beliefs.

Nora Beth Cochran-Gomez, a respiratory care practitioner, excitedly told me, "It worked!" She then explained that she had used my stories about different chronically ill patients feeling cheated out of good health when she'd spoken with the mother of an infant with chronic lung disease. The child had undergone frequent PICU admissions, and the mother was angry, brittle, and difficult to work with. Nora, when she began oxygen therapy for the baby, asked if the mother felt cheated of having a healthy baby. I was aghast and feared the worst (preoccupation with failure, I guess).

The mother began crying. That morning, she had been in the park with her baby, sitting on a bench. At the other end of the bench were three mothers sharing their babies, holding them, and laughing. She could not join in because her baby, connected to an oxygen cylinder, was quite thin and frail and not very active. She did feel cheated that she could not share her baby.

Through Nora, we acknowledged what the mother could not openly express. We accepted the mother's emotion as normal and one that we might have if our circumstances were reversed. Afterward, the mother's demeanor changed, and she became loyal to the unit, working closely with us to give the best care possible to her baby.

—Daved van Stralen

(2). In the first few days of a critical illness, a patient's family tries to make sense and understand a disease and treatment plan that have taken healthcare professionals years to learn. Their grief is somewhat ambiguous—they grieve the potential loss of their loved one, combined with the hope that medical care will now find an effective treatment. They also see the limits of this hope, however, because their loved one is not rapidly improving. The immediate caregivers may wonder which of them is responsible for the accident, or for not taking the patient in sooner. Often, a family will decide that one of them must be blamed. Friends and family will ask questions about what people missed, why they didn't go to the hospital sooner, or what they had done to contribute to the illness or injury. Anger begins to grow toward one of the caregivers when blame is sought, or toward the healthcare team when family and friends question the care that is being provided.

The following two vignettes describe common presentations of anger in patients from the sudden occurrence of a serious illness or injury. The first vignette describes anger directed at a family member felt responsible. The second vignette describes anger directed at healthcare givers.

Typically, in near-drowning events, the parent who has custody at the time is blamed for the accident. In our experience, this often appears to contribute to divorce within a year. In this case, Leigh Aveling, our chaplain, took the parents into a side room and reiterated what I had said: that this drowning could not have been prevented at the time. We told the parents that they will blame themselves but that family members will also blame the parent who had responsibility for the child at the time of the drowning. We've seen spouse turn on spouse from this family dynamic. Because they were forewarned, when this did occur, the parents physically clung to each other as the grandparents berated the parent. The other parent responded with a loving defense. Over time, we watched the parents draw closer together; counterintuitively, the grandparents also changed their initial view and accepted them both.

    —Daved van Stralen

Over time, in the ICU and the long-term care facility, I often encounter parents who express anger at the care team as soon as their child has arrived with us. We have not yet taken any actions, but they clearly express this anger toward us.

    When I hear these criticisms, I ask the parents if their family members or friends had told them that they had missed something, or that they should have gone to the doctor sooner, or that it was their fault in some way. Or if their family and friends were saying that their child was doing poorly because the doctors, nurses, or hospital were not doing a good job. Inevitably, they say yes.

    I generally tell them that they have done everything possible and that they have done what I would have done. I tell them what the staff in the referring hospital and the ICU are doing and the heroic efforts that are being made on behalf of their child. Then I say that these comments will continue, because no one wants to believe that a child can suddenly become so ill. They do not want to believe that it can happen to their child. They must believe that the parents did something or that the medical team missed something. They must blame someone so they can feel safe. This same dynamic underscores the need for having someone to blame in HRO events.

    —Daved van Stralen

Reducing the Fear Responses

When we recognize these emotional responses as being neurochemically mediated, they become easier to self-regulate, to deal with in an objective manner, and to intervene either with ourselves or with others. Our experience is that focusing on an objective helps self-regulate the fear response before the event. If that objective cannot be reached, then we decompose the objective to an objective we can more readily achieve.

Driving a force function into the prefrontal cortex can reduce the anger response. For example, asking the question, "How can I help?" may drive someone into the prefrontal cortex function and away from the amygdala. On the other hand, asking "why" or "what" questions frustrates people, driving them further into the amygdala. If you can keep an angry person talking, without increasing the person's frustration or anger, then he or she is less likely to become physically belligerent. On the other hand, we can use physical activity to reduce the anger-fight response by asking people for information that is only available by physical activity or by asking them to perform a task or function in their area of specialty. This request *must* be related to the person's expertise and must be germane to the activity, or it might be seen as dismissive.

Modulating the tone of voice also helps. Responding to an angry person with a louder voice and faster speech, whether as defensive action or to intimidate, accelerates the anger cycle. Speaking softly and slowly, in a normal cadence, can decelerate the action. Care must be taken, as speaking softly and slowly in a tone that can be taken as condescending can almost be worse than raising your voice.

Instrumental anger (see "Fear as Attitude" in chapter 5, "Cognition and Affect") is anger with a secondary motive extrinsic to the situation and directed toward manipulation. Someone who exhibits this type of anger may burst into anger out of proportion to the situation and then rapidly return to an outwardly calm state. Here, anger blocks discussion and questioning. With practice, these people operate on the staff to the degree that they see these early heralds of instrumental anger and act to avoid the outburst. Seen from within this social interaction, it appears that peacekeeping works, although this may be difficult to observe from outside the social group. After a tragedy, those who use instrumental anger can readily stay outside blame or causation.

Plausible avoidance, which is a flight response, responds to redirection: for example, assigning a relatively straightforward physical task, particularly if it appears not to be associated with the emergency, can bring someone back into the team. This strategy also works for the freeze response. Stress is associated with cortisol release and has effects on working memory. In stressful situations, we must filter information for relevance and retrieve stored information, all of which is processed and recalled in our working memory. Though acute stressors can improve working memory, severe stressors more often impair working memory (Sandi and Pinelo-Nava 2007). The freeze response can be rapidly induced from sudden, stressful circumstances. When recognized, this response can be just as rapidly resolved by carrying out a simple, thoughtful task.

> During one two-month period, three pediatric residents came to me and described their experience during a resuscitation, when they had felt the freeze they had earlier experienced on rounds with me. (Reciting the months of the year in alphabetical order to demonstrate the cortisol-induced freeze response.) Each one had found that checking the endo-tracheal tube for patency brought them back to thinking clearly. I now teach this exercise and use it when I observe someone freezing.
> —Daved van Stralen

Perceiving threat as negative has adaptive benefits for safety. Over prolonged periods, though, negative appraisals have deleterious effects on our psychological and physical well-being. Resilient people use positive emotions to recover from these negative experiences.

Humor—A Special Case
Humor can be an adaptive or maladaptive response to fear. Knowing some of the models of humor can help us interpret where people are in their developmental growth or if they are in a stress response. Three primary theories have been described in humor research: relief theory, incongruity theory, and superiority theory. Relief theory is an emotion theory that holds that humor releases physiological tension; incongruity theory is a cognitive model that singles out discrepancies as a target for the humor. Superiority theory examines successful moments or, in the worst case, looks at people who become elevated at others' expense. Having positive emotions, finding positive meaning in events, and using positive forms of humor all contribute to resilience and people's physiological recovery from negative emotional arousal (Tugade and Fredrickson 2004).

Humor also serves in communication. Two humor functions unite groups, and two divide groups (Meyer 2000). Unity comes from (1) mutual identification and (2) the clarification of functions and shared values, while division comes from (1) the enforcement of group norms and (2) the differentiation of acceptable versus unacceptable behaviors or people. As a form of social knowledge, humor delineates social boundaries. We must be aware when people use humor to create division, whether intentionally or unintentionally, and address it immediately.

These functions also align with styles of humor that are potentially beneficial or detrimental to our well-being. *Affiliative humor* is similar to humor for mutual identification, in that it facilitates relationships and minimizes interpersonal tension. *Self-enhancing humor* is similar to the clarification of functions and shared values. Self-enhancing humor maintains a cheerful outlook and functions to regulate emotions and cope with adversity. Coping with adversity is similar to using humor as a sign of mastery (see below). *Self-defeating humor* uses self-disparaging humor to amuse others at one's own expense as a means of ingratiating oneself or gaining approval; this form of humor can be a positive form of differentiating unacceptable behaviors. Self-defeating humor can also serve as "role distancing" during an error in the presence of a severe authority gradient. Erving Goffman (2005) described the use of humor in role distancing to reduce tension in his discussion of role theory. Role distancing is not the denial of a role but, rather, a person's "claim" they are not "just the role." *Aggressive humor* (sarcasm, teasing, or ridicule) is a form of humor used in both enforcement and differentiation. Using humor to demean or manipulate others to advance one's needs is similar to the instrumental use of anger (Martin et al. 2003). Humor, as social knowledge, delineates social boundaries.

Tension and Humor
Members of an HRO commonly find themselves in situations that cause mental or emotional strain. Humor is one way to release the tension. Pent up nervous energy or anxiety that rapidly resolves can give pleasurable physiological relief. The sudden release of psychological energy that had been used to regulate or repress socially unaccepted beliefs or desires produces psychological release.

Duchenne de Boulogne identified the difference in smile expression between fake joy and one "only put in play by the sweet emotions of the soul" (Duchenne 1990, 276) Involvement of the cheeks and eyes in the smile, and a quicker upturn of the lips, indicate an emotional or spontaneous smile, also called the Duchenne smile. The social, or cortical smile, uses different facial muscles controlled by different brain circuits. The response to humor as a tension release reveals to the leader the level of tension that people continue to experience after the resolution of an event—genuine relief or continuing tension (Ekman et al. 1990).

Dan Kleinman, retired chief of operations at the National Incident Management Organization, has served as incident commander for some of the largest and most complex wildland fires. He would monitor his rookies for signs of stress, particularly by asking, "Are we having fun yet?" He watched their smiles for genuine relief smiles or forced smiles revealing underlying stress. From this simple act, he could monitor his team for early intervention and support.

Incongruity, Mastery, and Humor

We find humor in the pleasurable recognition of placing the familiar against the unexpected or meaningless. Children's humor marks their mastery over a stage of development, such as in Jean Piaget's model of development (Inhelder and Piaget 1958). After their initial understanding or mastery of a physical task, children derive pleasure from the incongruity of jokes which play on a discrepancy with the task. This humor comes only after the child learns control of the task, such as potty training. While this situation is not studied after adolescence, we do see this dynamic in high-risk organizations: as novices gain mastery over major tasks that mark a landmark in their progress, they begin to use the task as a basis for humor (McGhee 2013, 69–71).

Superiority and Humor

Finding pleasure from sudden, unexpected success produces positive humor. Finding pleasure at the expense of someone, or to aggressively downgrade someone, is negative humor that lowers the performance of others, their effectiveness in social communication, and the overall operations of the organization when a crisis occurs. We may not think that we participate in this form of negative humor, but it is not that uncommon in healthcare, whether it takes the form of humor directed at a patient's unreasonable request, a professional's judgment and actions, or the situation of "stupid mistakes" often discussed in safety lectures.

What this form of humor does is to separate the group from others. No one can learn from a safety lecture when the pointed barbs separate the subject of the humor from the audience. In effect, the person in the vignette, a victim, becomes a buffoon in the story. We sit, separated from the target of the ridicule, and believe that "since I'm not a buffoon, I wouldn't have done that." Therefore, no learning occurs.

The Threat Response

This is the physiological fear response but in an adaptive form. That is, the amygdala maintains focus and the motivation to act. The threat response is not the sense of feeling afraid, which is mediated through the prefrontal cortex. LeDoux (2014) now separates what operators have long distinguished: fear is an emotion that impairs our response to threats, while the threat response is the focus and drive to engage the threat.

In his book *Thinking, Fast and Slow*, Daniel Kahneman (2011) focuses on the speed of decision-making and *cognitive* biases. In our experience, however, fear and situational cognitive distortions augment, if not amplify, the cognitive biases.

For this reason, we discuss cognitive biases, but in context with fear responses. "Fear responses" here does not refer to the fear responses of failing an exam but to the magnified fear responses associated with live-or-die situations or those with acute, severe, complex demands. These responses are not amenable to laboratory study, so we must obtain our information from our informed personal experiences, reflective experiences from others, and from those who have crossed the liminal threshold, learned how to perform in dangerous environments, and then developed the language to describe their experiences.

Models that academically describe what happens in these situations can help us understand and interpret outcomes and the actions that are taken. They may, however, be of less use in conditioning for decision-making or teaching us how to perform. We seek an approach that is of immediate use, much like that used by the Connecticut paramedics in the opening vignette of chapter 7, "Decision-Making in Healthcare." The approach must be pragmatic and based on daily practice. While VUCA is a useful description, we must remember that it goes along with very real and immediate physical danger, thus making it VUCA-T. Our approach must incorporate the effect that threat, and the associated fear response, has on thinking and decision-making. We must create decision-making skills that are immediately applicable, rather than having scientific discussions about how the decisions are made.

Emotion can mean the strong, idiosyncratic responses from fear, which is the definition neurobiologists use. Emotion can also refer to a feeling, which is the definition that laypeople more commonly use. We use "emotion" in the sense of the fear response. We also use "affect" as another term for emotion, hence our distinction between the cognitive domain and the affective domain in decision-making.

In decision-making, it appears that a divide occurs between rational thought and cognition in the prefrontal cortex and irrational thought, anger, and emotion due to fear arising from the amygdala. This duality seems at first glance to be firm and fixed: we are either rational, using cognition, or irrational because of fear.

We do not accept this dichotomy. In the real world, the fear response tends to heighten our senses and drive our responses, to a degree. We cannot, however, let fear control or capture us. We have seen the effects of overreliance on cognition as well as the denial of the fear response. What we need is the ability to moderate the fear response—in effect regulating our emotion—to give us access to the cognitive abilities of the prefrontal cortex as needed, with the fear response giving us the drive, motivation, and focus we need when engaging a threat.

Late at night, resident physicians would treat patients who had difficulty controlling seizures. The choice of drug and the dose to administer always confounded the residents. Of itself, this is not too difficult of a decision. The problem was the next morning, when the neurologist would criticize the choice of drug based on the underlying neurology. After several years of this happening, the criticism stopped. I discussed this with an associate, who told me, "It was simple. One morning at two o'clock, I called the neurologist and asked him what drug to use. He never criticized me again." The extreme emphasis on cognitive problem-solving had provided the unintended consequence of delayed treatment.

—Daved van Stralen

Several regions of the brain modulate the amygdala and provide alternative decision-making approaches to the prefrontal cortex. One region is the anterior cingulate cortex, which modulates the amygdala, identifies error, and is one of the sites where adaptive decision-making occurs. Another part is a specific region of the prefrontal cortex. Decision-making in the prefrontal cortex is binary: it is either/or.

We know the structures in the brain that can bring rational thought and fear responses together, but it is not perfectly clear how to do this in an operational manner. For this we must look to the experience of people who have learned how to bring their rational thought and fear responses together. While it is beyond the scope of this book to re-create these programs, we can assure you that the principles discussed above have demonstrated the ability to prepare people to make decisions in the face of threats.

Conclusions

(1). Failure *is* an option.
(2). HRO approaches are readily translatable to conventional environments.
(3). HRO supports homeostasis in unstable, adverse environments.
(4). Adrenaline distorts thinking and cones attention to create unsafe performance.
(5). Humor, as a response to stress, can mitigate or increase stress responses.
(6). Fear responses are neurochemically based.
(7). The brain processes perceptions of the novel and the familiar in different hemispheres.
(8). The anterior cingulate cortex modulates the stress and fear responses.

CHAPTER 10

SENSEMAKING OF NOISE

T he "sensed" patient, or the patient whom we evaluate for the purposes of management, does not exist later for review. Only the "monitored" patient does; this is the patient who is reconstructed later from monitored and recorded data and from caregiver notes for diagnostic, heuristic, or legal reasons. The two patients are not identical (van Stralen and Perkin 1994).

The Problem of Sensemaking

"Sensemaking" means to give meaning to the environment, which is made difficult when the environment appears unstructured, random, and disordered. The lack of structure may be real, emerging from active nonlinear interactions, or a product of inexperience, when we have never encountered such a situation. Beliefs provide meaning for sensemaking in these unstructured environments; specific beliefs such as rules, laws, principles, and models; or more general beliefs such as attitudes.

Beliefs brought to the unstructured environment, however, can create difficulties of their own making. Beliefs can conflict with one another, or the environment can conflict with closely held beliefs. Holding resolutely to certain beliefs may reduce discomfort but at the risk of committing errors driven by this cognitive dissonance.

In High Reliability, we are more likely to reduce the discomfort of dissonance by questioning and changing our beliefs. That is, we use the situation to learn and to acquire knowledge. We also engage the environment and improve our perceptions of the situation while changing the environment. By doing so, we increase our adaptiveness and capture error as it occurs while we are changing our beliefs and the environment. Not to approach sensemaking in this manner is to risk the problems of sensemaking, which is having conflicting beliefs.

A belief may conflict with the reality of the situation, or, more accurately, the reality of the situation may conflict with a belief. One may readily dismiss a situation or process in the environment that conflicts with a particular strongly held belief. This is made easier when the situation has no effect on current operations, or its trajectory is not predicted to cause damage. While this mode of sensemaking reduces the dissonance between what is believed and what is perceived, it can become a habit that contributes to missed heralds of impending failure. When we face threats, strongly held beliefs can be deadly.

A belief may conflict with another belief. We then decide which belief is useful, which to adjust, or which to abandon. Engaging in thoughtful deliberation is not an option when time is constrained or compressed. Holding resolutely to selected beliefs reduces the discomfort of dissonance, at the risk that a strongly held (but false) belief will drive errors.

A few fundamental beliefs may take precedence, to the degree that they do not interact with other beliefs or the environment. The rigorous linear application of only a few beliefs reduces the discomfort of dissonance but constrains sensemaking; weak signals or early heralds of failure are interpreted as noise. Sudden, catastrophic failure results.

> "The clash between a mistaken old belief and an updated belief would seem to be a form of dissonance…The more you engage in dynamic reasoning [processes], the less chance there is for dissonance between the old belief and the updated, [improving] belief to develop, the fewer errors you make, but at risk of a new set of cues being neglected."
> —KARL WEICK, PERSONAL COMMUNICATION

We experience our environment. Our perceptions are the sensing of stimuli and sensory input; we then, from our beliefs, give meaning to those perceptions. Beliefs come from the cognitive and affective domains; in fact, we can easily hold beliefs independent of the environment. The inferences we make from the environment follow a logic of environmental stimuli, how they develop and what they mean. We can only sense a stimulus when the stimulus is above a threshold of signal strength and can only perceive a stimulus depending on our attention level and its salience. Then we can give the stimulus meaning from our beliefs. This process is the creation of sensemaking.

Experiencing the environment through close interaction (i.e., being a participant) differs from experiencing the environment from a distance in time or space (i.e., through retrospective analysis by the observer), as noted in the opening and above quotes.

The differences in distance from which two people experience and analyze the environment create different conclusions. It is not that either is wrong, only that their sensemaking operates at different levels of analysis. Operating at different levels of analysis creates a false debate (MacDougall-Shackleton 2011) unless we recognize and acknowledge the sources of these differences. Levels of analysis differ between objective sensing (physical stimuli) and subjective sensemaking (beliefs), between digital data and analogue measures, between description and explanation, or between discrete categorization of concepts and the continuum of the environment. This is also discussed in chapter 3 "The Logic of Practice and the Logic of Operations: Levels of Analysis."

Worse than false debate, we may accept sensemaking as normative. "How I see / experience / understand the circumstances is closer to reality than another person."

Justification is a common, though maladaptive, means to reduce dissonance. People may justify the sense they make of a situation, the decisions they make, or the outcomes. In any event, justification not only prevents open discussion of missed information and maladaptive thought processes, but also entrenches maladaptive beliefs and attitudes.

Not all discrepancies and disruptions are equal. We either learn or are taught what is salient, then we learn the effect of context on salience. This occurs as we learn what works for particular discrepancies, disruptions, and contexts. Some people argue for the primacy of the situation (environment) and others for the primacy of the concept or belief (cognition); we argue for the duality: each contributes characteristics independently and interdependently.

This approach guides people to have vigilance toward those gaps that have salience to them—that is, what they can detect, what will affect the future, and what they can do something about. In Karl Weick's version of cognitive dissonance, our discomfort is caused by contradictions in which we have a stake; since this is what arouses our attention, he asks the question, "Could contradictions in which we have a stake be the crux of sensemaking?" (personal communication).

If this is true, then the duality of sensemaking helps explain the acceptance of belief over the situation and the resistance to change we see in some people. This is most marked in planning and preparation for a crisis and is also present at the beginning of the crisis, when beliefs that conflict with the future possible worlds can still be comfortably held, with the discomfort reduced by holding more tightly to these beliefs.

> "Contradictions in which we have a stake are the
> source of discomfort in cognitive dissonance.
> This could be the crux of sensemaking."
> —KARL WEICK, PERSONAL COMMUNICATION

The two quotations from Weick immediately above appear similar but came from distinctly different conversations with one of the authors (van Stralen) about the discomfort from dissonance. In the earlier quote, Weick responded to van Stralen's observation that new information generated during an event, particularly if unexpected or disconfirming, creates cognitive dissonance. That some people will reduce the discomfort from dissonance by rejecting the new, or updated, information would explain their failure to respond to changes. Weick, referring to observations from his doctoral dissertation, wondered if engagement reduces the dissonance but brings in the risk of neglecting new cues. The second quote describes how cognitive dissonance from contradictions drives sensemaking -we want to make sense of the contradiction. Returning to the first quote, contradictions from the unexpected quickly "outdates" beliefs and the individual can reject the beliefs or engage to create sensemaking. Acting is how we think, how we make sense, and how we enact. Sensemaking and enactment, in response to the unexpected, reduces the discomfort of dissonance.

This nature of sensemaking as serial dualities is similar to the problem of light having characteristics of both *discrete* mass (photon) and *continuous* wave (electromagnetic radiation), the wave-particle duality of light. Either partially explains the nature of light but at the expense of the other. Albert Einstein's resolution of this duality of light led to his winning of the Nobel Prize in Physics in 1921. Duality of sensemaking arises from the two contradictory pictures of reality. To paraphrase Einstein, cognitions and the environment separately do not fully explain effective operations for uncertainty, time compression, and threat, but together they do.

Sensemaking in the VUCA-T environment has similarities to this duality. The *discrete* concepts of categorizations and cognitions combine with the *continuous* characteristics of the environment to produce the cognition-environment duality of sensemaking. Therefore, we will look at sensemaking through its various functions, acknowledging the various dualities of sensemaking. According to Albert Einstein and Leopold Infield (1938, 263),

> Duality can confound us or it can lead us to more elegant models of sensemaking. As with theories of light, Einstein describes how "It seems as though we must use sometimes the one theory and sometimes the other, while at times we may use either. We are faced with a new kind of difficulty. We have two contradictory pictures of reality; separately neither of them fully explains the phenomena of light, but together they do."

Sensemaking can consistently have the same structure, but different frames of reference change the appearance of a situation to those outside the frame.

This idea is not the same as duality, where sensemaking combines contradictory features; it is more similar to Einstein's principle of relativity. Sensemaking depends on where you stand and what you do, which is the experiential or existential aspect of sensemaking. An outside observer, without the immediacy of engagement, relies on passive, observational sensemaking alone. Salient but transient data points and the proximity of threat are not detectable or are disregarded.

Sensemaking, whether shared or individual, has (or can be described by) conscious and unconscious components, cognition and affect, continuous or discrete characteristics, and, as described by Orton and Weick (1990), order and elements.

Categorization itself has different approaches of finding similarity versus describing differences. For example, in the Linnaean classification system for taxonomy, "there are 'lumpers and splitters.' Lumpers emphasize similarities in categorization, grouping, or lumping together, to reduce the number of species. Splitters search for differences, splitting groups to increase the number of species," Jules Crane, Cerritos College, Norwalk, California (1971) (personal communication with Daved van Stralen). Charles Darwin (1857) recognized this dilemma, it "seems to me one of the most important arguments I have yet met with, that varieties are only small species—or species only strongly marked varieties. The subject is in many ways so very important for me... *It is good to have hairsplitters & lumpers*" (emphasis from the authors).

The use of these different aspects gives sensemaking its duality, which can confound us at the same time giving us the ability to describe sensemaking and create models. As in the duality of light, looking from one viewpoint but at the expense of another creates contradictory "realities" or different "possible worlds" (see chapter 3, "The Logic of Practice and the Logic of Operations").

The duality of sensemaking is also found in the structure of the brain. "Cortical bilateralism" describes how the right cortex receives novel stimuli and the left cortex receives familiar stimuli. Sensemaking is how the brain combines these two opposing features. The brain has a system to combine cognition and affect. Cognitive functions take place in the prefrontal cortex, and the amygdala rapidly processes threat perceptions, thereby impairing the prefrontal cortex. The cingulate cortex in effect combines these two brain regions with its own adaptive functions. The brain also combines experience and memory (cortex and hippocampus) and assurance and fear (prefrontal cortex). Each word set is descriptive of distinct axes of brain function combined in the act of sensemaking. Sensemaking is how our brain combines thought and experience.

What Does Sensemaking Do?

In a crisis, people may act in a way at odds with their strongly held beliefs, hidden biases, or maladaptive attitudes. Their action changes the way they make sense of the situation and may change their opinion or belief.

> "How can I tell what I think till I see what I say?"
> —ATTRIBUTED TO E. M. FORSTER QUOTING SOMEONE
> CONTEMPTUOUS OF LOGIC, *ASPECTS OF THE NOVEL* (1927, 152)

> "How do I know what I think until I see what I say? "
> —KARL WEICK DESCRIBING ITERATIONS TO CREATE CUMULATIVE
> UNDERSTANDING, *SENSEMAKING IN ORGANIZATIONS* (1995, 25)

Logic is the method we can infer new information from known information; professionally this is how we think. E. M. Forster presents a phrase that contests this method of inference: he tells us he must see what he is saying, that is he must see his acting, before he can think. We cannot infer in order to think, we must act in order to think. This is an insightful admission that actions create thinking. Our beliefs and thinking do not *precede* actions. This is a different logic of practice-that we act *in order to* think rather than think *before* we act.

Karl Weick's highly quoted phrase "How do I know what I think until I see what I say? " is easy to misunderstand. In discussions, Weick describes how the four verbs, all action verbs, can enact higher reliability.

Consider the process implied by the phrase, "How can I know what I think until I see what I say." There are four verbs, four actions, in the sensemaking recipe: to know, to think, to see, and to say. Organizing around those four verbs can be done in ways that enact higher reliability. Think carefully about what actually happens when someone asks you what the story is, or what your opinion is. Many times, when you start describing your opinion, you listen to what you are saying and discover that your opinion is actually a little different than you thought it was. You and I do this all the time when we try to make sense of things. When we make sense, first we talk, next we look back over what we said, and finally, we discover what we were thinking. People need to act in order to discover what they face, they need to talk in order to discover what they think, and they need to feel in order to discover what things mean. When you say something, that involves action and animation; when you see what you said, that involves directed observation; and when you draw conclusions about what your words mean, that finally tells you what you've been thinking.

Usually we assume that we think and then we act. We do that less often than it appears we do. Instead, we often make sense using the opposite sequence. We act in order to think, we think while acting, our thoughts are defined by what we do. If you substitute planning for thinking, you can see the relevance for this gathering. How can I know what I've planned until I see what I've checked off? Plans reflect the words you use to describe something and what you see in those words. You act your way into plans rather than plan your way into acts. This is why sensemaking is not the same thing as decision-making. And this is why sensemaking affects your decisions.

—Karl Weick (personal communication)

Iterations of sensemaking and action, driven by circumstances, become interactive, muddling the almost artificial separation of belief and behavior yet underscoring that one can bely the other. The iteration of sensemaking and action driven by circumstances, the contextual interaction of belief and behavior, enact higher reliability.

Sensemaking communicates what one is thinking and doing. The change in sensemaking during the dynamic event reflects more than intrinsic change in circumstance or changes caused by actions; the change in sensemaking also occurs from the change *caused* by acting. Open communication with changes in sensemaking increases the fidelity of reports generated in real time, a social construction of sensemaking. Sensemaking as a social construct increases stability though it can also create sensemaking that is less effective in a situation (Maitlis and Sonenshein 2010).

Sensemaking is a continuous search for salient information and not a quick observation of things. Sensemaking, compared to observation, classifies things into categories to simplify a complex situation for the purposes of mental function. Sensemaking identifies gaps where, in the unstructured environment, we must create new categories; it also makes the situation more complex by revealing hidden linkages and new information. Sensemaking makes the complex simple and the simple complex. This is not mindless, if we recall Ellen Langer's recipe for mindlessness: rigid categorization creates mindlessness. To prevent a mindless rush to judgment, the HRO principle *reluctance to simplify* slows the creation of simplicity from the complex and drives us to create complexity from the simple. It is in complexity where we find opportunity, and it is through sensemaking that we recognize that opportunity.

Sensemaking is both kinetic and a goal. But to relegate sensemaking to simply a goal—a step toward understanding, explanation, or knowledge—diminishes the elegance of its role in thought and action and minimizes its many functions. Sensemaking as action makes it a step forward; by guiding engagement, sensemaking also becomes the outcome, or how we see the situation after it is over. Our sensemaking drives our actions, which enact what we are making sense toward. To summarize: (1) sensemaking is kinetic and a goal; (2) sensemaking is interactive and retrospective.

Sensemaking is the immediate antecedent to engagement. As action, sensemaking enacts toward the desired end-state. HRO is to change the environment more than adapting to it. While it may be possible for the organization to adapt to an adverse environment, it is less likely to thrive. Sensemaking is a form of awareness, of asking different questions, or of taking actions that change the circumstances as we make sense of them. In this manner, sensemaking is the early step in enactment.

Sensemaking as a Function

Different discussions and lines of research develop with (1) *sensing as input*, or sense as perception; (2) *sensemaking as a process* to develop meaning from belief that can be modeled; (3) *sensemaking as a produced output* for decision and action; and (4) *sensemaking as an outcome*. The purposes of each differ, though they overlap. Their functions, how those purposes are attained, also overlap.

Academically, sensemaking is discussed with different models, each model coming from an academic domain for a specific purpose. Examples include library science and information gaps (Dervin 1983), social psychology and attention management (Langer), and computer science and external representations (D. Russell); rather than discussing sensemaking as different models, we are better served to describe its functions (see table 12).

A function has a purpose and performs a process, operation, or set of actions by taking some input to create some output. Sensemaking, considered as a function, brings out discussion of how we use it and its purpose(s). The inputs of sensemaking come from the environment, mingled with noise, weak signals, and salience, among other things. The process of sensemaking involves the mental processes of interpretation, decision-making, actions, and the like. The output is not sensemaking but the process. The output is decision, action, and enactment.

We constantly make sense of our surroundings, even in familiar situations. We do this for responsiveness to changes in the environment. In fact, the brain is hard-wired for certain threats such as a particular face in the crowd (Hansen

Function	Purpose
Teaching	Affective domain- what helps, how it helps
Signals	To identify information in a noisy environment as content, meaning, and value
Communication	Shared sensemaking and conceptualization
Update	Changes in conceptualization and performance
Homeostasis	Identify drift
Environment	Identify structure
Threat	Identify threats and safety
Risks	Identify the direction of action
Engagement	Identify where to start What works and what does not
Friction	Path of least resistance
Causal reasoning	To produce prediction during event
Existential	Meaning to the individual
Resilience	Adaptiveness during event Reappraisal after the event
Gaps	Identifies gaps in planning Identifies gaps in training & performance
Learning	Change from error and experience
Emotional memory	Creates rapid, intuitive responses May interfere from disproportionate response

Table 12—Table of sensemaking functions

and Hansen 1988; Ohman et al. 2001) and noxious smells. The proximate cause of sensemaking is survival, to identify threat for immediate response, and there is an ultimate cause, for understanding, communication, and learning. Academics bring a third "cause" for sensemaking: that of building a model, which produces multiple functions of sensemaking,

Meaning—particular or situational meaning—comes from beliefs. Beliefs that people hold or that are connected to the situation we call "internal beliefs." Beliefs received from higher in the hierarchy, held by the culture, or specific to this action we call "external beliefs." Internal beliefs act in sensemaking as the proximal cause, giving bottom-up influence; external beliefs act as ultimate cause, giving top-down influence (see figure 9).

It is hard to know when belief ends and reality begins.

Two levels of analysis for sensemaking generally occur, the cognitive level of the individual and the social level that includes social psychology and social constructionism. The vignette below describes a situation with multiple parallel sensemaking amongst individuals and the difficulty in attaining socially constructed sensemaking.

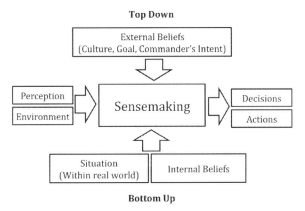

Top Down

Figure 9—Sensemaking

A man is trapped in a car on a major road, impeding rush-hour traffic into downtown. His door is damaged; the opposite door is blocked. My driver for the rescue ambulance tells me the man has no injuries. This was one of my first experiences in charge of the fire department rescue ambulance.

My driver, a new firefighter, is working to pry the door open with help and equipment from the tow-truck operators. He tells me that a full alarm for this physical rescue (a ladder truck, two engines, and a battalion chief) would completely block the road. A heavy utility vehicle carrying the Jaws of Life for extrication is at least twenty minutes away, one of two the department had at that time. The man is turning gray and does not talk as much—an early sign of a heart attack that may have led to the accident or occurred after the accident. Paramedics are also at least twenty minutes away. It seems we can pry the door open before any assistance can arrive.

Well, we can't, so we call for the physical rescue assignment. We remove the man and transport him to the hospital emergency department. He dies fourteen hours later from a heart attack.

That evening my captain calls me into the office, thanks me for my work, then tells me I'm the most qualified rescue ambulance driver the fire department had for the call and that the department would support me and everything I did. Then he asks what I would do differently next time. He gives me several reasons for each different decision point. He explains why it's OK to call out too much equipment; that is not an over-reaction. He tells me again that I'm the most qualified rescue ambulance driver the department has. But he adds, others are more qualified, others are more experienced, but they weren't available. So, at that time, I was the most qualified rescue ambulance driver for that assignment, so the department would stand behind me and my actions.

Then he tells me, "There are a thousand things happening at a scene. You can only see a hundred. You can only act on ten. I may see a different hundred. I may act on a different ten. That doesn't mean I'm better than you; only that I'm different." Even if engaged side by side, people experience different forms of sensemaking in unexpected events.

"This remains, to me, one of your more powerful, rich experiences. One can dwell on its implications for a long time." Karl Weick, personal communication.

—Daved van Stralen

Throughout the day we experience many environments and situations, and our sensemaking must perform in each. We can share sensemaking, but we do so at the risk of suppressing the idiosyncratic nature of sensemaking described in the vignette. Sensemaking as experience is peculiar to the individual.

In this chapter, we focus more on individual sensemaking for a specific reason. We choose the individual as the level of analysis because it is the individual who encounters the unexpected situation and who *must engage and communicate.* People who must act in uncertain situations or who encounter an immediate threat are alone with their thoughts. What they do will make sense to them, if not at that moment then later as they justify their actions to make sense to themselves and/or defend themselves from criticism. No authority can demand specific behaviors in a time of uncertainty or danger, since you cannot tell someone how to make sense of events. During routine times, the effective methods of sensemaking people develop within themselves will create effective decisions and actions for High Reliability situations. Development of sensemaking in the individual, rather than as a normative or standardized process, is more likely to create an organization that performs at a high level of reliability. Organizational sensemaking emerges from individual sensemaking.

We all act for reasons in ways that will make sense to us within our perceived limits. Our decisions make sense to us, since we do not intend to make errors or mistakes. Any other belief from others sows suspicion and mistrust, thus corrupting honesty about thoughts, perceptions and action that will and preventing learning. Recognition and acceptance of idiosyncratic actions is essential when evaluating and analyzing rare or uncommon events.

The idiosyncratic nature of sensemaking places some limits to reason that affect sensemaking (Herbert Simon's bounded rationality), no ideal decision-making environment exists, and decision models developed in ideal conditions are not relevant under the constraints and limits of the VUCA-T environment. Actors are "trying to reach their goals within the limits of their perceived scope of action…This is the logic of action behind all mechanisms…Only assume that actors behave in accordance with the situation and its logic and nothing else" (Bengtsson and Hertting 2014).

This, however, does not mean that we cannot generalize from make use of this idiosyncratic nature of sensemaking. Bengtsson and Hertting (2014) offer the assumption that, based on *thinly rationalistic social mechanisms*, similar actors will use similar mechanisms when operating in similar contexts. This assumption, that actors will in most cases do things for a reason, they call *thin rationality*. We can then examine a single or a few cases, develop ideal-type mechanisms, and then use "thin rationality" to bridge to other contexts where similar actor constellations exist (Bengtsson and Hertting 2014). Doing so allows HRO to generalize from the single case.

This strategy also makes sensemaking vulnerable to errors. For example, thin rationality, people act for a reason and their reasons will be fairly similar, and bounded rationality, perceptions and cognitive processes place a boundary on an individual's rationality, can be predictive in more routine circumstances. This is the logic behind the training and many of the protocols for emergencies. But we do not know how an individual will behave when encountering an emergent event with novel properties. The individual may have an inaccurate representation of reality due to training and protocols based on thin rationality, how people can be expected to respond from a small number of occurrences.

> "Can you make an error and know you are making the error?"
> —KARL WEICK (PERSONAL COMMUNICATION)

The principle of relativity, discussed above, and the potential mismatch between discrete cognitions and a continuous environment—particularly when the continuum of time includes action-response sequences—will cause errors. Here we define error as the distance from the desired state or end-state. Actions are not mistakes; actions *become* mistaken (Paget 1988). HRO, by accepting the inevitability of errors, is vigilant for errors and builds in early error detection and correction. But this is the trick: "How do you tell when you are wrong?"

"A mistake follows an act. It identifies an act in its completion. It names it. An act, however, is not a mistake; it becomes mistaken. Seen from inside of action, from the point of view of an actor, an act often becomes mistaken only late in its development. As it is unfolding, it is not becoming a mistake at all. It is moving and evolving in time" (Paget 1998, 45). The paradox of mistakes is that "the errors are errors now, but weren't errors then" (Paget 1988, 56).

This is a similar problem as that identified by Niko Tinbergen (1963) with animal behavior. The field observer cannot observe antecedent behaviors or triggers because the animal is not noticed until the desired behavior occurs. Any antecedent behavior that is observed may not always precede the behavior of interest. We cannot know when actions or sensemaking become uniquely mistaken because we cannot observe until the mistake is identified. We cannot necessarily conclude that any observed antecedent behavior or sensemaking will always precede mistaken actions.

The identification of a discrepancy between our experienced reality and our beliefs can lead us to change our beliefs—we grow. On the other hand, when the discrepancy conflicts with a strongly held belief, we may consider the source of discrepancy an error or misunderstanding; we keep our belief. Remember: sensemaking is how we change; sensemaking is why we don't.

When people make errors, we can learn about their cognitive and affective processing by assuming they acted in a way that made sense to them. We often hear them say "I would have done that." We can then seek to understand what situation or thinking would make their decision correct. This will illuminate what people may have seen and how they interpreted it, their knowledge, and their objective. We can ask ourselves, "What would it take for me to make that decision or take that action?"

> "A story always sounds clear enough at a distance, but the nearer you get to the scene of events the vaguer it becomes."
> —GEORGE ORWELL (2008, 31), *SHOOTING AN ELEPHANT*

In conventional situations, one can continue to observe the situation or others even when in close proximity. For the High Reliability Situation (HRS), to the contrary, inherent threat forces the observer to become a participant with increasing proximity to the threat. Moving closer in High Reliability creates a conundrum in making sense of the story, with the precise clarity of observation melding into the more accurate ambiguity from participation. During participation, one encounters the paradox of well-crafted plans; complex situations inherently contain indications and contra-indications for every plan. The participant must discern the most favorable plan for that situation, making sense of both the situation and plan. In a constantly changing situation, we may believe we are making an objectively sound choice rather than being deceived by a sense of satisfaction from our choice. Precision and observation come at a distance; accuracy and participation come from proximity.

> In an after-action review, starting with the premise that "I would have done that" changes your viewpoint toward what was observed, or observable, that would have driven the action in question. Doing so also adds a separate viewpoint of what knowledge and decision skills would have made the action in question appear rational. This is a procedure I bring in when others begin the process of criticism.
>
> When intensive care physicians criticized our management of mechanical ventilation for long-term care, we were able to identify the source of discrepancy: they treat oxygenation and ventilation problems, while we treat sensation. Even though we use the same technology and evaluation, we have different problems and dynamics.
>
> —Daved van Stralen

Thus, the conundrum of sensemaking: the integration of the clarity gained from a distance with the nuance and ambiguity gained at close proximity. At a distance, events are clear and can be defined, categorized, and studied objectively. Up close, however, events are subjective, ambiguous, nuanced, and subtle, and they evolve as an uninterrupted progression of change. This is also the paradox of sensemaking: planning, and then carrying out that plan. Understanding and planning come from clarity of definitions and discrete boundaries of categories, which are more readily made at a distance. Meaning, which is necessary for effective operations and personal performance to carry out the plan, comes from the newness of events and experience; the lack of clear boundaries creates a continuous spectrum of possibilities. This can only be known up close.

Finally, there is the deception of satisfaction in sensemaking. We believe we are objective, cognitively thinking beings. Without a doubt, this can be true in a well-controlled, protected, comfortable environment. We must not forget that humans have also developed effective means for performance in constantly changing states with complexity and threat. This effectiveness comes from the amalgamation of cognition and affect, which is possibly more responsible for our survival, adaptation, and evolution than our cognitive abilities alone. As we evaluate the situation, we may rely more heavily than we think on preformed ideas and latent prejudices. For example, we may place more weight on false information because it comes from a person we like and place less weight on disconfirming information because we do not like the person. When we make sense of a situation sufficiently to make a decision and act, we must be aware of the deception of these biases and prejudices. Our decisions may be dangerously derived from our misplaced sense of satisfaction rather than from the questioning attitudes necessary for accuracy in sensemaking. Making sense and feeling satisfaction are not equivalent.

Sensemaking: From the Lab or the Field

The intellectual activity involved in developing models and improving sensemaking through modeling and games has a certain allure. But we risk adjusting and refining models for their internal coherence and perceived applicability to life rather than their accuracy to human performance under profound stress or fidelity to a complex, time-compressed, and threatening environment. Through the control of variables, we study the effect of time-dependence and uncertainty. The definition of other specific variables measures human performance. Both require the control and manipulation of the environment. But time-dependence and uncertainty in a steady environment are not necessarily causative of profound stress, and profound stress is not equivalent to serious life threat. Fear is ethically difficult for researchers to manipulate. Although we know that fear, emotions, thermal stress (i.e., cold and heat), and (unrecognized) dehydration impair cognitive function, we rarely acknowledge these effects on sensemaking or decision-making.

Sensemaking models may be a product of the researcher's sensemaking, not of the operational environment. To explain data and concepts, one may reason to the best inference, which is abductive reasoning, or reason to a possible world that the researcher understands or is familiar. Then, when researchers reach a subjective understanding, they stop developing their theory and begin refining it, polishing it, and offering it to others. Validation may be obtained from those with limited or no experience in the specific operational environment or who have been away sufficiently long that the immediacy has waned. With this, we lose fidelity to reality or existence. Models are developed in a controlled, structured, predictable environment based on research studies that are observational or experimental, with the manipulation of a single variable. Such models do not have fidelity with the uncontrolled, unstructured, unpredictable environment. Inaccurate models in such environments can kill.

We appreciate models of sensemaking for what they can help us learn. But models developed in a controlled environment are not fully equivalent to the profoundly stressful environments where sensemaking occurs. The experimental situation itself creates expectations to "do it right" or "follow procedure." ("Proceduralization" may be an artifact of experimentation or come from organizational expectations placed on, or assumed by, novices.) Fear may be impossible to measure in a study environment. As Mitchell Berkun has written, "Subjects who are aware that they are subjects, that they are being tested, and that they are, quite naturally, in the protection of the responsible experimenters may be quite different people from the same subjects responding to unexpected threats to life and limb" (1964). This results in models that are not sufficiently accurate for real-time use and that have limited fidelity to real-world operations. Inaccurate models quickly become a matter of life, and even death, in the uncertain, time-compressed, hazardous environment.

As Sally Maitlis and Marlys Christianson state, "Sensemaking is the process through which people work to understand issues or events that are novel, ambiguous, confusing, or in some other way violate expectations" (2014, 57). The sensemaking literature has little comment on impending threat.

> Sitting in the restaurant, I asked my lunch companions what concerns they would have in an emergency here in the restaurant. I was curious about the concepts of sensemaking and situational awareness, and how they manifest in different people.
>
> "I'm looking for the rear exits. In an emergency, people go out the way they came in. I'd then go out the rear exits, because they'd be less crowded," said Gary Provansal, the deputy fire chief.
>
> "I'm looking for wall sockets and electrical outlets. If a child who's dependent on a mechanical ventilator is here and the battery dies, I want to know where I can plug it in quickly," said Racquel Calderon, the respiratory care practitioner.
>
> They both had situational awareness, but specific to their domains. One is not better than the other, only different.
>
> —Daved van Stralen

Sensemaking is not a normative process, since there is no ideal way to make sense of a complex, changing world or situation. Creating standards, firm rules, or models of sensemaking may give comfort for confusion or failure, but doing so comes at the cost of creating expectations and consequent gratuitous stress in real-time sensemaking. Reliance on *prospective* plans developed from *retrospective* knowledge, then used to engage volatility, uncertainty, complexity, ambiguity, and threat (VUCA-T), is seductive. Normative sensemaking, a "proceduralization" of experience, interferes with a person's openness to new experience, embrace of the novel, efforts to balance order and chaos, and use of paradox to synthesize new interpretations.

Yet, it remains intuitive to many authorities that an engineering model—no matter how well crafted, structured, and designed and incorporating signal versus noise and rulemaking—will prepare us for emergencies. The only support for this approach is hindsight-based. We advocate what Robert Bea, Professor of Civil Engineering, University of California, Berkeley, describes as "interactive, real-time risk assessment and management" (personal communication). This creates sensemaking in real-time performance toward enactment, described by Weick (1995) in his description of sensemaking as an iterative process of sensemaking and enactment, improvising when encountering the unexpected (Weick 1998).

Sensemaking has functional uses we are at risk of overlooking. People make sense of events for a reason (actually numerous reasons). As a never-ending, iterative process, sensemaking influences our concepts of understanding, knowledge, and explanation. While sensemaking occurs in various environments, at the most granular level it is most confusing and complex in the VUCA-T environment consisting of uncertainty, time compression, and threat. Here, environmental disruptions and noise affect our physiology and brain function. We must describe and critique models of sensemaking for use in live-or-die situations. Finally, we must bring into open discussion obstructions and interferences to sensemaking, which is important, as we cannot easily critique our own sensemaking—it makes sense to us.

Four themes are found in definitions of sensemaking (Maitlis and Christianson 2014). First, sensemaking is dynamic, concerned with the transient. Second, cues and environmental signals play a central role to initiate sensemaking. Third, people make sense of the situation within the social context in which they operate. Fourth, sensemaking concerns engagement and actions we take to further make sense of a situation, thus enacting the new environment (Weick 1979: 130).

Sensemaking in High Reliability Organizations

Sensemaking in High Reliability Organizations developed in response to dangerous situations, either for prevention or engagement. This may be why sensemaking appears to have common features across various HROs, though there appears to be a nontrivial difference between sensemaking to *prevent* system failure and sensemaking in *response* to system failure. Our experience is that people who have experienced extreme vulnerability, to the degree of a threat to life, will more readily accept High Reliability organizing methods and sensemaking than those who have not.

The experience of extreme vulnerability, or enculturation into high-risk operations, creates a threshold between routine operations and High Reliability operations. This threshold marks the boundary to an environment where death can be immediate and the systemic effect of failure increases by several orders of magnitude. We can better understand this environment, whether it is a potential or actual "death zone," as a liminal space, and the threshold we cross into HRO as a liminality (both concepts are borrowed from anthropology).

Liminality is an anthropological concept that describes the ambiguity or disorientation one experiences in the middle stage of rituals, here is where participants have lost their pre-ritual status but before they have the acceptance they will have after the ritual is complete. This liminal stage is where the participant stands at the liminal threshold before the new identity or acceptance into a new community. This rite has a symbolically destructive nature that represents the death of the old identity and rebirth into the new. The participant experiences disorientation, confusion of the senses, isolation, and fear bordering on the sensation of death. This qualitatively describes either the extreme operations of an HRO or enculturation into an HRO.

Liminality creates the difficulty of translating the culture of High Reliability into the general culture of business. Besides the behaviors and beliefs of an HRO, the importance of the syntax and semantics of language for high-risk operations must be considered. Events and dangers exist independently of our language, but this creates difficulties in describing these dangers in a manner meaningful for executives and managers, though the difficulty is surmountable. Sensemaking facilitates appreciating these dangers.

Liminality and Everest: A Management Story
Tempest, Starkey, and Ennew (2007) describe the 1996 Mount Everest disaster through the lens of liminality, illuminating the detrimental effect liminal team members can have in an organization. This also reveals the effect of faulty sensemaking in a "death zone."

In high-altitude mountaineering, the death zone, at an altitude of about eight thousand meters, describes the altitude where the human respiratory system cannot reliably maintain human physiology. A drop in barometric pressure from weather changes or the absence of supplemental oxygen can lead to death. Mountaineering culture, from a century of high-altitude experience, has developed behaviors and beliefs to increase the safety of major mountaineering climbs conducted as a full-scale operation. Deviation from accepted practices is recognized as foolhardy and courts death.

Commercial climbing organizations now escort novices into this death zone for the purpose of scaling high-altitude mountains such as Mount Everest. This is not necessarily a problem if sojourners follow the directions of the experienced mountaineers or if ideal conditions persist. Difficulties arise when sojourners disregard critical elements of mountaineering culture. Dynamics similar to this operate as limits to management practice when the drive to succeed in an organization exceeds the abilities of managers. Just as these mountain-climbing customers—sojourners into a liminal environment—did not recognize their limits or the dangers of the extreme environment when the weather changed, managers entering extreme conditions may not recognize new environmental dangers or their limitations.

The authors defined four key categories of limits to management practice pertinent to the use of liminal team members in extreme management conditions.

Temporary organizational teams. Temporary teams can operate with flexibility, agility, speed, and more rapid responsiveness. Organizations may rely on contractual workers to create these temporary teams. Individuals in these teams may feel disconnected from the other teams or from the organization and work beyond their capabilities. During a crisis, these people may act as individualized actors rather than cooperating as team members. Temporary teams may be poorly suited to extreme conditions when mutual understanding and trust are requisites.

Strategic intent. People aspire to great heights of achievement but do not discuss how to do this. When a team overstretches near the goal or is overly influenced by ambition, they can overfocus on opportunities and disregard limitations, going for success at any cost. This can lead to a ruthless, irrational drive to achieve goals by whatever method. In mountaineering this is called "summit fever." Reaching the peak is such a drive that "a rational understanding of reality is unlikely as perceptions become distorted and characterized by bravado—a lethal cocktail in a high-risk context" (Tempest et al. 2007, 1053). We must achieve goals without threatening our survival and work to a broader agenda.

Competence. Some uncommon competencies offer a unique and reliable basis for program development. The combination of having false assumptions about personal competencies and inadequate knowledge of others' competencies encourages individualism and bravado. We must know our own competency limits and those of the people we work with who are new to high-risk operations. We must also ask if the competencies of these new people, the sojourners, are relevant for extreme conditions. All too commonly, managers and executives do not recognize the genuine limits to competencies when they enter an extreme operation or time period (if they can even recognize the unique competencies necessary). At worst, they may assume that more experienced people can easily support the less experienced members the team. This requires the experienced people to know their own competence limits and assumes that the liminal team members acknowledge their personal limitations and are willing to subordinate themselves to the experienced people. This is particularly a problem in a hierarchy-based system. People may work too far into a high-risk operation without recognizing their limits; at that point, failure has already occurred, even if it is not recognized. There is a limit to how far experienced team members can leverage their expertise for the benefit of the organization. At this point, tacit knowledge cannot be translated into shared competence and action.

Strategic leadership. Conventional organizations rely on strategic leaders to provide vision and motivate workers to change direction toward achieving a new goal. In the extreme environment, liminal members may lack the self-direction necessary and will rely too heavily on leaders for this direction. Liminal members may not have the questioning attitude necessary to work in dangerous environments, particularly those situations that change after orders and directions are received. In these cases, the direction the leader takes may no longer confer an advantage, and liminal members, at the point of contact, may likely be the first to know. At this point, it might be best to move forward, withdraw, or wait. Some will argue the need for people to take on leadership roles, or "reciprocal interdependence." We cannot expect this type of leadership from liminal members who have not had experience in extreme environments and have never functioned as true team members in a crisis. It is in these situations where one must be certain of others' competencies and weaknesses. It is in these times of challenge when liminal team members expect more from their leaders than they do in benign conditions, and it is in these conditions where leaders are already overstretched.

Reliance on a strong central leader for the extreme environment follows the *myth of the heroic leader.* This refers to leaders who help us strive for the extraordinary and move beyond our limits. The myth is that to do this we need appropriate, strong leadership. In the feedback between leaders and followers, leaders become lulled into a false sense of their strength and invincibility, while followers are lulled into a false sense of security that if they do what they are told, the leader will take care of them, and the organization will succeed. This is almost a Confucian belief.

Initial success can generate the "paradox of success" when the success feeds into the leader's sense of ability to overcome limits and control events. Attributing personal expertise and organizational prowess to the leader ensures against catastrophe. The mission must be completed; there is no turning back; failure is not an option. But these leaders cannot control events, which led to the preventable catastrophe of 10 May on Mount Everest.

Tempest et al. (2007) describe the liminality between conventional operations and the crisis. They further describe the problems of leading liminal members, even when the leader has experience in a crisis. This situation describes the contrast in behaviors and beliefs between people in the HRO and those who are not in the HRO. Not having HRO characteristics poses little threat to conventional management in the non-extreme environment.

The authors use a single environment, extreme mountaineering, in two weather patterns (with and without a weather crisis) and three styles of behavior. They describe the liminal member as a sojourner into the extreme environment who is expected not to have the cultural elements necessary for a crisis. The extreme mountaineer does have the cultural elements necessary for this environment and any crisis that may occur. Then, a subgroup of extreme mountaineers brings liminal members onto a mountain. This can be done safely in extreme environments without a crisis, but during a crisis, liminal behaviors will kill. The extreme mountaineers are faced with the difficult task of not giving in to the expectations of the liminal members and guiding the liminal members safely through this crisis.

This describes the purpose of HRO and the difficulty in teaching it. HRO is for uncontrolled environments, regardless of the magnitude. People do not always recognize the extreme characteristics in their environment, or they do not believe a crisis will occur that they cannot somehow control. People will not recognize their overstretching during the ambitious expansion of an organization. This situation makes the case for sensemaking and for the use of HRO in routine operations.

Being Wrong Still Works: The Example of Biochemistry

Just because we are experiencing success during an operation does not mean we are right. Some of our actions are self-correcting or are corrected but go unnoticed by other actions or operators. During World War I, for example, Germany developed methods to manufacture explosives using biochemistry. Their model was wrong, though it supported research for twenty years. During the war, German biochemists adapted yeast fermentation, normally used to create alcohol, to turn sugar into glycerol. ("Glycerol" or "glycerin" are different names for the same molecule, which also acts as the backbone for triglycerides.) Replacing each of the three alcohol groups of glycerol by a nitrate group converts the glycerol to nitroglycerin. This is the explosive used in dynamite, invented by Alfred Nobel. A naval blockade prevented the importation of glycerol into Germany during the war.

Metabolism converts a six-carbon sugar to carbon dioxide and energy. Incomplete combustion of the sugar produces a two-carbon alcohol (ethanol), aldehyde, or acid. Carl Neuberg discovered that the addition of bisulfite interrupted the metabolic process to create two molecules (glycerol and pyruvate), but each with three carbon atoms instead of two. Chemists could not understand the pathway that would create glycerol, a three-carbon molecule.

To explain this, Neuberg in 1913 proposed an equation where a molecule with one carbon would add to a molecule with two carbons. Though wrong, his model formed the basis of productive research for two decades (Barnett 2004; Lenzen 2014) and for the production of glycerol for Germany's war production. It was the strength of Neuberg's position in the field of chemistry that maintained this error. He was one of the founders of the field of biochemistry and, more important, was also the editor of the leading chemical journal of the time (Nordwig 1984). His analysis, however wrong, allowed production of glycerin during World War I.

Gustav Embden identified fructose as a different intermediate six-carbon sugar that was split into two three-carbon sugars and then modified to the three-carbon glycerol. He published this result in 1933 but, because Neuburg was editor of the major biochemical journal, Embden used a different journal.

Progress had been delayed by the persistence of many wrong leads and the influence of a well-respected researcher. Within six years of Embden's discovery, only one reaction was missing. But that required ten more years of work, because another well-respected researcher, Nobel laureate Otto Warburg, made his pronouncement that there was only one possibility for the reaction. This also threw investigators off track (Oesper 1968).

While being wrong may delay getting to the truth, it does not stop research activity. One or a few highly respected intellectual leaders who insist they are correct can have a profound effect on research. (Dr. Donald Simonsen, biochemistry professor at California State University, Long Beach, taught this lesson over the course of one week; at the end of the week he announced, "It was wrong. But if it was good enough for science for twenty years, it's good enough for you over the weekend. On Monday, we'll learn the correct equation.") We can succeed and reach our goals, even though we are wrong.

High Reliability Sensemaking

Sensemaking differentiates High Reliability from other methods of organizing. Like other aspects of HRO, High Reliability sensemaking seems counterintuitive and inconsistent with rationality and normal operations, but it makes possible the intensity of interaction necessary to engage extreme events. In this section, we will discuss the outlier of disrupted rationality as well as concrete thinking, paradox, and the experience of time flux.

The core of sensemaking in High Reliability is the *outlier* and *short-feedback interaction*. Taken as a random, independent event, the outlier is readily disregarded, a belief founded on statistics, probability, and the normal distribution. The outlier, however, rather than being an extreme, independent, and random value, is, in High Reliability, identified as a precursor of a new process, an early herald of system failure that indicates a previously unidentified performance deficit or identifies a gap in our knowledge of the system. But High Reliability is more than recognizing the outlier; it also describes the organizational response. HRO is not a state of an organization but the dynamic of an organization, a dynamic rooted in actively making sense of outliers.

In these events, we are sensemaking for a moving, nebulous target while at the same time being exposed to hidden and unrecognized threats. Even observation is continuous as we sense what is moving and what is interacting. Probing through interaction identifies structure but most importantly identifies what is responsive to our efforts and what is not. Sensemaking sometimes directs us to the path of least friction and sometimes leads us to identify the strongest impediment.

There are dangers in taking a reductive approach to sensemaking, and there are dangers from being intimidated by its complexity. Our approach is to dignify several principles of sensemaking that interact in a nonlinear fashion, from which sensemaking will emerge. These principles come from the environment, perception, cognitive processing, affective responses, and communication.

Science is empirical because it relies on experience and observation; the most reliable and valid observation is a *randomized, controlled, prospective study*. This type of study, which represents *experimental* empiricism, serves us well in predictable situations but is not reliable in VUCA-T environments. But empiricism also includes what Bertrand Russell calls "knowledge by personal acquaintance" (B Russell 1910), where the individual, in a sense, creates knowledge on the fly through sensory perception and interaction, which is a form of *experiential* empiricism. It is this type of sensemaking that differentiates conventional sensemaking in more controlled and predictable environments from High Reliability sensemaking. To avoid confusion, we distinguish *empiricism* (as knowledge from sensory experience) from *rationalism*, where knowledge is derived from reason alone. Rationality describes the exercise of reason as the explanation of beliefs, and it commonly incorporates experience and perception, which are not a part of rationalism.

This is an important digression, because many criticisms derive from people's reasoning in situations they found confusing or threatening. They will not recall their reasoning (and rapid changes in reasoning), and the behaviors may appear to the outsider as irrational behavior. This represents the pursuit of sensemaking without having access to the full view in a rapidly changing situation. What is logical in the ephemeral moment will not appear logical in sequence or upon later review. This *disrupted rationality* occurs not only from limits of perception and cognition (the bounded rationality described by Herbert Simon) but from impaired cognition due to stress, physiological deficits (for example, more than 2 percent dehydration), and the physical environment (thermal stress from cold or heat, and ambient light or sound).

> The effects of fluid loss are easily observed in younger children playing organized sports in the heat. One summer I observed a ten-year-old boy playing on the opposing team in baseball, standing then sitting in the outfield. I told my fellow coaches that his coach would soon pull him off the field. When this happened, I told them that his coach would give him water, and the child would throw up. After this happened, I told the coaches that we needed to keep our team hydrated.
>
> We made the team drink water before the game, then throughout the game. In the last few seasons, the opposing team made increasingly serious mistakes that contributed to our team winning several games. Unfortunately, there was still a climate in that league among coaches of "being tough" to handle the heat.
>
> I described this experience to Jonathan Seals, a professional ballroom dancer. He began drinking more water throughout his day-long dance competitions—and was especially vigilant when working in Las Vegas—but his partner would not. She believed they had no performance decrements during their competitions in Las Vegas or otherwise. Jonathan found that her fine motor control, necessary for many of their dance steps, deteriorated over the course of the day. Only from videos could she see these changes.
>
> —Daved van Stralen

We can easily identify the loss of abstract thinking from fear and disrupted rationality by the presence of *concrete thinking*. The person becomes docile, regressing toward childlike thinking and behavior. One author (van Stralen) learned this in his early ambulance work. It was necessary for the ambulance drivers to know this when working with people in the first minutes of a crisis. Anyone new to emergency work would take it for granted that people would operate with abstract thought and reason. This expectation often leads to confusion on the scene. Veterans stressed this early and made further observations that the more regressed people become, the more afraid or stressed they are and, likely, the more serious the situation is. This observation was a gauge for seriousness and acuity. People sincerely believe they are being prudent and have not regressed to concrete thought.

Regression to the concrete has an important place in planning and operations in the "first light" of an emergency, which refers to the moment before the person or system has fully shifted from routine operations to an emergency condition—the period of least efficiency in emergency-response programs. This lack of efficient performance is derived from variations in sensemaking that are meant to recognize the change and the effect of regressing to concrete thought and interference with the use of abstract plans.

Stress impairs thinking and other cognitive functions but experience in the field also demonstrates stress leads to concrete thinking. We may conjecture that stress causes reversion to lower levels of Piaget's operations, that is, reversion to concrete operations. Several examples have been given in this book.

The belief of regression to first-learned behavior in the face of stress likely derives from identification in laboratory environments. People believe they will strongly maintain their capability for abstract thought. It is counterproductive to point it out in an emergency. Rather, speaking in concrete terms is more efficient.

People are also resistant to accepting impaired rationality, because everything, in real time, appears to make sense. In a group situation, this severely impairs communication when not recognized.

A respiratory care practitioner (RCP) told me how angry she was with me when I first arrived to help create an intensive care unit. I had told her that people think concretely in emergencies, so we must recognize that and work with it. If we assign a task, it must be concrete in terms of performance, when to start, and what to do if it doesn't work. She had years of experience working in emergencies and took offense that I was telling her what would happen and what to do.

During the resuscitation of one small infant, the resuscitation team prepared to place an endotracheal tube (a long, narrow plastic tube to protect the airway and assist artificial breathing) through the trachea to allow them to assist the infant's breathing. Both of the smallest endotracheal tubes they needed fell on the floor. The resuscitation team urgently needed another tube, so she sent an RCP to obtain one. After an extended period, she went to obtain the replacement tubes herself. She saw the RCP arrive while she was in central supply, housed in the medical center basement. Angrily, she asked him why he had not quickly obtained the tubes and brought them to the resuscitation. He answered that she had told him to get the tubes, so he went to the ICU on the floor. They had none. He went to the neonatal ICU, but they also had none. Then he went to the operating room, but they had none as well. So he went to central supply, where he met her.

That was when she no longer was angry with me. Had she been more concrete in her directions, such as specifically saying where to go or what to do if he did not find the tubes, then they would have obtained the tubes sooner and not have lost two RCPs in this quest.

She did return in time to safely treat the infant who recovered after a prolonged hospital stay.

—Daved van Stralen

Regression in behavior is a clear sign of severe stress or fear. More commonly discussed are fear reactions such as fight, flight, or freeze; less well known are the docility and acquiescence that also occur, which in some ways are similar to the flight response. Disrupted rationality, impaired cognition, concrete thinking, and regression to docility all affect our perceptions and how our brain is *capable* of processing perceptions for sensemaking. This is unrecognized by those who lose their abstract abilities, including the use of concepts, principles, and time (both past and future tense).

One of the first things ambulance men taught me was what to expect from people on scene: "They'll think concretely because of stress. They'll act like children when they're afraid. You can judge a scene, their level of stress and fear, by how concrete they are and how much like a child they act. This immediately gives you an idea of how serious the call is. Then you work with them on that level."

—Daved van Stralen

Extreme events involve interactions between multiple forces. For example, a serious infection involves human physiology, the person's specific physiology, the invasiveness and severity of the pathogen, and any physiologic deficits due to the situation or specific time. This makes predictability of any trajectory impossible. It also reveals how treating one problem can make another worse. In these events, it is not uncommon that what worked last time will hurt this time and what hurt last time will be a benefit now. This is the paradox of intervention; that is, we titrate opposing forces to subdue a dynamic, rapidly changing force.

A dynamic time course means more than simply rapid change. As in paradox, objects in the environment can have opposing purposes and changing purposes.

Every item in the scene has a past, present, and future, and experienced High Reliability practitioners often regard them simultaneously. That is, a vase on a headboard may reflect close family ties, and its presence may make the person in the room feel loved, yet it can be dangerous if it falls. Experienced High Reliability practitioners sense all these things simultaneously.

Paradoxically, what makes High Reliability safe is doubt, which is equivalent to the inquiring mind that is driven to question, even when the question remains at the back of your mind. You can never be certain until after you take the action and observe the result.

> Simply verbalizing that something is not making sense can cue the team into higher levels of sensemaking. Many times, others are experiencing the very same concerns but have not said something because they we unsure if others shared their concerns.
> —Spence Byrum

We must exercise caution in this sensemaking and be aware that we may include a trajectory we cannot predict or include overconfident judgments based on past experience.

High Reliability can be found in the details. The novice or layperson will see noise where someone with experience sees signs and signals. It is this salience that separates signal from noise. This differs from the concept of a weak signal, that is, a signal with less energy or strength. We are concerned that a signal with unrecognized meaning will be discounted as noise. Signs, signal, and salience build from details in the event and environment. Paying attention to these details brings events to notice when still in the compensated state and when the system does not show any disturbance.

> Craig Davenport, a respiratory care practitioner (RCP) in long-term care, reported to me one morning that he had changed the settings for a child because of agitation. Our standard is to hand-ventilate first to identify what calms the child, place the ventilator at those settings, and then call the physician. I asked him if he'd done that, and he said no. I asked if he knew that we work that way, and he said yes, so I asked him why he hadn't followed our standards.
> Craig immediately laid out every problem that had happened overnight: the action the night RCPs had taken, what had worked and what had not, and the response of the child to each intervention, including the time of event and the interval time between events. In detail. He knew

what settings made the child calm and the reason the RCP at the time had not continued the treatment. He used the settings that had been demonstrated to work earlier and that had been described in his documentation as having had successful results.

Craig is also a former US Army military police officer and Vietnam veteran. He uses his experience and has retained the necessary attitudes. He and I then brought this up on rounds, when we asked the staff what had made Craig right. It was the details…but the appropriate details.

—Daved van Stralen

Details alone are insufficient for sensemaking. When taken in that manner, the observation of details can be used in an abusive manner. Using "details without context is micromanagement," according to Weick (personal communication). Using discrimination and the judgment of details require salience and context.

Sensemaking and Outliers

The distribution of events in complex, nonlinear interactions is better described by the power distribution, sometimes called the Pareto distribution. This fits our experience in High Reliability situations, which is that most outliers resolve themselves or are minor. Occasionally, some of our interactions generate more attention or there may be greater severity, but we can still handle them. It is when these interactions become extreme when we absolutely take notice; these are the events for which we prepare. However predictable they are, the moment they will occur is not predictable, so we are not immediately ready to engage. This is the power distribution: most events are minor, some are larger and require attention, and some are extreme and have the potential for catastrophic failure.

> "If it happens once, it will happen again. If it
> happens again, it will happen worse."
> —DAVED VAN STRALEN

We all have the same brain as a processing unit. The way in which an experienced veteran engages extreme events is not significantly different neurologically from that of a novice or beginner. We can use this situation as a strength in our system to model how to approach uncertainty. Young people entering the workforce, newly hired employees, new managers, and so on will at some point enter an environment they have not encountered before, do not know the unwritten rules for, and have not developed sufficient tacit knowledge about. This represents liminality on a smaller scale than extreme events, but this liminality can prepare novices for crises. In this way, we can use the routine to expand our procedural knowledge for novelty. Any novel encounter and every new experience becomes practice for extreme events.

> "What you do in an emergency is what you do every day."
> —JAMES P. DENNEY, PARAMEDIC, LOS ANGELES FIRE DEPARTMENT

We cannot leave it to novices to learn how to make sense out of confusion. When we do, they will make sense of their experience with what they know and, most critically, from others who have similar levels of experience. The authority gradient is too great for a rookie or beginner to approach a senior team member for counsel. Jim Holbrook, educator and professor of Emergency Medical Services (personal communication), observed that "this is also seen in sex education of adolescents. They are more likely to ask questions of another adolescent than to ask an adult." Making sense in this manner can effectively shut out knowledge transfer from more experienced or senior staff.

We must help the student interpret new experiences and develop methods to think about the situation and act. It is the hallmark of an HRO to take pride in the improvement of students who pass through any section. Unfortunately, it often becomes a practice that people find students a burden, complain about their performance, and consider it the student's fault if the student performs poorly in the next rotation. This is not to say that some students are not misplaced, which is a problem that can be identified when the student does not improve under different mentors and in different situations.

We must identify what information is salient for our purposes and teach to that salience; we must ensure that the beginner knows the purpose of the organization and group. By knowing what information is salient, people are more likely to be vigilant for and to recognize the early heralds of system failure. By clearly knowing the purpose, they're more likely to take initiative and act on the information they develop.

The Sensemaking of Outliers
Sensemaking motivates the engagement of uncertain situations, and it is through this engagement that HRO sensemaking is created. In a series of short feedback loops, people not only develop sensemaking but also create more easily transmitted information. Providing descriptions of what they believe is happening or stating what they believe should be done will carry less information than a simple

statement based on the OODA loop (see chapter 6): "I did [action] and then saw [response]."

When we act, we act in a manner that makes sense to us. We make sense of our environment, make a decision that makes sense to us, and then act from that decision. Sensemaking, then, drives us to act or not to act. "Not deciding" or making "no decision" is a decision; "not acting" or "no action" is an action. As straightforward as this sounds, we must state it to novices.

When a veteran does not respond, a novice may make sense out of the nonresponse to conclude that the situation is not important. The veteran may have distinguished a particular problem that can be ignored from a problem that might become serious. Experience creates a form of mindfulness distinct from neglect or ignorance; it is *mindful indifference*, which Olivier Berthod and Gordon Müller-Seitz (2017, 5) defined to denote a reflexive lack of concern over potential problems. This is not reckless disregard or sloppiness but the "capacity to distinguish particular problems that might turn into serious ones from problems that can be ignored."

Sensemaking creates abstract concepts from concrete information, then uses these abstractions to make a decision for performing a concrete action. Our environment is in a concrete form that we must translate into abstract concepts; then we must translate concepts to perform concrete tasks. *Sensemaking takes you from the concrete to the abstract and back to the concrete.* One way we can look at this is the sensemaking-action loop:

Concrete environment > abstract concepts > concrete action
Concrete action > feedback > shapes the concrete environment

Sensemaking, as a process, gives purpose to our thoughts and actions. We perceive pertinent information from the environment as signals that we differentiate from noise. By giving meaning and value to this information, we categorize it and turn its content into an abstract form. According to Weick, "HRO may be significantly about categories and categorizing" (personal communication). This may be a significant contribution to operations in an environment without structure or internal logic: the "sensemaking of noise."

Finally, we use these abstract conceptualizations to perform some concrete action. This process draws from multiple domains: *content* from information theory, *meaning* from the cognitive sciences, and *value* from our affect.

Information theory, specifically Shannon's concept of information (Shannon and Weaver 1949), considers information in a statistical way as unexpected signals in an observed source. Too many unexpected signals, and the information becomes corrupted. In Shannon's concept, information is a measure of uncertainty, something unexpected. Certainty and predictability do not give us new knowledge; therefore, they do not constitute information to us. This is also congruent with our concept of information as a signal with meaning or predictability; sometimes we do not expect meaning, and predictability can be a surprise to us. Information as structured content only—how various information signals are related to each—is the *syntax* of information.

Information has significance only when it has meaning within a context, neither of which are necessarily part of the transmission of information in Shannon's information theory. It is at the semantic level that information has meaning. Pragmatics is the intent or the purpose of the information. To be made significant, we must also add value to the information. Value is both valence (good or bad) but also the degree to which the information can be used or the degree to which it will do harm.

Sensemaking involves content, meaning, and value—we cannot assume it is part of communication. Sensemaking in its most basic function drives action. Our decisions, and thus our actions, always make sense to us, even if only at that moment. In VUCA-T environments, sensemaking has other vital functions. Sensemaking tells us if our environment is safe and if danger is approaching. We use sensemaking to combine our knowledge and our situation for reasoning and to infer knew knowledge. Sensemaking is the basis of communication as we make sense of our environment and transmit this information to others, or we receive information about the environment from others.

> In the 1970s, as the first paramedics, we often encountered physicians who were unfamiliar with a concept or rule. They might not order morphine for myocardial infarction, for example, and we could not diagnose. We couldn't say the patient had myocardial infarction, and "chest pain" was too nonspecific to trigger treatment. Ron Stewart, our training physician, always stressed description over diagnosis or the use of slang or jargon. He taught us to accurately describe something like "crushing substernal chest pain." This phrase drove the physician to act, order the necessary drugs, and to ask for any further information that might be pertinent.
> —Daved van Stralen

When we enter any situation, the unconscious mind processes environmental stimuli through the amygdala for threat identification. This is an ongoing and constant process. Through the amygdala, primates have a strong inborn response to sinusoidal curves: such as the shape of a snake, for example, and humans have one for a face with a frown. One severe threat to people's existence that we do not commonly discuss is the lack of structure in the environment. Oddly, this same response by young novices who enter the workplace for their first day is also experienced by veterans who encounter unexpected environmental events of great magnitude. More commonly, sensemaking is used for reasoning. In this discussion, we will describe the importance of sensemaking both for action and for protection.

Sensemaking plays a role in communication when we encode information in the environment for the purposes of transmission by the signaler. We place another role for sensemaking on decoding transmitted signals by the receiver. Sensemaking and communication in a noisy environment differ significantly from a quiet and focused environment where management and research are conducted.

Sensemaking functions include action, protection, reasoning, and communicating. Because HRO came out of effective emergency operations, we will first discuss the change in sensemaking that appears to develop after we experience a grave threat and the loss of recognizable structures. A veteran or threat-experienced person makes sense of events differently than a novice or threat-naive person. In these circumstances, the brain must continue the conversion of perception to thought, but it also must take perception to action. This sequence produces a sense of knowing and contributes to learning. Knowledge, understanding, and explanation give meaning to our experience but may be more subjective than we realize. With that background, we can discuss the functions and modes of sensemaking with greater clarity. To create the HRO, initiates must make the transition from being threat-naive to threat-experienced, a process that involves modeling, social learning, and incremental change.

We will end this chapter with short descriptions of commonly used sensemaking models: situational awareness (Endsley), human-computer interaction (D Russell), cognition and metacognition (Klein), "Cynefin" (Snowden), library and information science (Dervin), mindfulness (Langer), and organizational behavior (Weick).

Sensemaking and the Post-Trauma Experience

The sensemaking for High Reliability emerged from, and is continually tested by, extreme events. We have discussed how we have found the principles of HRO to be more readily accepted by people who have felt their own vulnerability or the salience of their own mortality. Researchers have identified similar sensemaking approaches among people who have survived extreme experiences. One discussion in that literature debates whether the beliefs and sensemaking of such people protect them from psychological trauma (Westphal and Bonanno 2007) or are a result of their experiences (Tedeschi and Calhoun 2004).

We have described context dependence, regulation of emotion, and the use of short feedback loops in order to engage a given situation. These are also elements of "emotional flexibility," which may support the successful adaptation to trauma (Bonanno and Burton 2013). Emotional flexibility is comprised of three components operating in sequence: (1) the person is sensitive to context, (2) the person has a diverse repertoire of emotion regulation strategies available, and (3) the person is responsive to feedback from the environment.

Surveys of people who have faced major life challenges have identified several characteristics described as post-traumatic growth, or PTG (Tedeschi and Calhoun 2004). People who experience PTG are more likely to embrace novelty, are more open to experience, and are more accepting of paradox. These people use paradox for synthesis to balance order and chaos and to integrate complexity (Calhoun and Tedeschi 2014). Changes in core beliefs and in relationships with others may occur; most strikingly, people recognize the personal strength they acquire *because of* their experience of vulnerability.

Whether these characteristics prepare people for traumatic events or develop in response to the events is of less importance to us than the fact that these characteristics are found in common with people who have experienced extreme situations. Within extreme environments, these people are sensitive to context, embrace novelty, and appreciate paradox as being important for sensemaking in complex environments. Internally, they regulate their emotions and are open to experience. During the interaction, they are sensitive to feedback and seem willing to synthesize new ideas. These are shared characteristics with veteran operators in High Reliability systems.

We would think there would be a difference between experiencing a near-death situation and contemplating one's own death. Near-death experiences have led to the controversy described mentioned above about whether one changes one's beliefs or actions and whether growth comes from interpreting the experience or if one is resilient beforehand. Contemplating one's death, or "mortality salience" (Burke, Martens, and Faucher 2010), has been studied in terror management theory, or TMT (Greenberg and Arndt 2011). In their study of PTG, chronic disease, and mortality salience, Cozzolino et al. (2004) found that people can reach a positive growth state in each of these situations.

TMT initially addressed the source of motivation to protect self-esteem and assert group authority (Greenberg and Arndt 2011). This feeling of mortality now has been found to motivate members toward intergroup hostility. On the other hand, tolerance, open-mindedness, and shared humanity can arise from the mortality salience of TMT. Both defensiveness and inclusion can buffer the anxiety of death awareness.

Sensemaking Functions

Sensemaking is a multifaceted, multipurpose, and ongoing activity we cannot reduce to a singular situation with a singular viewpoint. Through sensemaking, we identify whether a situation is safe and observe the effect of our actions. Communication in a complex and dynamic situation is a dynamic interaction between people striving to make sense of what others are experiencing. Using sensemaking as a continuous reappraisal keeps us updated to changing situations and afterward can help reduce disabling stress reactions. It is difficult to fit these functions into a single model.

Identify Change

Not only is sensemaking *dynamic*, but we also do not know what is changing or when. As events change and demands on us continue, we must update not only our information from the environment but also update changes both in our conceptualization and in our internal milieu of the state of our mind and body. This adapts us for change and to change. "Thought sensemaking" can be thought of as hindsight in preparation for the future, but it also must be interactive with the situation. How you make meaning *during* an event tells how you will perform and how you will recover.

Bloom's Affective Domain of Learning

We *teach* sensemaking through the affective domain of Bloom's taxonomy of learning domains (Krathwohl, et al 1964). The cognitive domain of facts, concepts, models, and theories forms the basis of an educational program in which we use objective measures for progress toward competence in the subject or discipline. The ability to structure knowledge in the cognitive manner makes for easier presentation of new material to students. Lectures are more easily organized in a logically developed, linear form, with distinct categories, building to a comprehensive review of the subject matter. The cognitive domain also advances the science of a discipline.

The cognitive domain provides our common verbal knowledge, knowledge organization, and cognitive strategies, which are the facts, models, concepts, and theories we need for sensemaking. This represents declarative knowledge to know information about *what*, procedural knowledge to know information about *how*, and tacit knowledge to know information through experience. Focusing on the more easily and objectively measured cognitive domain risks the creation of normative sensemaking and the rejection of knowledge elements when entering the field. You might hear, "I know this is what they taught you, but let me tell you what really works."

Lecture and teaching material may be organized to make sense to the instructor, which leaves the student alone to make sense of the world, a potential fatal flaw when experiencing an unexpected threat or entering an unstructured situation. The cognitive domain softly avoids uncertainty and ambiguity and does not completely describe how to use knowledge in particular situations, which is necessary for proficiency, expertise, and mastery of a field or domain.

In the affective domain, in contrast, we focus on "how this will help" and provide the context necessary to give meaning to information. Doing so also increases our motivation to learn and to better understand the knowledge we have gained. Motivation, as affective learning, describes responsiveness to phenomena, the valuing of knowledge, and the worth applied to an object or idea.

There are two motivational dispositions: *performance orientation* and *mastery orientation*. In performance orientation, which is found in the student who does well solely in order to be positively evaluated, learning tasks are fixed and cannot change. This idea of a correct way to do things creates a normative approach, which is hazardous during extreme events (Kraiger, Ford, and Salas 1993). This is a common structure in formal education to produce competent students, but this happens at the risk of creating a ceiling of knowledge: competency becomes the goal of the organization and of the employees.

When I began teaching, I knew that what I taught would be lost once someone told my students, "I know this is what you were taught, but this is what works," or "this is how we do it." I tried teaching what works, but the students wouldn't know that unless they had used the knowledge. The educator Jim Holbrook told me, "It's simple. Tell them how it will help them."

From that point on, I taught what helps and how it helps. This became my "seventy-two-hour" rule: what I teach today must explain yesterday or be used tomorrow. Soon my students returned to me and told me what I had taught that had worked and how it had worked; or they told me about experiences that had long puzzled them, but now they understood. Over the years, this body of teaching knowledge has grown, including input from students sharing what they learned as many as thirty years earlier.

I did worry that my students would not learn the rest of the science or other important knowledge. My experience quenched that worry, as I found that having a basis of practical knowledge would drive the students to learn more, "fill in the gaps," or study to gain a stronger foundation to what I had taught. Jim later told me that what they were doing reflected Bloom's affective domain of knowledge.

—Daved van Stralen

Mastery orientation increases students' competence. Students have a tendency to make internal attributions for success and failure, thereby increasing their independence for better performance during tumultuous events. Skills and abilities can be improved, and goals are flexible and individual rather than normative (Kraiger, Ford, and Salas 1993). This is the method to move into proficiency, expertise, and mastery of a subject.

Mentoring, Affective Learning, and Tacit Knowledge
The VUCA-T environment is too varied and unpredictable to rely on rationality, cognition, tacit knowledge, and cognitive concepts. To gain independence in a high-risk environment, people must learn attitudes, values, the application of general ideas to specific situations, context-dependent knowledge, and how to understand knowledge that is difficult to codify. These abilities are described in the Dreyfus model of skill acquisition (Dreyfus and Dreyfus 1980), Bloom's affective learning domain (Krathwohl 1964), and Polanyi's tacit knowledge (Polanyi 1966). While it is possible to develop these abilities through individual action and practice, high-risk environments are too dangerous for this type of on-the-job training. A trusted veteran working alongside the student within the work context and in real time can model and teach this material. This is the role of a mentor.

In common educational and training programs, students generally graduate at a competent level with generalized, cognitive knowledge. Proficiency develops as they gain practical experience, thereby becoming more experienced with the particular. The affective domain of learning includes awareness, responsiveness, attitudes, placing value on information, and internalizing values. Sensemaking in the affective domain develops from responsiveness to novelty, the valuation of information in context, and appreciation for how certain kinds of information will help. This type of sensemaking is more readily taught by modeling the attitudes, processes, and tacit knowledge we desire the novice to learn. Tacit knowledge is not codified knowledge; it is context-dependent knowledge that is acquired through practical experience.

Mentoring for the practical application of knowledge is done in real time at the time. The mentor is present as an expert and observes the novice's performance in the actual domain for learning and performing domain tasks. The mentor then shares his or her specific expertise and sensemaking using both behavioral and cognitive modeling processes, which gives the student the social component of knowledge. *The mentor draws attention to signals, makes them salient, and gives context to the signals.*

The mentor creates a scaffold for learning. Mentoring is to teach the student practical knowledge for a discipline or in a community of practice as a means to communicate. Embedding tacit and social knowledge increases communication and coordination (Brown and Duguid 2001). The mentor, in effect, creates disorientation to the world, only to guide reorientation with a new identity.

The disorientation and reorientation of students to a new way of thinking is a vital function of High Reliability mentoring. The mentor also creates in the student an identity as a practitioner of the particular discipline, and the student gains acceptance in that discipline or practice. This is something that is only accomplished through sensemaking from a participant, not from an outsider (hence "I know what *they* taught," with emphasis on "they"). The ability to cut through the clutter with sensemaking is what it means, for example, to be a good physician or nurse. The practice of a good mentor is to know how to transfer tacit knowledge as guided sensemaking, or Bloom's affective domain of learning (Krathwohl, et al 1964). This identity then shapes how people interpret the world (Daft and Weick 1984).

Mentors are the repository of organizational knowledge as stories. As oral tradition, stories are person-specific and can be applied to or modified for particular situations. Stories that are meant for knowledge transfer to give organizational and situational context for sensemaking serve several purposes (Swap et al. 2001). First, knowledge that is rich in tacit dimensions about managerial systems, norms, and values can be readily communicated to newer staff; these stories tend to be concrete and readily identified with. Second, a single, richly contextualized story communicates tacit knowledge about the organization's capabilities and problems, which are likely not recorded in physical form. Third, stories that support explicit statements of the organization powerfully reinforce members' buy-in; these stories include negative stories, which do not necessarily harm the organization. (The sense in which we are using "mentor" refers to someone who is informally, physically, and situationally present, rather than referring to the formal use of the word as a position or teacher.) Stories and anecdotes are vital to teach tacit knowledge and to acculturate students to the culture of the industry and organization. We learn tacit knowledge through performing and modeling veterans. The difficulty arises because we "know more than we can tell" (Polanyi 1966, 18).

Signals

Sensemaking, at its most basic, processes *signals* from the environment for information and filters out noise. This requires judgment to determine if the stimulus is actually noise and not a signal with weak strength or something salient that goes unrecognized. This is the problem of using the concept of "weak signal strength": the phrase truncates the conversation about unrecognized meaning and context. The cognitive aspect of the signal is its content and meaning, while the affective aspect is value in the face of threat. The term overlaps with "signal strength" used in information theory and "signal meaning" from cognition and affect. Although information theory is not really concerned with meaning, we must acknowledge the role of affect in identifying threat and the role of cognition that gives meaning. This is necessary as we try to understand the threat.

> I'll share one concept you [van Stralen] taught me that stands out. I think you called them "OODA loops." Learning to look for what's going on under the surface, and recognizing to look for the less obvious signs of what's truly going on with patients, has been a valuable tool for many years for me (25 years). I learned much more, but that stands out the most.
> —Michele Grainger, educator for Respiratory Care Practitioners

Homeostasis

A control system maintains *homeostasis* by monitoring distance from a set point; then, through feedback control systems, it returns the system to that set point. This may occur when a change in external environment takes place or when the internal system has changed the set point (i.e., the external milieu balancing with the internal milieu). *Negative feedback* is a deviation from the desired, to be offset by a corrective action in the opposite direction. We commonly use this system to maintain the temperature of our homes and offices and to maintain driving speed and direction in a vehicle.

In High Reliability, the environment is more extreme, and we may not recognize if our *internal* set point has been reset or is not properly matched for the external environment. When immersed in these situations, we experience homeostasis through our interactions with the situation. Negative feedback corrects deviations from our desired state, and positive feedback supports our strength and resilience. To an outside observer, this method of homeostasis may appear to be one of constant or repeated error rather than the identification of deviations and negative feedback loops.

The correction of negative feedback may be classified as error, but it is a mark of safety, resilience, and adaptability. As we operate in this unstable environment, we will also test the boundaries between our performance capabilities and the limits for safety and harm. These boundary checks can sometimes only be performed in real-world situations in real time. Failures are useful in these situations, because they mark our performance *boundaries*. The outsider, not appreciating the exigencies of the situation, may have a different, negative interpretation of this level of operation.

Emotion and Arousal

Once a discrepancy or disturbance is detected, it arouses attention. This arousal can either lead to perception of the event as a challenge, which will directly lead to engagement and further enactment, or to cause aversion, with subtle and unrecognized fear responses. Neurologically, this attention mechanism is processed through the amygdala. Emotion, then, accompanies any aroused state and influences sensemaking and behavior. People may disregard the signal because of missed salience, distraction, or aversion. A second reason is one of expectant management: they have noted the signal but watch for further activity, or they have mindful inattention, in which they recognize the signal but recognize a harmless trajectory (Berthod and Müller-Seitz 2017).

Sensemaking enmeshes arousal, emotion, and cognition by combining the threat response and emotion of the amygdala-dorsal thalamus-cortex axis, moderated by the cingulate cortex, with brain laterality between the right hemisphere and novelty and left hemisphere and the familiar. Positive arousal can develop when the anterior cingulate cortex moderates the amygdala, and the stimulus is taken as a novelty. This leads toward challenge. Negative arousal develops when the amygdala unconsciously suppresses the cortex and cognition, and the arousal is consciously sensed as fear. Perception that is taken as novelty in this state may also contribute to the fear response. Negative arousal contributes to problem identification, which is a necessary component for the identification of threat (Maitlis, Vogus, and Lawrence 2013).

Emotions can influence sensemaking to be either *generative* or *integrative* (Maitlis, Vogus, and Lawrence 2013). Generative processes construct a more novel, creative account of the event and increase agility, while integrative processes give heightened sensitivity, whether new cues are consistent or inconsistent with what we expect. Positive emotions tend to foster generative processes, whereas negative emotions tend to foster integrative processes. Taken together or to create sequences, "emotion sensemaking" generates new ideas and integrates new experiences into what is known. Creativity can be enhanced when generative sensemaking and positive emotions follow integrative sensemaking and negative emotions.

In crisis situations, extreme positive or negative emotions can become a handicap, just as panic can be as destructive as overconfidence (Berthod and Müller-Seitz 2017). Sensemaking under these conditions will change from abstract thought to concrete thinking that is unrecognized by the individual. It can become difficult to disengage, either by relinquishing one's tools and protocols and leaving the situation mentally or physically or by the embodiment of the situation. At this point, making a conscious reappraisal and doing some physical activity may break the cycle before deterioration cascades into irreversible failure.

Cognitive Dissonance, Arousal, and Missed Opportunities

Cognitive dissonance describes the discomfort between two opposing cognitions. In High Reliability situations or VUCA-T environments, the discomfort develops between the cognition of a strongly held belief and the cognition of perception of the environment. Some people reduce the discomfort of High Reliability cognitive dissonance by accepting belief over perception (environment), thus delaying engagement. Because many events are self-resolving or amenable to minor intervention (power or Pareto distribution), we can see Weick's enactment error from failure to act. The reduction of discomfort guarantees the absence of arousal and missed opportunities to intervene, as noted by the "Systems deteriorate rapidly" or "No one could see it coming" factors. What people missed were the early heralds that occurred in the covert but compensated state.

New Environments

We want to identify structure when we enter *new environments*, which could be social interactions, physical activity, or sources of energy. If we are approaching a situation as an emergency, then we are observing for control of, or uncontrolled, energy and behaviors. Structure is distinct from threat; while a threat is something that may cause immediate harm, structure tells us how things come together and interrelate. If we know the structure, then we can better predict which interventions will work. People look to place elements into a category by using more easily identified, though superficial, characteristics. Sensemaking of the structure leads us to identify the mechanisms or principles underlying the situation. At the same time that we are making sense of the situation for structure and threat, we are also looking for *safety*. We must make ourselves and others safe in order to engage dangerous situations.

Risk Assumption

Our sensemaking allows us to take *risks*. We can only enter a dangerous environment if we can make sense of it as we go. Safety culture not only *prevents* error but also identifies when we err at the earliest possible moment. In order to work with danger and to prospectively work with hazards or threats, we must identify when the problem is not responding to our actions. By doing so, we can ensure threat separation. HROs never have a consideration that we can prevent all error or remove all threats from the environment.

Safety

Sensemaking tells us if we are safe and identifies whether or not the environment has identifiable structure. The most dangerous situation is when we do not know the structure or whether or not it is present. This is true for a new hire walking into the office or an experienced veteran engaging a life-threatening crisis. Predicting the trajectory of events is also a matter of safety, a result of structure, and the function of sensemaking. In sports, ball players will sense the trajectory of the ball and place themselves into a position to gain control of it; they do this by identifying the trajectory. In the same manner, during an event, we note small changes in an effort to identify the trajectory.

Friction

Sensemaking allows us to identify the least resistance in a dynamic state so that we can move ahead; we also identify any obstructions, which we will then decide whether to go around or engage. We will identify threat and respond appropriately. This situation has to do with *friction*. To move forward toward our goal, we not only think in terms of forward motion but also in terms of taking the path of least resistance toward our goal. We are also sensing friction while acting, which is something that comes from the environment or from our team and colleagues.

Friction describes situations where our actions are timely and efficient but produce noticeable negative feedback. When this interferes with operations we may want to update our plan or change direction to an approach that will have less friction. Internal friction develops from team dynamics but also from performance decrements and people who are overwhelmed by the situation. In the HRO, seasoned veterans have already evaluated team members for their expected performance under stress (Haas 1977; Ashforth and Humphrey 1995).

Another source of operational friction is the lack of shared sensemaking, or overreliance on explicit knowledge and context-independent information. The use of shared tacit knowledge reduces the amount of information that must be transmitted in an emergency, thus reducing the possibility of corrupted communication occurring. Context gives meaning to information—to knowing the context of the situation—and then gives meaning to the information that is being transmitted.

Causal Reasoning

Sensemaking is done for *causal reasoning*. Interacting with the situation helps identify what preceded the incident in order to act as a guide for further actions. Probing the situation and sensing the response will identify effective interventions.

Causal reasoning changes by level of analysis (see chapter 3, "The Logic of Practice and the Logic of Operations"). The distinction between proximate and ultimate causes have more strategic value and have an important place in after-action reviews. We further discussed causation in chapter 3, but we noted that the closer one is to an event, the greater the importance of individual sensemaking.

Causation as a level of analysis is important in consideration of the chain of events that led to the incident. Doing so guides intervention but can be misleading if the focus on distal, extraneous, or resolved causes becomes too intense. Causes can be considered as a series of reactions following fixed laws and principles—a linear deterministic causal model. In such cases, simple interventions to disrupt the reactions can quell the incident, and operators can use quantitative analytics. Mechanistic models of causation reflect the belief that, rather than immutable laws, some mechanism drives the incident. Events will continue until the mechanism runs its course. Quantitative analysis is of limited use in these models. Nonlinear reactions confound the clear identification of antecedent events and predictions. Plans, algorithms, and predetermined decision maps rely on linear processes. People who are heavily invested in linear models, processes, and plans may find it difficult to shift to the idea of nonlinear causation.

Communication

Sensemaking means *communicating* in order to share information. We must make sense to other people when we share what we have perceived. We also must make sense of what they have sent us as a message. We identify, interpret, and translate; we are objective, articulate, and succinct.

Identify, Interpret, and Translate

We *identify* information in the environment, which is influenced by our knowledge and experience but also by our purpose—why we are involved. We must *interpret* this information not only for its meaning and value but also for how to use it. Multiple people may use this information, but in its raw form, they may not realize its importance. For this reason, we must *translate* the information into a form they can use.

Objective, Articulate, and Succinct

Being objective with information is more difficult than it sounds. Too easily we add our interpretation or give value to something rather than allowing the context to speak for itself. This sometimes comes from a desire to help, but it may also represent a desire to persuade someone to your point of view. Even the order of presentation is subjective, as people typically place more emphasis on what they hear first. Tying this clear information together is critical for making sense. We must have a well-connected, meaningful, and articulate presentation. We sometimes tell a story with a beginning, middle, and end, while in a moving crisis, we more often want a scene. In theater, a scene carries one or two-story arcs from the previous scene to the next. Too much information distracts us, but too little may leave us more confused. Succinct information is enough to provide meaning without distracting excess; it has a level of information specific to the situation and to the specific parties involved in the communication. The key is to provide the right information at the right time; clear, concise, solution-driven communication separates the wheat from the chaff.

Action

Action and sensemaking are iterative processes that can be interactive, real-time feedback loops or more reflective hindsight-laden thought processes. Actions not only generate information, but actions also evaluate the responsiveness of environmental elements. Actions also test abductive hypotheses. In this manner, our actions enact new environments as they create experience (Weick 1979, 130, 148; Weick, 1988). The presence of someone in a situation is the first action, and it changes the environment. The person then becomes part of the problem, but not in the negative sense of causing problems. We become part of the problem in the existential sense that our presence changes our perceptions and changes the environment. In unsafe environments, those who engage the problem must be protected by those who are outside the situation through the use of resources—to stand by for rescue or for the rescue itself.

Identity and Existential Action

Wieck (1995) distinguished *identity* as one of the seven characteristics of sense-making. People respond to threats or challenges to their identity by trying to understand the challenge; by doing so, they enact a new situation and construct a new account of themselves and their organizations (Maitlis and Christianson 2014). This action restores their identity, in a similar manner of reducing the discomfort of cognitive dissonance.

Sensemaking, as an *existential action*, gives meaning to the individual, particularly through decision-making and action. Sensemaking, decision-making, and action merge into a smooth flow through acts of engagement, which moves enactment toward the more desired end-state. Any one element, separated from the others, becomes lifeless and even dangerous. Relying on the sensemaking of a subordinate for a decision gives meaning to the subordinate's efforts and position, thus changing the subordinate's identity. This increases the quality of sensemaking by the subordinate because then the sensemaking becomes personal to the subordinate. The subordinate comes to feel like a valued member of the team. In this sense, sensemaking and decision-making are existential actions.

> Early on in my EMS work, I found I could almost immediately identify college students. When communicating with us, they were slow to make decisions, looked for guidance, and were easily influenced by our authority. In contrast, teenagers who worked in environments where they made decisions were more confident and engaged.
>
> Later, as an attending physician in the PICU and a subacute care facility, I found the same dynamic. By migrating decisions to the bedside caregiver, the quality of decision-making increased, we saw an increase in initiative, and overall the quality of sensemaking improved. When working with staff from units or programs that retained central authority and

339

decision-making, I witnessed more docility and less confidence in their sensemaking.

—Daved van Stralen

Preventing decision-making infantilizes staff in how they make decisions. Excessive scrutiny and micromanagement create docility and decrease initiative. Significant trauma can undermine one's identity and, in High Reliability environments, interferes with resilience. The values of humility and empathy drive our support for colleagues. Veterans' modeling of how to respond to these traumas acts through the affective domain and the ideas of social learning theory to help the victim. When our image is entwined with our identity, even the suggestion of challenge, real or imagined, creates a threat to our identity, which results in a quarrelsome personality and gratuitous conflict with colleagues.

Resilience

Sensemaking is a source of *resilience* through reevaluation and revision of our environment, situation, and capabilities during an event. The identification of changing boundaries while taking action reduces overstretch.

Sensemaking, as part of social learning theory, helps underexperienced people model behaviors, beliefs, sensemaking, and decision-making from more experienced seniors in preparation for an event. Afterward, the same social learning sensemaking assists novices in placing meaning on the event and facilitates learning. This sensemaking, modeled from more experienced people, creates growth, a sense of community, and preparation for coordinated group action in the future.

Sensemaking after the event *creates a narrative* that has meaning that links events to a person's personality, identity, and personal growth. When faced with unexpected and uncertain events, we expect performance deficits. The personal narrative that develops after an extreme event can incorporate these deficits into learning and growth or it can become negative, leading to a decrease in self-worth and impaired resilience. Reappraisal changes the way we perceive situations and can decrease the emotional impact, for example by reinterpreting an emotional event in more objective terms. Using reappraisal as a regulatory strategy contributes to this resilience (Bonanno and Burton 2013).

Meaning-making is difficult to define. For our discussion, meaning-making connects events within the situational environment with the external environment and the person. In effect, meaning-making transcends sensemaking in the moment and situational awareness. Meaning-making is of greater importance for internalizing extreme experiences and to some degree protects us from isolation, which speaks to *global meaning* and *situational meaning*. Global meaning represents beliefs that are broader views as well as internal representations of what is desired, modified by personal experience. Situational meaning is the meaning in the context of a particular situation. The discrepancy between appraised situational meaning and global meaning can drive post-event distress. It is this distress that drives our efforts to make sense of the situation, accept the situation, or reevaluate our personal identity or beliefs. Reappraisal, a form of sensemaking, is also used for the events, causes, and meanings of the experience (Park 2010).

Error

Through sensemaking, we discern *errors* in our knowledge, design, plans, decisions, and performance. But we can become fooled if enough errors come together and form a pattern, which can create controversy when people disagree over whether the pattern represents a norm versus inconsequential effects versus a deeper, structural problem. These patterns, and other isolated errors, would not become visible as errors without the extreme environment. Trauma does not always destroy; it also reveals.

> "Two expert knitters described in *Vogue Knitting* their contest
> to identify who could knit a sweater with the most mistakes.
> The difficulty of this contest surprised them: too many
> mistakes, and the knitting began to look like a pattern."
> —DAVED VAN STRALEN

We can use the extreme event as a form of real-time "destructive testing" of the system. Models can overestimate performance or underestimate strengths. Testing the models and plans that we use in a system simply shows whether they can perform their functions correctly. Conventional testing does not necessarily demonstrate what the system looks like before the break, the limits of the system before it breaks, or its performance while breaking. The extreme event, as a form of destructive testing, produces qualitatively and quantitatively more and better information that will be useful to the program. The use of an open and inquisitive mind to study the system failure and the circumstances surrounding the failure can identify "occult" risks, risks that are not manifest or detectable by clinical methods alone and are hidden properties of the system. Besides yielding more information, failure in operations can be easier to interpret than during conventional testing. The caveat is that the justification of people's behaviors, particularly of management and higher, will mislead reviewers, while the use of

reductive processes to identify a single root cause will dismiss important contributors to failure and missed opportunities for success.

> Forget your perfect offering
> There is a crack in everything
> That's how the light gets in.
> —LEONARD COHEN, "ANTHEM"

Engaging in sensemaking to identify these gaps in real time during failure is the
duty of each participant to improve the quality of the system. The purpose of this
is not only to identify weaknesses but also to identify unrecognized strengths,
which may be found in the paradox that knowing one's weaknesses creates
strength.

Learning

Sensemaking also refers to how we identify and *learn* from error (Maitlis and
Christianson 2014). Sensemaking is critical for learning from novel events and
from errors in more routine operations. Such sensemaking starts with real-time
situational learning, including the emotional response to the error. We share error
as a social construct with our team. Learning through sensemaking can only move
up within the organization when senior members and leadership accept ambiguity, maintain an inquiring attitude, and accept the actions of their subordinates.

Error is retrospective sensemaking. In real-time sensemaking, where we look
to the present while thinking of the future, it is difficult to label an action as
an error; actors are more likely to say that "it" did not work out or call "it" a
mistake. Mistakes and errors are expected in stochastic situations; in fact, they
mark boundaries for prudent action. The use of error as an operational or moral
construct is more likely borrowed from organizational theory but now carries a
moral tone associated with blame.

Error and mistake appear to have different meanings and purposes on opposite sides of the liminal threshold. In predictable, structured environments, error
is a measure from the expected or desired, and mistakes are a mark of performance decrement. In unpredictable and unstructured environments, error is a
feedback signal for real-time learning that indicates when to correct or update
conceptualization, and mistakes guide performance to increase effectiveness.
Error and mistakes are also signs for us to recheck our regulation of emotion. As
William J. Corr, Captain of the Los Angeles Fire Department, has stated, "If your
body is moving faster than your mind, you must slow down. If you feel your eyes
glaze over, slow down" (personal communication).

Emotional Arousal and Learning

Extreme events elicit more extreme emotional arousal than routine operations. The farther one is from the context, the less arousal one experiences. Emotional distance can come either from finding a microclimate within the event for safety or from having greater distance because of time, space, or position in the hierarchy. This situation creates serious problems when evaluating error sensemaking, because sensemaking in the middle of uncertainty, time compression, and threat differs significantly from sensemaking in a protected, well-controlled environment. In the latter environment, sensemaking tends to be normative and rule based; it is commonly derived from models that have not been validated in the VUCA-T environment. In the healthcare field, people can be over-reliant on rules derived from academic papers, particularly those with a prospective, randomized, controlled research design.

We look to routines, procedures, checklists, and protocols to reduce error, yet these elements can contribute to error in the confusion that occurs at the beginning of extreme events (Catino and Patriotta 2013). Cognitive routines can cause mindless behavior, which starts a chain of events that can lead to error. As described by fighter pilots in the Italian Air Force, the danger of flying a fighter jet can, in itself, cause emotional responses, but negative emotions also come from the fear of being judged by one's colleagues. More easygoing people reduce their negative emotional responses, while more angry or unforgiving people increase their negative responses. These responses from others directly affect our sensemaking during an event and our ability to later learn from errors (Catino and Patriotta 2013). Having a culture of mutual support and respect, though, can cause pilots to fly in a manner that will pass the scrutiny of their colleagues (Ron, Lipshitz, and Popper 2006).

Learning from error through sensemaking is a cultural process (Catino and Patriotta 2013). Error, and how we view error, during an extreme event is based on our individual sensemaking and how the group culture views error. When error is an expected discrepancy or disruption, the individual or team will engage the error as sensemaking. The resolution of the error is processed and reappraised for learning to be shared with the larger organization. The sharing of lessons learned is one of the most important attributes of an HRO.

Unrecognized justification enmeshed in sensemaking serves to protect the person who erred, which is more of a sign of organizational pathology that people cannot be honest. In some cases, though, such justification represents people who feel a threat to their self-identify and are protective of their image, which they do as an alternative to blaming others.

We must capture sensemaking across the liminal threshold and translate it into a form that liminal people, those who sojourn into the death zone, can use to protect themselves and one another. This form of sensemaking makes existential sense out of the discrepancy or disruption: Is it a threat to the *survival* of the person or organization or is it a threat to the *image* and identity of the leader and organization?

When we encounter a discrepancy or a disruption, sensemaking creates linkages between the operators, paradoxes during the event, belief structures, and reconceptualizations during the event (Maitlis and Christianson 2014). In this way, individuals and organizations learn novel responses to extreme events, which is most important when faced with high levels of ambiguity, unclear cues, and multiple choices of actions. Sensemaking is how we identify the relationship between actions and the outcomes (Maitlis and Christianson 2014).

Emotional Memory

In extreme environments, where we find High Reliability, people experience highly arousing events that create *emotional memories.* The amygdala processes highly arousing rewarding or aversive experiences to create persistent and vivid memories. Emotional memory is a form of episodic memory, which is a type of autobiographical memory from our lives. Episodic memory contains our unique experiences and specific objects, people, or events, while semantic memory contains general knowledge and facts about the world. Once formed, emotional memory enhances the salience and priority of later stimuli.

Learning to identify life-threat from a single experience, emotional memory, improves survival in the wild. Ecologists have also identified the effects of this traumatic stress in wild animals as being similar to post-traumatic stress in humans (Boonstra 2013). This is due to the need for prey species to rapidly learn predator threats without the lengthy time period needed for learning with operant or classical (Pavlovian) conditioning. Because this neural circuitry is conserved in animals through predator-prey interactions, it is likely adaptive.

Conserved in this setting describes a trait that is unchanged despite evolutionary pressure. It indicates a trait essential to the organism. The fact emotional memory is conserved indicates it is important for human survival.

In VUCA-T environments, the stress response is similar to this ecological predator-induced stress. While the stress response of emotional memory is adaptive, it can become maladaptive from severe threat or a more extreme stress response. HROs attempt to proactively institutionalize adaptive responses and limit the maladaptive psychological injury that results.

An environmental cue associated with the original experience can involuntarily trigger an emotional memory. Any of the senses can act as a cue. Though we more easily think of sight, other senses can also act as cues. The pathway for the perceptual cue travels through the amygdala, causing reflexive emotional, visceral, and behavioral responses. Everyone has memories of some emotionally charged experience, which is a product of life in general. The recall of these memories can be pleasant or unpleasant. A more emotionally charged experience creates more severe emotional memories, from aversive behaviors to the extreme experience of post-traumatic stress. This involuntary recall of emotional memories benefits us by its protective function by warning and preparing us of danger.

Emotional memory, then, can help and hurt us. Rapid and early recognition of a previously experienced threat is invaluable when entering a dangerous situation. On the other hand, hypervigilance can become exhausting and debilitating. The arousal response through the amygdala in more severe forms decreases cognitive function. The arousal can prepare us or cause aversion. We have all met old veterans, a bit crusty, who warn us about things when we are working. We are never sure what has upset them, but something in our actions or the situation has quickly caught their attention. In our youth, we resent this intrusion; in midcareer we envy it and want to learn more; at the end of our career, we are doing it ourselves.

The trigger is from today; the response is from the past. We can recognize this in our colleagues when their response is out of proportion to the event. Sensemaking is heavily influenced by the experience of emotionally charged events. Emotional memory as sensemaking has two faces: the rapid and visceral identification of an occult threat or overreaction to a benign event.

Sensemaking Models

The remainder of this chapter lists several sensemaking models, including their authors, their domains, and other pertinent information.

Model	Information systems, 1983
Author	Brenda Dervin
Domain	Library science, communications (journalism)
Purpose	Information is to be used; gaps lead to information needs
Direction	Bottom up
Expertise	Novice to expert
Process	"Methodology between the cracks"; reality is not continuous but has gaps; information is a process of observation; all information is subjective
Reference	Agarwal, N. K. (2012); Dervin, B. (1983)

Model	Mindfulness, 1989
Author	Ellen Langer
Domain	Social psychology
Purpose	Attention management; danger of automatic thinking; experience formed by the words and ideas we attach to them
Direction	Bottom up
Expertise	Novice to expert
Process	Create new categories on the spot; be open to new information; be aware of other perspectives; evaluate information in relation to context; pay attention to process (doing) rather than outcome (results)
Reference	Langer, E. J. (1989, 2014)

Model	Human-computer interaction, 1993
Authors	Daniel Russell, Mark Stefik, Peter Pirolli, Stuart Card
Domain	Computer science, cognitive science
Purpose	Externalize representations of knowledge for machine computation
Direction	Top down (goal-directed, representation search); bottom up (encoded schema representing a concrete entity, "encodon"
Expertise	Expert
Process	Degree of effort, degree of structure, foraging loop to seek information, sensemaking loop (representation search) for best fit
Reference	Russell, D. M., M. J. Stefik, P. Pirolli, and S. K. Card (1993) Pirolli and Russell (2011)

Model	Situational awareness, 1995
Author	Mica Endsley
Domain	Human factors, ergonomics
Purpose	Integrate people with technology
Direction	Bottom up
Expertise	Expert
Process	Local data input; develop meaning and trajectory
Reference	Endsley, M. R. (1995a; 1995b).

Model	Cynefin, 2003
	"Cynefin" is Welsh for habitat, describing the five decision domains simple, complicated, complex, chaotic, and disorder
Author	Dave Snowden

Domain	Business decision-making, systems theory
Purpose	Challenges assumptions of cause and effect: order, rational choice, intent
Direction	Top down (strategy)
Expertise	Expert
Process	Diagnostic for type of complexity; normative
Reference	Kurtz, C. F., and D. J. Snowden (2003)
Model	Cognition, metacognition, 2006 (Cohen 1996)
Author	Gary Klein
Domain	Psychology, cognitive science
Purpose	Apply mental models to uncertain, tie-dependent events
Direction	Bottom up, internal
Expertise	Expert
Process	Recognition-primed decision-making
Reference	Cohen, M. S., J. T. Freeman, and S. Wolf (1996); Klein, G., B. Moon, and R. R. Hoffman (2006)
Model	OODA loop (mid-1970s)
Author	John Boyd
Domain	Aerial combat
Purpose	Maneuver
Direction	Bottom up
Expertise	Novice to expert
Process	Rapid feedback cycling
Reference	Hammond, G. (2012)
Model	Sensemaking, 1979
Author	Karl Weick
Domain	Social psychology, organizational theory
Purpose	Uncover what is not known; use enactment to keep moving toward end-state
Direction	Top down
Expertise	Novice to expert
Process	Interactive
Reference	Weick, K. (1979, 133-137).
Model	Operational sensemaking, 1995
Author	Daved van Stralen

Domain	Public safety, neuroscience
Purpose	Synthesis of sensemaking articles; operation in dangerous situations
Direction	Bottom up, top down
Expertise	Novice to expert
Process	Interactivity; responsiveness to environment
Reference	McConnell, M., and D. van Stralen (1997)

Conclusions

(1). Sensemaking is how we change; sensemaking is also why we don't.

(2). Sensemaking is how we tie together experience with knowledge.

(3). High Reliability sensemaking is a method for simultaneously identifying and creating structure and predicting ability in VUCA-T environments.

(4). An outlier, as a discrepancy or disruption, is an early herald of a system failure and should be used to initiate engagement.

(5). Sensemaking is how we identify errors and learn from error, both in real time and retrospectively.

(6). Emotional arousal and fear alter sensemaking.

(7). Sensemaking does not make sense to those who do not understand it.

CHAPTER 11

OTHER SYSTEMS

Hospitals have been focusing on improving safety and processes for over a hundred years. The genesis of healthcare performance improvement can be traced back to the efforts of Florence Nightingale and her team during the Crimean War (1853–1856). They realized that infectious diseases killed more soldiers than war wounds. Nightingale and her team focused on improving cleanliness, sanitation, nutrition, administrative order, and patient care, which drastically improved the conditions for the care of soldiers and reduced the death rate among patients by two-thirds. Her careful data collection and analysis and reasoned conclusions were instrumental in her success, along with her leadership skills and aristocratic connections (Inozu et al. 2011).

Over a hundred years later, in the fall of 1987, Donald Berwick and Joseph M. Juran made history with the launch of the National Demonstration Project (NDP) to improve hospital performance using total quality management (TQM), a variant of continuous quality improvement (CQI). Twenty-one American healthcare organizations joined as members of the NDP. Project participants experimented with using TQM tools, which other industry leaders such as Toyota, Mitsubishi, Honda, Sony, Xerox, and Motorola were successfully implementing. During the following decades, healthcare organizations across the world began to embrace new tools and methods as they evolved to improve safety. These include (but are not limited to) Lean, Six Sigma, Theory of Constraints (TOC), checklists, human factors studies, SBAR (situation, background, assessment, recommendation), TeamSTEPPS (the trademarked "Team Strategies and Tools to Enhance Performance and Patient Safety"), the incident command system, crew resource management, operational risk management (ORM), and resilience engineering. These methods and tools all have value and have been implemented with varying levels of success. These tools and methods also provide a basis for the understanding of the foundational elements of High Reliability.

HRO expands and enhances all of these key attributes to organizational culture to a new and higher level. Although HRO is not isolated from these attributes, taking them out of context or not integrating them for a coherent program can lead to danger. Often an organization takes one of these attributes as the talisman or focus, neglecting how it fits into the organization or how it acts when put in motion (compared to static, independent use by an individual or group). The medical field also has a tendency to take these elements as initiatives and not integrate them into a process for engaging unstructured situations or events, thus leading them to become lost, discarded, or marginalized. In this chapter, we will review these methods and discuss how they fit under the HRO umbrella.

Approaches for Standardization and Improvement

The following sections discuss several leading approaches to standardization and improvement: Lean, Six Sigma, Constraints Management, Checklists and Protocols, and Human Factors.

Lean

During Japan's recovery from World War II, the automobile manufacturer Toyota developed the Toyota Production System, a system that describes a more effective and efficient organization over time compared to similar organizations. Doing so would produce a "lean" organization (i.e., with the absence of fat), which became "Toyota lean" or simply "lean" in the 1980s, with a systematic approach to eliminating waste. A lean organization's primary orientation is to give value to the customers and build sustaining relationships. In the seventies and eighties, American industry became fascinated with Japan's qualityand job security.

A lean organization considers people to be more valuable than machines. This respect for people builds relationships both inside and outside the organization. The organization relies on the resulting highly motivated people within the company, because such employees will more likely identify a problem and speak up to fix it. This situation is comparable to the HRO's deference to expertise. While high Japanese morale and the use of distributed decisions were initially thought to ensure productivity, this was later disproven.

Lean organizations constantly look for ways to improve, often by maintaining vigilance for problems, much as an HRO would with preoccupation with error. Lean organizations use flow for their processes rather than "batch" steps, which is a source of the just-in-time delivery method that replaces the warehousing or stockpiling of materials. Identifying obstructions to flow will uncover sources of waste and identify areas for improvement.

Kaizen, a term used in lean, refers to a Japanese philosophy of improvement through all aspects of life. Kaizen is the process that lean uses to improve the system and give value. Value, relationships, motivation, and flow make a lean organization. Value is defined by the customer; Toyota would study and provide that value. An organization that uses lean understands that it is selling value and must add value to the product or process. Numerous hospitals in the United States and around the globe have embraced lean.

HRO and lean have potential conflicts between the two systems. The waste-minimization processes of "muda, muri, and mura" reduce what does not add value to the organization's product or service, which is reasonable in routine, more stable production environments. (*Muda* is wastage of resources that do not add value to the customer; *mura* is wastage from unevenness or irregularity in the operation or process; *muri* is wastage from overburdened work or excess demand on people and machines, the result of an imbalance between muda or mura.) Planning and preparing for the unexpected may muddle what is muda, muri, and mura and what is not. That creates the question of what plans and preparations only add value if an unexpected event occurs. Some resources, or specific quantities, are only necessary for an unexpected event; the same is true with education and training. The HRO philosophy gives the future and the idea of possibility importance in defining wastage.

Jidoka is the expectation to stop the process immediately upon discovery of an abnormality in the product or process. In lean manufacturing, people then notify the operator or a supervisor. In HRO, we expect people to make sense of the situation and engage the problem for enactment. Engagement may mean leaving the area to seek assistance. HRO, in jidoka, goes beyond lean manufacturing.

Keiretsu is an alliance of companies, a form of conglomeration created after World War II that replaced family-owned or government-sponsored companies. Toyota is a vertical keiretsu, a group of companies surrounding one company (Toyota). Keiretsu governance relies on trust between companies to coordinate productivity. In fact, mutual trust is a primary method Toyota uses to develop mutual benefit in partnerships, with the aim of having mutually beneficial, long-term relationships with suppliers (Kerber and Dreckshage 2011). This high-trust, long-term cooperation reduced new model development time in the Japanese auto industry (Ahmadjian and Lincoln 2001).

Keiretsu and high or mutual trust developed starting in the 1950s, when technological knowledge was transferred from auto assemblers to suppliers. Over the years, the suppliers and vendors who developed greater expertise contributed to the design process, transferring their knowledge to auto assemblers (Ahmadjian and Lincoln 2001). Even the best mechanisms of knowledge transfer do not, alone, guarantee the successful transfer of knowledge, however. Having high levels of trust is crucial for the transfer of tacit knowledge (MacDuffie and Helper 1997), the type relied on in lean manufacturing. But even the best transfer mechanism, applied to a highly absorptive and responsive recipient, is not sufficient to guarantee successful knowledge transfer. The fundamental lesson of Honda's BP experience (BP for "Best Process," "Best Performance," or "Best Practice") is that a supplier-customer relationship that generates high motivation for learning and high trust between provider and recipient is a crucial condition for any transfer of a complicated, largely tacit body of knowledge like lean production (MacDuffie and Helper 1997).

Six Sigma

Believing that reliability comes from consistency, Motorola developed this approach to reduce variation and eradicate defects for internal quality of control and to increase the company's return on investment. Motorola found that, because of the complexity of its products, the specific level of 3.4 defects per million products (see discussion below) was a small enough number of defects that this exceptional performance dramatically reduced complaints about the company's products. GE later adopted and successfully used the system in the 1990s.

Six sigma (6σ) is a statistical term that refers to 3.4 occurrences per one million events. Statisticians use sigma (Greek letter σ, represents a standard deviation) to measure how a sample deviates around the mean (average or norm). Through a mathematical equation, the distance between sigmas (standard deviations) on the x-axis is the same, but the area under the curve changes. The area under the curve represents the number in that portion of the sample. When graphed, this area forms a curve called a "normal curve." (The technical name for this is the normal Gaussian curve or linear distribution.) Six sigma describes the area of the curve that is six standard deviations from the mean, or 0.00034 percent. Because of the nature of the curve, six sigma refers to 3.4 occurrences per one million events, while five sigma is 233 occurrences. The system has the assumption that risk and errors develop from variation in processes that will propagate through the system and reduce the quality of the product. The organization will then benefit by identifying and controlling variation in those processes that most affect performance and profits.

In mechanical processes, inputs, transforming processes, and outputs are related in a deterministic manner, with each directly determining the outcome.

Cause and effect are direct and have great importance in identifying where to intervene. If you determine the cause of the problem, then you can fix it. The cause will come from variation (i.e., deviation from the expected) in the process that has resulted from error.

In the Six Sigma system, variation, or error, is to be identified and mitigated; it is represented on the normal curve as being wider than the desired curve. A wide curve represents a larger number of products or processes in the sample that vary from the expected. This variation prevents parts of the system from working with one another, just as you would see if people came to work with different training, clothing, and expectations and speaking different languages.

To identify and reduce variation, Six Sigma programs will analyze the root cause and develop corrective action. Six Sigma applies a five-step method called define-measure-analyze-improve-control (DMAIC), with each letter representing one of the steps in the methodology. The methodology includes the application of a full range of statistical tools. Six Sigma enables the identification of the root causes of complex problems and the reduction of variation, both of which are central to the improvement of processes. Examples include reductions in infection rates, patient falls, and missed appointments as well as enhanced medication reconciliation and coding.

The goal of Six Sigma is to reduce variation. Because an HRO must prepare for unexpected, more variable events, a wider variation is necessary. In confusing situations, however, narrowed variation in the processes that are used adds to the reliability of performance. This system strikes an important balance between what must have a wide variation to respond to variability and what must have narrow variance to ensure dependability in operations.

Constraints Management

Constraints management is a management philosophy encompassing an integrated suite of techniques used in operations and supply-chain management, project management, conflict resolution, and strategic planning. Eliyahu Goldratt began its development in 1979 and has led its evolution in logistics/production, performance measurement, and problem-solving/thinking tools. Goldratt introduced the basic concepts of constraints management to the public as the Theory of Constraints (TOC) in his landmark 1984 book, *The Goal.* In the book, Goldratt details a systematic approach to managing complex organizations by identifying and controlling key leverage points within a system or process. By managing these key control points, healthcare organizations can focus on areas that drive system-level improvement instead of trying to manage every element of a process, which can lead to local optimization without systemic impact.

Constraints management has been applied to manufacturing, project management, retailing, supply-chain management, and process improvement in various industries (including healthcare) with breakthrough results. System improvements under constraints management seek to identify (1) what system variable to change, (2) what to change to, and (3) how to cause that change. This follows a "process of ongoing improvement" (POOGI) comprised of two prerequisites and five steps that underlie all constraints management production techniques. The prerequisites for constraints management process improvements are (1) define the boundaries of the system and its goal and (2) determine a means to measure goal attainment. After satisfying the prerequisites, system improvement proceeds according to five focusing steps:

(1). *Identify* the system constraint. What limits the performance of the system now? What is the weakest link in the system?

(2). Decide how to *exploit* the system's constraints. How can the most performance be achieved from a constrained step in the process without additional investment? (*Exploit* in this context means "use, develop, make use of, take advantage of, and make the most of.")

(3). *Subordinate/synchronize* everything else to exploit decisions. Set up and implement rules to maximize the capacity of the system based on the speed of the system's constraint.

(4). *Elevate* the system constraint to physically increase the capacity of the system through the acquisition of or investment in more resources. Always remember to predict where the constraint will be after elevation and its resulting impact on global performance. This decision will definitely affect an organization's "elevate" strategy.

(5). *Go back* to step 1. This will ensure that improvement is ongoing and never ceases. This step also helps to avoid inertia by keeping the relentless tendency to accept established precedent at bay. Even the most transformational improvements, once established, become the status quo.

Goldratt also developed several Thinking Processes, two of which are particularly relevant to the science of decision making: The Evaporating (or Conflict) Cloud method and the Change Matrix method. These two methods form the basis of the "Change Matrix Cloud Process" recently developed by Dr. Alan Barnard (Barnard 2016).

Lean and Six Sigma are known as process-improvement approaches. Constraints management, in contrast, takes a systems perspective by looking at the interdependencies among processes and their dynamics for system optimization. Although each of these three methodologies has its merits, a careful integration of them promises much more effective results than practicing any single methodology in isolation. When separated, lean tools cannot bring a process under statistical control, and Six Sigma cannot improve cycle time dramatically, as Michael George states in his book *Lean Six Sigma*. Lean promotes the elimination of waste everywhere without necessarily focusing on the overall system, and Six Sigma has an inherent risk of local optimization. Constraints management highlights where to *focus* improvement efforts for system-level impact by offering a dynamic, holistic view of where bottlenecks and the weakest links of healthcare organizations (among others) become not only visible but also manageable.

Lean Six Sigma and other continuous-improvement programs have been widely integrated into HRO deployments at hospitals. The Joint Commission Center for Transforming Healthcare and its participating organizations use the trademarked Robust Process Improvement (RPI) methods and tools to improve the quality and safety of healthcare as one of three critical features in HRO deployments, as shown in figure 10. RPI tools include lean Six Sigma, change-management processes, and other change-management methodologies and tools. The Joint Commission coined (and trademarked) the phrase "Robust Process Improvement" because they recognize the advantage of having a variety of approaches to address complex work environments (Chassin and Loeb 2013). HRS Consulting, Inc. has trademarked the term "Reliable Process Improvement" as a means of further emphasizing the need for any process improvement to be truly "reliable", or it will not be sustained.

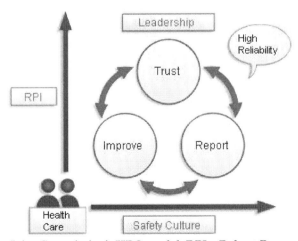

Figure 10—The Joint Commission's HRO model; RPI = Robust Process Improvement

Checklists and Protocols

Checklists are static; protocols flow. Both ensure thoroughness while constraining activity. They are a control on action. In complex environments and situations, checklists and protocols act as accessory, objective monitors and increase safety and reliability. Scrupulous adherence during cascading failure, however, introduces risk to the system.

What problem does the checklist solve? This is the central problem for use of a checklist, the checklist's usefulness and interference during unexpected events, and its acceptance by operators. Karl Weick asked, "Who writes the checklist?" (personal communication). Different writers create different checklists for different vulnerabilities. The checklist must serve a purpose to the operator rather than solely act as a tool to migrate control *over* the operator, independent of the situation or context.

Preflight checklists came into aviation during World War II as the complexity of combat aircraft increased. This singular intervention reduced air crashes and deaths. Dr. Peter Pronovost and his team used this concept to reduce infections in central venous catheters. (Because the large veins in the trunk of the body do not have valves, bacteria have the freedom to rapidly spread, making the presence of a catheter especially dangerous.) Following their success, they applied the checklist to operating room briefings with some focus on the site of operation to reduce wrong-site surgery (Berenholtz et al. 2004). They again achieved success.

Atul Gawande (2010) advocates for wider use of checklists to reduce error in complex tasks. Specifically, he believes checklists will identify when information is not being used (even though it is available) and when information that is available is not used properly. Checklists can further reduce memory lapse, contribute to thoroughness, and build cohesive teams.

> Checklists are greatly misunderstood by many people in medicine. The checklist is not designed to think for you. Checklists are not a replacement for teamwork and professionalism. They are simply tools to aid the practitioner in caring for patients. There are countless instances in HROs where the checklist has helped avoid an oversight, so how is it possible that there is such resistance to checklists in healthcare when the applicability is so real?
> —Spence Byrum

The overreliance or misapplication of checklists can contribute to failures. Once the item is checked, people may not recheck it if circumstances change or if there is a need to start over. Rigidity in the use of lists can increase harm when emergent circumstances drive other behaviors or change the value of select items. James Reason has identified the "strong-but-wrong" rule as a source of error. Checklist use can become strong but in the VUCA-T state could be wrong.

Human Factors

The field of "human factors" (or HF), earlier known as human engineering or ergonomics, is concerned with the design of machines to facilitate their interactions with people; the field deals with the human-machine interface. Decentralized decision-making and focus on the work group over the individual as personnel are not isolated atoms but work together. HF engineers use engineering psychology as a background with the human/machine interface, but there are not always direct parallels as human beings can be isolated.

The field of HF and ergonomics is a *systems approach* for the *design* of equipment, processes, and systems for better integration with *human performance* (human body and cognitive abilities) within the *operating environment*. The field of cognitive ergonomics studies the mental processes for interactions among people and other elements of a system, including mental workload, decision-making, and stress in operational environments.

HF studies originated after World War II, particularly following several failures from poor interfaces between humans and machines. Failures could be found when no feedback existed between the consequences of design (which affects the consumer) and the designer. Design engineers then pushed what could be done to surpass the ability of an individual's performance.

HF has a broad meaning as an interdisciplinary profession that studies the interfaces between humans and machines. The field applies a blend of engineering and behavioral sciences to solve complex human/machine interface, human/complex systems control, human to human communications, and simulators. HF covers individual, team, and now organizational performance. HF also uses the public-health model of accidents, where human performance vacillates—which is also the basis of FRAM (the "functional resonance accident model," mentioned later in this chapter) in resilience engineering—and events will produce alternating task underload (i.e., complacency and dulling of skill) and task overload (i.e., overwhelming). That is, long periods of inaction will be interspersed with bursts of action.

Communication and Coordination

The following sections combine communication with coordination at several levels, from one-on-one to crew interaction to the Incident Command System that can, over hours to days, expand to manage the largest emergencies covering multiple states.

SBAR: Situation, Background, Assessment, and Recommendation

Doug Bonacum, Vice President of Safety Management for Kaiser Permanente, served eight years on active duty in the US Navy submarine force. He went to work with Kaiser Permanente in environmental health and safety work and then subsequently patient safety and risk management. During perinatal patient safety training in 2002, physicians and nurses discussed their disappointment in their communications. Experienced nurses did not feel the physicians listened to their recommendations, while physicians complained that the nurses did not focus and get to the point quickly. Bonacum believed the lack of structured communication contributed to this problem.

In the submarine fleet, submariners had to communicate important information across hierarchical structures—for example, from the lowest-ranking enlisted man to the submarine commander. The technique Bonacum developed codified this behavior for civilian healthcare use as "SBAR," which means to (1) describe the situation you are seeing succinctly; (2) provide some background information for context; (3) provide an assessment; your assessment is valued, and you then (4) provide a recommendation. The recommendation is inclusive and empowering of people. The senior officer retains the ability to say, "No, that's not right" or "We're going to make a change." SBAR flattens the hierarchy that is inherent in healthcare, which needs to be hierarchical, but in specific situations the hierarchy must be flattened. SBAR provides a very easy way to flatten the hierarchy quickly. While SBAR did not directly come from, and is not used in, submarine operations, it derived from this culture. (Kaiser Permanente 2002) (See http://www.ihi.org/resources/Pages/AudioandVideo/ProfilesinImprovementDougBonacumofKaiserPermanente.aspx.)

Incident Command System

The Incident Command System (ICS) is a command and control system designed to rapidly be created for a sudden, large event then expanded as the event expands or as new resources arrive. The ICS can contract as the incident resolves and resources depart; the system exists both in depth to maintain a manageable span of control and in breadth to match diverse needs and resources.

The ICS grew from the loss of sixteen lives, seven hundred structures, and five hundred thousand acres in less than two weeks. These fires occurred in or

near urban centers in Los Angeles County and were fought with close cooperation of several traditional structural fire departments. Even with cooperation and
resources, resource coordination contributed to less than desired effectiveness.
Several Los Angeles City and County fire departments began to work together to
develop a program for the coordination of resources. A later set of catastrophic
fires in California led Congress to task the US Forest Service with a similar goal.
This led to FIRESCOPE (Fire Resources of Southern California Organized for
Potential Emergency) and the creation of the ICS (Cole 2011; Neamy 2011). Later
ICS was broadened from fire and EMS to include law enforcement and all hazards
and now is a component of the National Incident Command System (NIMS).

The ICS has assisted with some major improvements in coordination, however some of the weaknesses that have been identified in incident management
include:

- poor communication from conflicting terminology and incompatible
  communication systems;
- lack of reliable incident information;
- unclear chains of command and command authority for supervision;
- poor interagency integration of a management structure.

Crew Resource Management and Aviation Culture

In 1978 a commercial jet with a well-trained crew ran out of fuel and crashed,
killing ten of the 189 people on board. The National Transportation Safety Board
(NTSB) identified a recurring problem in air crashes: "a breakdown in cockpit
management and teamwork during a situation involving malfunctions of aircraft
systems in flight…because their attention was directed almost entirely toward
diagnosing the landing gear problem" (Anon 1979, 26). Also contributing to the
crash were the failure of the captain to respond to the crewmembers' advisories
and the failure of the other two flight-crew members to successfully communicate their concerns to the captain. "Admittedly, the stature of a captain and his
management style may exert subtle pressure on his crew to conform to his way of
thinking. It may hinder interaction and adequate monitoring and force another
crewmember to yield his right to express an opinion" (Anon 1979, 27).

The NTSB investigation (Anon 1979, 28) revealed:

1. The flight crew was properly certificated and qualified for the flight.
2. The aircraft was certificated, maintained, and dispatched in accordance
   with Federal Aviation Regulations and approved company procedures.

Safety recommendations (Anon 1979, 28), fourth on list:

"Issue an operations bulletin to all air carrier operations inspectors directing them to urge their assigned operators to ensure that their flight crews
are indoctrinated in principles of flight deck resource management, with
particular emphasis on the merits of participative management for captains and assertiveness training for other cockpit crewmembers. (Class II,
Priority Action) (X-79-17)"

NASA then became involved and studied the question of how an experienced,
well-trained crew could run out of fuel in flight. This occurred, basically, because the
pilot refused to take recommendations from junior officers and narrowed his focus
to a single problem when under stress. Clay Foushee (Foushee and Manos1981)
studied this as a social psychologist with NASA's Ames Research Lab finding that
within the culture of aviation, even when the pilot is approachable, the copilot
does not call out disconfirming information and pilots had the habit of ignoring
copilots, checklists, appropriate acknowledgments, and cross-checking. Foushee
(1984) later found workload stress characterized many accident scenarios yet were
infrequently encountered in day to day operations, a characteristic of healthcare.

The social psychologist Robert Helmreich (1980) studied crew performance
and personality determinants under high stress for the US Navy and NASA. He
found a divergence in pilot attitudes toward CRM indicating pilot performance
could change (Helmreich 1984).

The corrective program NASA developed became "cockpit resource management," or CRM. Because of problems identified in the 1990s with communications between crews on the flight deck and passenger areas, it became known as
"crew resource management" (still CRM) (Helmreich et al. 1999).

CRM is designed to avoid, trap, and mitigate error through communication, leadership, and decision-making. The original problem involved extreme
authority gradients and coning of attention under duress, which CRM works well
to level the hierarchy and facilitate communication. Its success derives from a
change in values, beliefs, and behaviors. Because the changes required for CRM
cannot be imposed on people, it will fail when professionals do not accept and
internalize the approach. Officers can perform well in training and testing but
revert to maladaptive behaviors in flight or under stress.

CRM describes the social interactions of the crew, but decision making is
both individual and collective. The individual process of Boyd's OODA Loop
decision making does not impede CRM (Helmreich, personal communication).

Rather, the OODA Loop, as described in Chapter 6, The Boyd OODA Loop, can overcome resistance and enhance collective sensemaking.

Others who use CRM inadvertently reduce it to methods of communication (almost all using checklists) and change only a few behaviors. Doing so misses the methods that onerous leaders have of maintaining the authority gradient, such as by using intimidation by countenance or tone of voice, a practice still commonplace (senior flight attendant and senior pilot for two international airlines, personal communication). This use also ignores the difficulty of changing behaviors that have major social ramifications. These subtle or nuanced cultural changes may be the source of CRM's success. Helmreich and Foushee identified the essential place of attitudes, a prominent affective process, early in the development of CRM (Foushee and Manos 1981; Foushee 1984; Helmreich 1984; Helmreich et al. 1986).

Situational Awareness

Situational awareness (SA) appears to have developed in operational military aviation during World War I and increased with the use of jet aircraft during the Korean and Vietnam wars. Endsley's 1995 studies have characterized SA in three levels of local data, in which the meaning of the data is determined, and then the situation is projected into the future. Endsley's three levels of SA are:

- Level 1: Perceive the status, attributes, and dynamics of relevant elements in the environment.
- Level 2: Comprehend the situation based on the synthesis of disjointed level 1 elements:
  - go beyond simply being aware that the elements are present;
  - form or identify patterns.
- Level 3: Make a projection of future status.

The domains of origin are aviation, human factors, and cognitive ergonomics. In aviation, the pilot and crew are closely situated and have a common frame of reference in the cockpit. The objective is pilot and crew awareness of the situation interfaced with and assisted by technology. As noted earlier, the field of human factors and ergonomics is a systems approach for the design of equipment, processes, and systems to better integrate with human performance (i.e., human body and cognitive abilities) within the operating environment. Cognitive ergonomics studies the mental processes for interactions among people and other elements of the system, which includes mental workload, decision-making, and stress in operational environments.

The purpose of SA is to recognize the situation, give meaning to what is perceived, accept input from the environment into decision-making, and perform tasks that are primarily physical or perceptual but involve highly complex cognitive tasks (Endsley 1995a). Time orientation is meant to project the future into system states, while decision-making is for dynamic situations.

SA operates toward the expert level and is something that must be learned. In SA, people use pre-attentive processing and attention with a more involved process of information sampling, working memory, perception, long-term memory, automaticity, and goals. Novices lack the efficiency necessary for SA, partly because their search for information can overwhelm them, and they risk becoming reactive to information (Endsley 1995a and 2013).

The process of SA is dynamic and challenging while data is being taken in and rapidly evaluated. Elements of the environment are defined, and the list of data elements can be exhaustingly thorough. Delineated elements that are known, such as information displays, are disjointed in level 1, to be integrated for level 2. The goal of integration is to understand its significance toward goals and project that significance into the future for level 3 (Endsley 2013 and 2015).

Sensemaking is driven by perception of environment, comprehension of the current situation, projection into future status, and the barriers that are encountered; it is also influenced by strategies, goals, and objectives from higher levels of the hierarchy (Endsley 1995a and 2015). Sensemaking in SA is a process by which the awareness of information in the current state (level 1) is given meaning (level 2) and then projected into future states (level 2). SA does not clearly describe how to influence the move to future states. Sensemaking (SA level 2) is created from synthesizing information, building a story, and using mental models that account for and explain disparate data. Sensemaking can derive from deliberative thought or from the automatic process of situation recognition (Endsley 2015). Although SA is a forward-looking approach, it can also be used as a backward-looking approach to create sensemaking. Endsley (2015) considers sensemaking to be backward looking.

The projection of time in SA level 2 can detect and identify critical problems and threats, according to Endsley (1995a), but SA is passive in that it does not drive action. Given that we have awareness of a situation, SA does not say what we ought to do, which is significant, since stress diminishes SA. Expected stressors in flight include physical stress, workload, complexity, and social-psychological stressors (including fear, anxiety, uncertainty), all of which alter perception and cone our attention (i.e., beyond the desired level of focused attention). Errors can result from a breakdown in SA.

One of the limitations of SA in HRO was that SA was developed more to prevent system failure and maintain awareness *during* system failure, but it is not a model of how to act. Sensemaking in SA developed from use by small groups in shared, constrained environments and was not directed by strategy or command. The approach does not explain interactions that create and form information, such as collective mindfulness. Endsley (2015) considers sensemaking to be an endpoint (2015) rather than a continuous process. In our estimation, during time compression and threat, sensemaking must be done in real time and interactive by learning what works, and that is done through engagement.

To achieve good plans within a military command, the quality of the sensemaking process is more important than the quantity of the available information. In Eva Jensen's study from the Swedish War College, the majority of the research community endorsed sensemaking as SA plus understanding, while sensemaking (per Weick) was top-down and originated with the sensemaker's goals. In Weick's version, thinking was done for some purpose, and attention was directed to information that was deemed relevant to complete the purpose. In the author's study, Weick's form of sensemaking was found to perform better (Jensen 2006).

SA relies on individuals' ability for information processing, innate abilities, experience, and training. The system provides necessary information, and its form is a designed system. Together, someone who enters a VUCA-T environment can be seen as a "black box," with information entering and awareness exiting. The reason that information has salience, the actual processing of the information, and the ability to change objectives in mid-act are not explained with SA (Endsley 1995a). Endsley (2015), in describing the multiple interrelationships of SA, states that the model has several key factors; he lists sixteen items that explain the applicability of SA to various domains, not all of which are unique to SA. This complexity, while meeting academic demands for coherence, underscores the difficulty of a novice using SA or anyone under severe stress or in extreme danger. SA does not explain how untrained or inexperienced people acquire awareness of their situations or how they should process information in the immediacy of direct threat from the environment to the individual.

Just Culture

Some believe that certain industries cannot afford a blame-free culture, that some errors (those done with intention or recklessness) warrant disciplinary action. We contend that systems are already in place to address intention and recklessness. A system with someone who intentionally or recklessly commits errors must not only identify and remove that person but also evaluate the system's hiring and management processes that have permitted the continuation of this behavior. We have discussed error as an effect of decision-making and sensemaking throughout this book.

> "When you identify the person, then
> you begin your investigation."
> —CHRISTOPHER A. HART, CHAIR, NATIONAL
> TRANSPORTATION SAFETY BOARD

James Reason, expanding on his work in the field of error studies, addressed safety culture by asking if a safer culture could be engineered; he wrote that some argued that "a safe culture is an informed culture and this, in turn, depends upon creating an effective reporting culture that is underpinned by a just culture in which the line between acceptable and unacceptable behaviour is clearly drawn and understood" (Reason 1998). The "just culture" he mentions is a culture that supports a reporting culture; people will not report if they will be punished for doing so. A reporting culture supports an informed culture, where all participants understand and respect the hazards with which they work. This informed culture then supports a safe culture. In this manner, Reason answers his question of engineering a safer culture. Since trust is an integral part of these four cultures, then trust must be ensured; to do that, the organization must engineer a just culture.

These four cultures, folding into and supporting one another, are not independent cultures in the sense that they possess the anthropological elements of the culture, are a social response to an environment, or contain shared contextual knowledge that is passed on to new members. They are cultures in a less rigorous sense of social knowledge and behaviors but layered to build on one another. The just culture model addresses two questions: (1) What is the role of punitive sanction in the safety of our healthcare system and (2) Does the threat and/or application of punitive sanction as a remedy for human error help or hurt our system-safety efforts?

David Marx (2001) developed just culture as a culture that ensures fairness and the open reporting of human error. Accountability describes how both the organization and employees share responsibility: the organization for safe system and process design, the employees for safe choices and behaviors. People are not blamed for "honest errors" but are held accountable for willful violations and gross negligence. Marx identifies that some errors and mistakes result from normal learning, where no punitive action should be taken. Sidney Dekker (2008), working in the field of aviation human factors, developed just culture as a support for safety culture. Dekker found that the criminalization of error is more than culpability and retribution; it is also a matter of deterrence. If error is the crime, then punishment does not deter error among individuals, either directly or by example.

Just culture is a cultural belief that errors that occur in the course of work, without intention or recklessness, should not lead to punishment. The increase in trust that develops will then support more open reporting of problems and an informed workforce in a workplace with potential hazards or adverse circumstances. Just culture in this way can engineer safety culture.

Operation Risk Management (ORM)

Authors' note: the following section is by Major Randy E. Cadieux, US Marine Corps.

Operational risk management (ORM), a tool applied by US Navy and Marine Corps units, mitigates risks associated with tactical and nontactical operations. As with any High Reliability tool, it is also used in off-duty activities. Because of its use outside the tactical environment, ORM can be useful in other organizations by reducing operational risks to their personnel and equipment. ORM's use can raise the awareness of risks by the organization's leaders, which will influence and improve the safety attitudes of members within the organization. ORM may be viewed as an extension of other types of system-oriented hazard-analysis techniques.

US Navy and Marine Corps aviation units apply ORM to aviation operations at multiple levels. The ORM planning process attempts to mitigate operational risks through hazard analysis and risk assessment, risk control implementation, and supervision at the most appropriate level. ORM can also be thought of as a tool for mitigating risks associated with operations that involve human interaction with systems and equipment. ORM involves the analysis of hazards that affect the operational phase of systems and the development of controls to reduce risks to personnel and equipment during operations. Application involves a five-step process of (1) hazard identification, (2) hazard assessment, (3) the making of risk-based decisions about hazard controls, (4) control implementation, and (5) supervision of the results. Initially, hazards are identified and then assessed in terms of probability and severity. This assessment results in the generation of risk-assessment codes (RACs). The first RACs are known as initial risk-assessment codes, or "initial RACs."

After the identification of initial RACs, risk-control implementation is developed to reduce risk levels in a prioritized fashion, working from the highest to lowest risks. These controls include interventions to reduce the probability of occurrence, the severity of impact, or both. Oftentimes operational risks are controlled through the implementation of training, tactics, or procedures (including standardized checklists) and other procedural or administrative controls, such as standard operating procedures, the adoption of personnel protective equipment policies, and the use of warnings and cautions to raise the personnel's awareness of the potential for hazardous situations. After the risk controls are implemented, the risk analysts determine the final risk-assessment codes based on the probability and severity of hazard occurrence after control implementation.

Decisions about mission execution based on this residual risk (i.e., risk decisions) are made at the appropriate level within the organization, which is an important principle of ORM. At the lower end of the spectrum, risk-based decisions can be made by the operator and, as risk levels escalate, the level of the decision-maker increases. Decisions about operations with the highest "final RACs" are normally made by those in command of a unit. These decisions about operations must take into account the mission and acceptable levels of risk. The goal of ORM is not to eliminate all risks but to manage risks for mission accomplishment with minimum amount of loss. In other words, ORM helps to reduce risks to acceptable levels, considering the mission and operational environment.

There are three types of ORM: deliberate, in-depth, and time-critical. Deliberate and in-depth ORMs are used when people have adequate time to analyze hazards; these ORMs often use qualitative and quantitative analysis tools. Oftentimes brainstorming, what-if scenarios, subject-matter experts, and lessons learned are used to identify hazards and then rank the hazards in terms of probability and severity. "Time-critical ORM" is a method that shortens the analysis and decision-making process to counter threats or ameliorate hazards during time-compressed situations. Decisions can be made by rapidly assessing the situation, balancing options, communicating intentions to crew members, taking immediate action, and then debriefing the action. This is known as the A-B-C-D decision-making framework, for assess, balance, communicate, and do/debrief.

In addition to the three types of ORM, four principles of ORM exist to help guide decision-makers. These principles are (1) accept risk when benefits outweigh cost, (2) accept no unnecessary risk, (3) anticipate and manage risks by planning, and (4) make risk decisions at the right level. These principles help to guide ORM facilitators and unit leaders during the ORM process.

US Navy and Marine Corps aviation has demonstrated that operational risk management assists with the discovery of risks and with elevating risk decisions to the appropriate levels of leadership. ORM helps leaders foster a culture of risk awareness, which has a positive effect on safety attitudes in the unit. Through the proper use of ORM, units can reduce risks to acceptable levels for a given situation and, when risks outweigh the perceived benefits, top leadership has a decision-making tool to identify better courses of actions for high-risk operations. Time-critical ORM has been shown to be a valuable tool to aid pilots, aircrew, and ground units in the reduction of risks and in making rapid risk-based decisions in dynamic environments.

Normal Accident Theory (NAT)

As a sociologist, Charles Perrow contributed a sociological perspective to organizational analysis and organizational behavior studies, which had been heavily influenced by psychology. He studied decision-making in centralized versus decentralized organizations and presented a sociological view of the human-machine interface, particularly for decision-making under varying abilities and demands. After the accident at the Three Mile Island nuclear power plant, he became involved with the study of what happened. This study led to his description of a "normal accident," which he initially characterized as being unpreventable and unanticipated and therefore something that cannot be trained for or designed against (Perrow 1981). A normal accident has four characteristics: (1) signals are only noticed in retrospect; (2) multiple design and equipment failures occur;(3) some type of operator error occurs that is not considered error until the accident is understood; (4) "negative synergy" occurs, where the sum of equipment, design, and operator errors is far greater than the consequences of each singly.

His book *Normal Accidents* (1984) introduced the idea that people will interact with complex technological systems to create whole, or unitary, systems. Interactions occur within these systems over two significant dimensions of interactive complexity and coupling of components. The complexity and coupling, whether by design or happenstance, determine the system's susceptibility to accidents and make accidents not only inevitable but normal. Accidents then derive not so much from human cognition and behaviors or by engineered designs but from dynamic human-machine interactions. While these accidents may be predicted (and the risk accepted or identified in hindsight from missed data), accidents may also result from information that is undiscoverable until events unfold. In effect, the surprise reflects not what is cognitively missed but what is cognitively absent.

Interactive Complexity and NAT

Interactive complexity refers to unfamiliar, unplanned, or unexpected sequences of events in a system, particularly at the level of the working environment. (As noted earlier, the working environment is where people engage the organization's external environment, either at the executive or operational level.) These events may not be immediately visible or comprehensible. The measure of interactive complexity is the number of ways in which parts and relationships of the system can interact. While interactions may be linear by design or only when a few interactions occur, they easily become nonlinear as interactions increase in number or degree. Nonlinear interactions of only a few components can rapidly lead to complexity, new and unexpected properties of the system, and accidents.

Components of a system are joined together, or coupled, very loosely when the parts are not very dependent on one another. They are coupled tightly when the parts are highly interdependent, that is, linked to many parts in a time-dependent manner. In tightly coupled systems, a change in one part rapidly affects the status of other parts and influences the system's ability to recover. This situation allows small perturbations to rapidly cause large effects, while in a loosely coupled or decoupled system, the sparse links or less tightly linked links allow the absorption of perturbations and dampen destabilization. The speed at which one variable cascades through the system, thereby causing changes or the entrainment of other parts into the cascading events, is a measure of how tightly coupled the system is.

The interactive complexity of a system is the trigger, while tight coupling is the propagator of events that lead to normal or system accidents. Simple principles, when combined in a nonlinear manner, lead to complexity and to novel properties of the system. These novel properties may not be able to be anticipated. The solutions Perrow (1999) proposed include (1) abandon those systems where risks outweigh reasonable benefits, (2) identify where systems can be made less risky, and (3) enhance those systems that have the characteristics of self-correction or self-organization. The difficulty of using NAT as a guide to risk is that it increases the importance of possibility or the ease an event will happen versus probability or the likelihood that an event will happen.

HRO versus NAT

Among academicians, the source of uncertainty is an important consideration, whether the source is technical, organizational, or social. Uncertainty makes engineering difficult and occasionally unsuccessful. With new technology, technical uncertainties will come along that cannot be resolved. Uncertainty makes social interactions for problem-solving both challenging and satisfying. Uncertainty drives self-organization. NAT offers society the option to accept the uncertainty, bring resources to bear, or not use the technology. HRO offers society a challenge to move forward, which is part and parcel of High Reliability.

As practitioners, we see NAT and HRO as parts of the whole—how can we contain, react to, or interact with any uncertainty? We also see High Reliability as a collective response of people sharing common attitudes. Uncertainty, by definition, cannot be prepared for, so High Reliability teams prepare themselves to function in the presence of uncertainty as part of their daily operations. We are not ignoring arguments either way; we only believe that these arguments are specious. If a technology is necessary, can we respond to its uncertainties (the HRO argument)? If a technology is not necessary and we cannot respond to its uncertainties, then why assume the risk (the NAT argument)? The discussion then becomes, "How much can we respond to?" We may not know this until it is too late.

The danger is, at one extreme, not knowing the dangers to the extent possible; at the other extreme, the danger is developing the mind-set of "I told you so." Either serves as a death knell to innovation: one to creating innovation, the other to its use. Failure is not as much the accident but the failure to identify the accident sufficiently early in its birth. Early identification, in this covert state, allows interaction with fewer resources and greatest effectiveness. Before an accident, HRO brings the risk of cockiness, and after an accident, NAT brings the risk of blame. Either is deadly.

HRO and NAT arguments sometimes fall into the "top-down" or "bottom-up" discussion. Those who live with High Reliability see it as more of a centripetal and centrifugal flow toward and away from an event. Information flows away from an event and toward the organization's center for processing. Action moves toward an event, away from central authority, to interact with the situation. We learn what works through action, and the response to our actions tells us the structure of the problem. There is no top-down or bottom-up, only toward and away.

In this setting, we do not break rules. Rules are written in blood. Of greatest importance is to identify, and identify quickly, if the rule, or any rule, does not apply, or if it competes or conflicts with other rules. Then, we quickly move to interactive judgment. NAT is the environment of HRO. Society must judge the value of the technology, which is something that is not a zero-sum game, reached by equation, or decided by self-described elder statesmen. (See http://high-reliability.org/Normal-Accident-Theory.)

Resilience Engineering

Understand what goes right. The development of socio-technical systems has created a predominance of knowledge-intensive activities and cognitive tasks. In response to the idea that accidents, an effect, must have a cause (the cause-and-effect principle), Eric Hollnagel developed the concept of cognitive-systems engineering: the idea that we cannot understand what goes wrong if we do not know what goes right. He has taken this further into socio-technical systems to study how humans and technology function as joint systems. The study of normal variability is the beginning of safety studies. This is the basis for his "functional resonance accident model" (FRAM) briefly mentioned earlier, where accidents occur when resonance develops between functions of a system's components to create hazards that led to the accident. The premise of FRAM is that performance is never stable, so the system is expected to have internal and external variability. If performance variability is the norm, then we should then study what makes the system work—what goes right.

Other HRO-Related Models

High Reliability Organizing developed as a means to engage confusing, threatening situations with minimal technology, often by teams of less-experienced people led by people with greater experience. It is now being adapted to more diverse environments and situations for use by a larger array of organizations. Understanding the environment and the limits of cognitive function in these situations provides a better grasp of what HRO can accomplish. HRO is the only model that was derived directly from operators. Resilience engineering is a model from observation created by engineers.

Conclusions

Comparisons of other systems are summarized in the following pages.

Model	Lean
Purpose	Reduce waste
HRO link	People more valuable than machinery; builds relationships across authority gradients; constant search for ways to improve; process oriented; value, relationships, motivation, and flow make a lean organization.
Limitations	Decreased waste impairs robust structures needed for low-frequency, high-risk events; limits rapid response, burden on logistics; limits resources for unexpected, time-compressed states; no preparation for threat or adversity; impedes improvisation or constrained improvisation.

Model   Six Sigma

Purpose   Reduce defects, minimize variability, reduce errors

HRO link   Standardization for communication and predictability of internal response; frees cognitive capacity for the unexpected; familiar routines reduce fear response.

Limitations   Not adaptive to unstable environment and uncertainty; human behavior not amenable to this process; product, not process, oriented; when process oriented, regimentation reduces adaptability and agility; error-reduction focus rather than error identification; normal distribution, statistics, and *probability* versus power distribution and *possibility*; no variability, then no improvisation.

Model   Constraints management (Theory Of Constraints, or TOC)

Purpose   Manage systems for system-level impact; focus improvement efforts on constraints; buffer-management tools manage uncertainty in dynamic conditions.

Limitations   Requires innovation, with radical paradigm shifts; counterintuitive changes; difficult to accept and sustain changes.

Model   Risk management (from ISO 31000)

Purpose   Risk is the "effect of uncertainty on objectives"; identifying positive and negative consequences; identification, assessment, and prioritization of risks; avoiding identified risk; stakeholders are people who "can affect, be affected by, or perceive themselves to be affected by a decision or activity."

HRO link   Identify and characterize threats; assess vulnerability of critical assets to specific threats; determine risk and the expectation and consequences of specific attacks on specific assets; identify ways to reduce those risks, including risk avoidance; use a strategy to prioritize risk-reduction measures.

Limitations   Some risks cannot be identified in advance (unexpected or unknown risks); risk avoidance or risk averseness reduces participation in high-risk ventures; tendency to discount low-frequency, high-acuity events; difficult to prioritize uncertain or ambiguous risk; risk management is treated as a compliance issue, for obedience.

Model	Safety culture
Purpose	Prevent system failure; specific types of threats include invisible threat (hazard), delayed injury (damage), and irreversible and lethal (treatment).
HRO link	Prevention of system failure; use of processes and rules; recognition of human fallibility.
Limitations	Created in stable environments; not developed for adversity or unstable environments; counteracts response to system failure; antecedent behaviors to failure difficult to identify: we only look if a failure occurs.

Model	Just culture
Purpose	People do not report accidents for fear of punishment
HRO link	Reporting and studying accidents necessary to identify vulnerability; focus on the system rather than individuals.
Limitations	Too easily accepted as distinct culture or a co-culture with safety culture; redirects discussion to when, or if, the organization should blame or hold accountable.

Model	Resilience engineering
Purpose	Complexity alone causes failure; changes safety from hindsight *after* an accident to safety from proactive resilience.
HRO link	Coping with complexity when under pressure; analyze successes to identify normal sources of resilience; brittleness (the capacity for a system to break down).
Limitations	Engineering model of resilience designed into system; does not account for individual perceptions, bounded rationality, and the logic of practice.

Model	Incident Command System (ICS)
Purpose	Interagency collaboration in emergencies: specific rules, communication, procedures, command style.
HRO link	Integrate teams for convergent response to crises; build organizational structure in self-organizing manner as emergency expands then contracts as control is brought about.
Limitations	Structured; takes time and experience to coordinate; cross-agency training to use common processes.

Model	Crew Resource Management (CRM)
Purpose	Planes crashed despite well-trained crews, fully functional systems and good airframes; poor communication across authority gradient, particularly with disconfirming information; original problem involved extreme authority gradient and coning of attention under duress, for which CRM works well; success from change in values, beliefs, and behaviors.
HRO link	Small-team management; communication; recognition of the danger from authority gradient; reduction of authority gradient; avoid, trap, and mitigate error through communication, leadership, and decision-making.
Limitations	Developed for small units, enclosed space, common threat, likely threat is predictable; HRO, threat is more expansive in space and type of threat, greater likelihood of uncertain or novel event; span of control much larger; dependent on acceptance of supervisors (for example, passive aggressive).

Model	Team STEPPS
Purpose	Reduce poor teamwork in crisis management; errors from poor teamwork in healthcare.
HRO link	Elements of functional leadership, situation monitoring, mutual support, and communication.
Limitations	Does not: work at the level of the individual; account for individual perceptions, bounded rationality, and the logic of practice; describe decision-making.

Model	SBAR (situation, background, assessment, recommendation)
Purpose	Communication tool; poor communication across authority gradient, particularly with disconfirming information.
HRO link	Flattens hierarchy; standardizes communication across disciplines; improves vigilance for failure and vulnerabilities; empowers and energizes deference to expertise; brings to attention when to be sensitive to change operations.
Limitations	Communication is a behavior; SBAR does not address causes of a malignant authority gradient or rigid hierarchy; some

superiors do not allow it; intimidation by countenance easily prevents use; does not encourage information flow as much as enables it—if the person is willing.

Model	Checklists
Purpose	Thoroughness for complex procedures.
HRO link	Standardization; rule-based scheme (Rasmussen) allows freedom to think and problem-solve while handling less complex tasks (knowledge-based scheme); competency level of skill (Dreyfus model).
Limitations	Time-consuming to repeat; not repeated when circumstances change; risk for mindlessness or strict adherence; not adaptive to novel situation; sequential listing prevents skipping irrelevant items; complacency once completed; set up for rule-based error (James Reason), "the strong-but-wrong" rule; we stop at competency—easy to train high-turnover employees, rather than move to proficiency.
Model	Situational awareness (SA)
Purpose	Thoroughness for complex procedures
HRO link	Bottom-up sensemaking; perception of environment, comprehension of current situation, and projection into future status; occurs over time, recognition that things change.
Limitations	Sensemaking is not directed by strategy or command; used by small groups in shared, constrained environments; does not explain interactions to create information such as collective mindfulness; not a behavioral approach.
Model	Normal accident theory (NAT)
Purpose	The challenge for human control of risky, complex technologies
HRO link	Risk awareness and acknowledgment
Limitations	Gives a sense for the acceptance of failure or the rejection of the technology; does not discuss how organizations can purposely enter dangerous situations.

CHAPTER 12

LEADERSHIP, AUTHORITY, COMMAND, AND TEAM FORMATION

This chapter covers leadership when the emergency is present but the leader is not. A leader is someone who significantly affects the thoughts, feelings, or behaviors of a significant number of people. Direct leaders address the public face-to-face, while indirect leaders exert leadership through the works they create (Gardner 1995). In a discussion of leadership, a symphony conductor once reported that the conductor has no role during the performance; his or her presence is mainly for show. All of the conductor's work occurs during rehearsal. Leadership in an HRO must fulfill the conventional purpose of leadership in the organization yet lead across distances of time and place and, most significantly, across the emotional threshold of fear and threat.

Marine Recruit Training

In a series studies for the US Marine Corps to identify causes of recruit attrition, an academic group from the UC Irvine, led by Raymond Novaco and Irwin Sarason, studied the recruits and drill instructors over several years in the 1970s. They found that drill-instructor leadership, rather than the initial quality of recruits, had the greatest effect on recruit retention, increased stress capacity, and the internalization of "locus of control."

Traits of Drill Instructors
Drill instructors who had the lowest attrition rates from their training platoons had common traits. Successful drill instructors set the tone of the social environment and training situations. It was their beliefs,

expectations, and attitudes that influenced the recruits' self-appraisals and expectations (Sarason and Novaco 1982). They were significantly more job-involved, higher in internal control expectations, significantly less impatient, less prone to anger, and lower in physiological arousal. They also had more realistic job expectations and greater empathy for recruits (Novaco et al. 1983). To improve their success rates, the drill instructors developed training films for new drill instructors in which they demonstrated common problems, identified these problems, and shared effective solutions. All actors in these training films were experienced drill instructors (Raymond Novaco, personal communication).

Increased Stress Capacity in Recruits

Recruit training increased recruits' distress capacity through increasing demands in the training and from drill instructors who developed the recruits' capability for effective performance under stress conditions (Novaco et al. 1979). The training films the authors developed emphasized two key themes: self-control of emotions and the importance of task-performance effectiveness. After viewing these films, the recruits expressed more self-confidence in their ability to endure stress, control emotions, and live up to the drill instructor's expectations (Sarason and Novaco 1982).

It is important to note that the drill instructors and commanders supported this philosophy and reinforced the video by modeling the behaviors, attitudes, and values viewed on the video.

Locus of Control

The leaders encouraged the belief that successful outcomes result from skill and effort; the recruits then developed a greater internal locus of control by changing their perceptions to take responsibility for their own behavior. The locus of control became more external in high-attrition units, where drill instructors were more likely to shape the belief that powerful others, luck, fate, or chance controlled outcomes (Cook et al. 1980; Sarason and Novaco 1982). Even recruits with an external locus of control and negative or failed experiences in life (failure, rejection, emotional disruption) internalized their locus of control under good leaders (Cook et al. 1980). "Recruits who have had negative or failure experiences in life can develop a belief that success results from their own efforts if they are trained in units whose reward contingencies are favorable to the formation of internal locus of control expectancies" (Sarason and Novaco 1982).

Marine Recruit Retention

Unfulfilled needs for personal growth in the areas of education and training contributed to the marines' high percentage of decisions not to reenlist. The authors suggested several areas for further exploration: "(1) lack of positive feedback from superiors to Marines concerning work performed in an exemplary fashion and (2) a sense of alienation stimulated by the perceived complexity of and distance from Marine Corps bureaucracy" (Sarason, Novaco, Sarason 1981, 9).

We must disabuse ourselves of the belief that subordinates are solely responsible for their personal development. We must become cognizant that the tone of the social environment comes from the top and that embodied leaders have a significant effect on subordinates' performance and increased stress capacity.

Leadership occurs, and is most effective, during downtime, since little time is available during time-compressed action for communication. A good example is the symphony orchestra, as noted above. Countless other examples may be found of subordinates "picking up the flag" after their leader has fallen. This does not occur by chance. The leader's primary job in HRO is to instill a sense of vision and purpose that transcends the presence of the leader.

Leader-Leader; Leader-Follower

We expect a "leader-leader." When a novel, unexpected event occurs, we expect someone to engage in some manner. This does not have to be active engagement; it can involve close monitoring or seeking assistance; collaboration does occur in these cases, but it consists of collaboration about the problem with an objective rather than through followership behind the leader. In HROs, people lead the problem until they are relieved, which is an action that combines the HRO factors of "sensitivity to operations" and "deference to expertise."

We acknowledge that "followership" may be important to some leaders, some organizations, and in some situations. Followership is the *capacity* of following rather than the *willingness* to follow. Followership is difficult to describe without focusing to some extent on conformity, obedience, and submission. Except for these characteristics, the traits of High Reliability followers often appear to be the same traits we find among High Reliability leaders. Few, if any, traits are unique to followers that leaders do not also have. What many see as good followership may actually be good leadership for a problem viewed from a different angle or point of view.

The concept of followership occurred in the 1940s to 1950s. Eugene and Ruth Hartley (1952) described leadership and followership as the differentiation of power through status. Not until studies for the US Navy by Edwin Hollander and Wilse Webb (1954) did researchers characterize traits of followership. The authors introduced followership in relation to leadership to identify the "characteristics which would make a man a good group member capable of following a leader" and whether these qualities are compatible or incompatible with good leadership. They found that the more desired followers tended to have greater leadership qualities. Good leaders are also judged as good followers in the context of the US Navy. Hollander continued his studies of followership into the 1990s (Hollander 1992), describing how perceptions, misperceptions, and biases affect the leader-follower relationship.

Rather than going by the maxim "learn to follow before you learn to lead," the best advice may be to "learn to lead to become a good follower." Followership continues to be generally defined in relation to leadership, even when discussed as a co-creation between leader and followers (Uhl-Bien et al. 2014). Variables in followership studies now include traits, perceptions, motivations, affect, and power to certain specific behaviors to reach specific outcomes (Uhl-Bien et al. 2014).

Leadership is a transaction, if not a joint product, between leaders, followers, organizations, environments, and situations. In our daily and regular processes, stable environments and routine situations have a minimum part in these transactions. This leaves most transactions to occur between superior-subordinate, a relation where followership makes the leader's job more convenient. By seeding a large share of the effort to their subordinates to manage, effective leaders intentionally enable channels of communication to occur regardless of the absence of a command and control environment. Because we understand that a challenging situation may occur when the leader is not physically present, it is critical that these communication pathways be viable, or the team may be incapacitated until the leader arrives—a situation completely unpalatable in the world of HROs.

> "The greater the capacity for leadership, the
> greater the capacity for subordinate success."
> —SPENCE BYRUM

Howard Gardner (1995) described followers in several ways. One type is the follower who serves as an apprentice to learn the profession on the way to becoming an expert; this type follows a specific person for a specific reason. Some followers are attracted to certain features of the leader, such as strength and power or original ideas and spirituality. And some people follow because they do not want to lead or because they are chronic followers (we, as human beings, have a proclivity to follow others).

The danger when we use the followership concept is when we use it to explain failed leadership. Followership risks pushing responsibility downward to the lowest levels in the hierarchy, where people have the least knowledge, experience, and power.

"The Strategic Corporal," an article written by General Charles C. Krulak (1999) in *Marines* magazine, describes how leadership in what we call the VUCA-T environment (volatile, uncertain, complex, ambiguous, and threatening; see "The Environment," in chapter 2, "What Problem Does HRO Solve?") has devolved to the lowest-ranking member of the armed forces. The corporal in the fictional story first considers what he *does* know, then he considers what he *does not* know before making a decision. More significant in the VUCA-T environment is someone's character, a commitment to lifelong professional development, and leadership. A "zero-defects mentality" and micromanagement are detrimental to initiative and must be replaced with "freedom to fail," which, paradoxically, produces the *opportunity to succeed*. Supervision must be complemented with proactive mentoring. The quality of leaders is reflected in their subordinates.

Leadership in Unpredictable Situations

The Mount Pinatubo eruption of 15 June 1991 coincided with the arrival of a tropical storm. Because ash was expected to fall on Clark Air Base in the Philippines, all personnel and dependents had evacuated to US Naval Base Subic Bay. The tropical storm put the wet ash onto the naval base, requiring evacuation by land to navy ships. Internal communications were maintained by armed forces radio and television and through police and community meetings. Because of the diverse locations of the damage, neighborhood captains were identified. The situation also required the care and feeding of a diverse population, two-thirds of whom were from Clark Air Base.

Evacuation and recovery plans had been developed over the previous two months that would involve airlift and sealift operations, with the sealift requiring a three-hundred-mile trip because of the lack of available port facilities. A major contributor to the smooth response was the presence of several US Navy ships with recent operational experience from the first Gulf War.

—Thomas A. Mercer, RAdm, USN (retired)

Models of Leadership

Using a conceptual model or typology for leadership is seductive. Such a model becomes something to which we can aspire or teach while at the same time serving as a measure to judge others. For a conceptual model, we must create salient and discrete concepts, at the risk of the salience reflecting our own interests, creating concepts to fit specific models, or splitting concepts into artificially discrete groups. A typology may reflect the interests of the *researcher* rather than the practice of the *leader*. As such, rather than proffering a model for leadership, we will discuss four ideas about leadership and the need for reliability in leadership; we will then complete this section with a description of leadership characteristics.

Identifying leadership traits during a crisis poses several problems. Some traits are situationally dependent, while some are characteristic to the threat. For example, though facing imminent personal physical danger and danger to one's identity have similar neurological pathways, how we handle each is quite different. During the onset of a crisis, we do not see, recognize, or accept it as a crisis and can miss some of the antecedent character traits necessary for leadership. In a hazardous situation, some leadership traits may be situationally exaggerated or may not be present. Finally, leadership in an emergency is a transaction, and this transaction in the face of a threat is intimate, subtle, and nuanced.

Transformational-Transactional Leadership

Transformational-transactional leadership theory dominates the current thinking about leadership research. Transformational leadership is defined as a leadership approach that causes changes in individuals and social systems; in its ideal form, it creates valuable and positive change in the followers, with the end goal of developing followers into leaders. Transformational leaders offer a purpose that transcends short-term goals and that focuses on higher-order intrinsic needs.

Transactional leaders, in contrast, focus on the proper exchange of resources; they focus more on supervision, organization, and group performance. Transactional leaders promote compliance through both rewards and punishments. They are not looking to change the future but to achieve stability. Leaders interact with their followers for a transaction, generally corrective or disciplinary in nature. Compared to transformational leaders, who develop relationships during routine times, transactional leaders appear after failures or successes, after resolution of the situation, or during the situation if things do not go well.

The four dimensions of transformational leadership are charisma or idealized influence, inspirational motivation, intellectual stimulation, and individualized consideration (Judge and Piccolo 2004). The three dimensions of transactional leadership are contingent reward, management by exception (active), and management by exception (passive).

Indirect Leadership, Motivational Leadership, and Practical Wisdom

An organization's leaders can have profound, far-reaching, and long-lasting effects on their subordinates and novices. Indirect leaders exert leadership through the works they create and the stories they tell. The leader *relates* the story but does not *tell* the story. In this manner, the leader *embodies* the story and its elements, which gives authenticity to both leader and story (Gardner 1995). Stories, compared to principles, can be adapted to specific situations or for lessons that are adjusted to the specific follower.

People resist change because of ambivalence, not because of resistance or denial. Leaders identify discrepancies between current behaviors and beliefs and desired outcomes; from the discrepancy, they can then develop awareness of consequences, thus increasing people's motivation for change (Rollnick et al. 2008).

Through the priority of the particular, we find good judgment and practical wisdom. Practical wisdom is the first of Aristotle's four cardinal virtues, a virtue because we must use judgment in particular situations. This judgment can be a virtue, when done for the community good, or a vice, when done for self-interest (Bartlett and Collins 2011). People learn judgment from experience with the particular and by modeling themselves after those who are experienced in practical wisdom. It is the leader's position to model practical wisdom and mentor inexperienced people.

Production, Logistics, and Operations

An organization has the purpose of creating goods and/or providing services. We will discuss production, logistics, and operations as a prelude to how leadership may differ in a High Reliability Organization.

Production, as a business term, is the process the organization uses to create its output, goods, or services. It is the reason for the organization.

Logistics is the detailed organization and management of the flow of goods, services, and information from the point of origin to the point of consumption. When used as a military term, logistics refers to planning and executing the movement and support of forces. This involves the coordination, management, procurement, supply, and maintenance of equipment; the movement of equipment, facilities, and services; and the maintenance and transportation of all material, personnel, and facilities.

Operations are coordinated actions that are taken in response to a developing situation. Operations have a plan, even if it is created on the spot, and an objective or end-state. The end-state becomes the goal in complex situations, where problems cannot be clearly identified, multiple problems exist, or problems are intertwined. These are tactical situations rather than strategic maneuvers. In the military lexicon, the operational approach describes the "broad actions the force must take to transform current conditions into those desired at end-state." The operational environment is a "composite of the conditions, circumstances, and influences that affect the employment of capabilities and bear on the decisions of the commander" (US Department of Defense 2010).

The basic model of combat operations can help us understand the change in operations necessitated by an emergency or crisis. Orr (1983) describes five phases: (1) seek to acquire objectives; (2) allocate and orient appropriate assets (people are assets) for successful engagement of the enemy); (3) make decisions about the doctrinal approach to the engagement; (4) execute the plan through engagement; (5) conduct postcombat intelligence assessment of the success or failure of the operations plan.

Authority and Command

All members of an organization, at every level, make decisions about what is to be done. Those with ownership of the organization expect this of all members. Only certain people, however, have the authority to make decisions that will affect the survival of the organization, such as business strategy, financing, marketing, costs, or profitability.

We must not equate decision-making with authority. Decision-making determines a course of action; authority is the power to make judgments and determinations on issues and have control over subordinates. For example, a nurse may decide on a medical condition for a patient, but only the doctor has the authority to make a diagnosis. A bedside caregiver may decide how to carry out his or her professional duties, but it is the employer who has the authority to require those duties.

Having ownership of an organization, whether public or private, is to have the control necessary to secure survival of the organization. Any decisions about activities and the allocation of resources, however, must be made throughout the organization on a regular basis. Those who make these decisions may not personally have financial risk or receive the benefits of ownership. Though they are not nearly as important as market decisions, these decisions can still affect the survival of the organization. The separation of decision processes and risk-bearing functions is an effective approach to problem-solving (Fama and Jensen 1983). The authority to make decisions is delegated by the "owners" to the executive and management team. The ratification and monitoring of decisions is generally maintained by central authority, while the initiation and implementation of decisions is decentralized (Fama and Jensen 1983).

Authority

We can define *authority* as the power to execute the broad mandate from our superiors, coordinate the execution of that mandate by our subordinates, and monitor the activity of our subordinates (Bolton and Dewatripont 2011). Formal authority rests with the owners of the organization or, in the US federal government, the director appointed through one of the three branches of government. Authority can remain central or become decentralized through delegation or allocation, although how this authority is delegated is beyond the scope of this handbook.

Decisions are the manifestation of authority, which are almost interchangeable, to the degree that we can differentiate different types of authority by the decisions that are made. Within the operations of an organization, the decision process has four steps (Fama and Jensen 1983): initiation, ratification, implementation, and monitoring. Bolton and Dewatripont (2011) use the following four processes to define different aspects of authority:

1. a supervisor's power *to initiate projects and direct* subordinates to take certain actions;
2. the power to *exact obedience*;
3. the power *to ratify and approve actions* in a predetermined area of competency (a form of decentralization by delegation of authority);
4. the manager's duty *to monitor* subordinates and *reward* them for good performance.

There are three main types of authority: line authority, staff authority, and functional authority. *Line authority* derives authority from the owners by way of the chain of command and generally follows an organizational chart reflecting superior-subordinate relationships. In the superior's absence, the subordinate will assume the superior's authority. Because line authority develops a superior-subordinate relationship, this authority must be well circumscribed and credibly delegated. *Staff authority* is the authority to advise and support line executives and managers; examples of staff authority include legal counsel, finance, and human relations. Conflict can develop between those with line authority and those with staff authority, thus contributing to disruption within the organization. Generally, this disruption comes from overlapping authority and responsibility and from poor interactions between members. *Functional authority* is the authority over a particular function for staff personnel or a particular situation for line personnel. It is authority based on expertise and includes the ability to make decisions. It is the way things "really work" within the organization.

Command

In civilian life, we use the word "authority" rather than the military concept of command, likely because "command" seems more dictatorial. Studying the military concept of command, though, can shed some light on how we can make HRO operational. Command encompasses legal authority, the orders given from that authority, and the specific area, system, or group commanded (US Department of Defense 2010). By virtue of rank or assignment, military and public-safety officers exercise this authority over their subordinates within their organizations. Law enforcement and fire officers also exercise this legal authority over the public for public-safety needs.

An emergency or crisis may require greater local authority than was routinely delegated or allocated. Several reasons explain this situation. First, the unexpected and dynamic nature of a prevention strategy may demand immediate engagement. Second, decisions may require local or specialized knowledge. Third, allowing local control frees the attention of the more central leadership to continue the work of the organization, oversee other unexpected incidents, or direct operations in support of the emergency. While it is nice to plan for every contingency, not every situation fits a plan, and leaders may not be in a position to give direct orders. Local people must then make decisions on the spot.

"Commander's intent" is a concept that was developed in the military for use during operations when it is impractical to obtain direct orders. It is "a clear and concise expression of the purpose of the operation and the desired military end state that supports mission command, provides focus to the staff, and helps subordinate and supporting commanders act to achieve the commander's desired results without further orders, even when the operation does not unfold as planned." This concept has now become embedded in law enforcement and urban and wildland firefighting.

Command is not rigid or dictatorial but instead allows fluid operations. The commander's intent supports sensitivity to operations through the ability to immediately adjust to changing circumstances. Some have difficulty with deference to expertise—for example a physician delegating his or her decision authority. Another definition of command is "those duties the commander cannot legally delegate" (Mercer, personal communication). Physicians cannot legally delegate diagnosis, prescriptive authority, or surgical procedures unless they are preauthorized in a legal manner. Other than those three elements, a physician can otherwise delegate medical decision-making and actions.

The Incident Command System (ICS) discussed in the previous chapter developed from wildland fires in California and Arizona. Under mutual aid, various fire departments would come together to fight fires that had crossed political boundaries. To reduce the confusion of the command structure, fire chiefs met in Arizona to identify a better approach. The system became fully developed in the 1970s during a series of large wildland fires in California. ICS integrates equipment, personnel, procedures, and communications into a common organizational structure. The structure can then expand or contract as the incident changes and as resources become available to (or must be removed from) the incident.

Assorted Elements of Leadership

The following sections discuss various elements used by effective leaders that may not fit into a specific model or may be shared across models.

To Teach, You Must First Let Yourself Be Taught

To influence or study the hidden principles in a social system, one must become a student. Instead of studying the structures of a social system or environment, we prefer to ask how people define concepts in their own words, how they describe the function of their tools, and how they identify the relationships they have with other people. Most significantly, what are the duties people feel toward the group, and how does the group support them? These insights provide the insider's view, and by allowing yourself to be taught, you gain people's trust. As you learn, you will find yourself teaching.

HRO is not a universal principle or a generalizable concept. It describes the social response to a specific event, the "particular" in the environment, with the event developing over time. When the immediacy of a situation is uncertain or ambiguous (yet demands action), people must make decisions based on imperfect or inadequate information. This stress impairs our cognitive ability to interfere with what the leader wanted or expected. Leadership is commonly described in terms of traits and the function of the leader, who leads or guides people toward a common goal or performance. The leadership necessary for leading when the problem is present, but the leader is rarely discussed.

Command Climate

The command climate is the culture of a military unit, including its moral tone, and is set by what the commander says and does. The leader owns the story and must embody the principles, because subordinates watch their leaders and follow the examples they set. Leaders also articulate the core values of the unit. Expanding on the story of the "strategic corporal" from the title of Gen. Krulak's *Marines* magazine article mentioned earlier in this chapter, Maj. Teague A. Pastel (2008) identified three problem areas in the command climate: the zero-defects mentality, micromanagement, and risk aversion.

When people are working in an environment they have never before encountered, they will generally make decisions that do not turn out well. Someone who looks back in hindsight or from outside the environment may call these mistakes. How can people make mistakes in situations they have never before encountered? A zero-defects mentality prevents learning in real time in real situations; because it prevents people from identifying the boundaries of their abilities, they stay safely within the confines of what they know. We must recognize that these mistakes are part of a strong program; the program itself must be sufficiently robust that it can tolerate mistakes from people learning.

In his book *Fooled by Randomness*, author Nassim Taleb (2005) discusses why humans seek to determine cause-and-effect relationships for life events. He explains how this "Monday morning quarterback" heuristic or "hindsight bias" makes events appear to be more predictable after the fact than they actually were at the time of their occurrence.

We must also use caution with the concept of safety culture. For example, if the intent of the US Navy was to be perfectly safe, the Navy would not send its ships to sea or launch its planes. Working in a hazardous environment with uncertainty and time compression means to work on the margins of safety. If we want perfect safety, then we must work away from the thresholds of such environments. On the other hand, we can use operations to ensure safety, and we can use safety to ensure operations, as discussed below. HROs do not make a distinction between safety and operations.

Safety through Operations; Operations through Safety

Safety concerns can lead to risk-averse behavior. When leaders become aware of risk, they may attempt to manage distant events from their central position.

This situation creates *micromanagement*: managing details without knowledge of the context. We must be aware of details in an HRO, but these are details within a specific context. Another cause of micromanagement is *risk aversion*, which is to think of worst-case scenarios. Everyone has encountered people, either leaders or subordinates, who believe it is their duty to identify problems and risks beforehand. What makes them different is how they stop the discussion and do not offer any solutions; they seem to try to block the action when they do not provide alternatives. We may also have difficulty understanding the logic behind their concerns or aversion, because their rationale for their behavior is to either block movement or to express their fear. Their ideas often sound improbable to everyone but them.

This discussion all comes together with the concept of "zero preventable accidents." The combination of zero defects, micromanagement, and risk aversion contributes to an atmosphere of justification and second-guessing. "Risk" needs to be replaced by more specific terms that we can address and measure. Rather than saying that something has risk, we can be more specific about the source of risk, whether from the participants, the environment, or the breach of duty (which is also an element of liability).

Expert Level of Performance

Who you compare yourself to tells a lot about your ambitions to reach expert performance. In his book *Outliers* (2008), Malcolm Gladwell popularized the idea that expertise takes ten thousand hours to attain, which is actually a fairly minor issue and one we have little control over. Reaching expertise, however, also involves who you compare yourself to as well as working on what is hard, which leaders do have some influence over. Leaders identify industries and other organizations that people can compare themselves to; they help address areas that can be difficult to accomplish and improve upon.

Failure Is an Option

Learning from experience, particularly experience where failure is an option creates expert performance. Fear of stress and the effect of stress can lead people to avoid engagement in these situations.

One of the results of our experience developing a pediatric ICU is that the pediatric residents told us that the PICU was their hardest rotation in residency, but the least stressful. Problem-solving releases dopamine in the brain's locus accumbens. This release provides pleasure and satisfaction; having low levels of dopamine is associated with depression. Leadership reduces the gratuitous stress that interferes with performance. (There is a form of depression associated with low levels of dopamine but through a different mechanism.)

Failure is isolating. We are social animals, both physiologically and psychologically. Bullying isolates a child, and the same behaviors and responses are also found in adults. One unrecognized form of bullying is social isolation, which itself is very stressful. No one should feel isolated in an organization, particularly an organization that works in high-stress situations and strives to be an HRO. A leader should ensure that everyone feels a connection to others in the group and, however directly or indirectly, to the leader.

Life is not a movie—failure happens. Todd LaPorte, former Marine fighter pilot, sociology professor at UC Berkeley, and leader of the UC Berkeley HRO project, wrote about complex organizations that "the organization not prepared to fail, will fail." One purpose of leadership is to prepare the organization for failure *as a method to prevent failure*.

Self-efficacy supports acting when failure is an option. The individual with high self-efficacy believes personal effort can influence events and improve outcomes. In an HRO, the leader must develop self-efficacy among rookies and novices, which may come through accepting results that are not optimal but are sufficient. Gaining confidence that one can effect change is critical for engagement.

Lead with Distance from the Action

In firefighting and fire EMS, the most important person on scene is generally a firefighter at the end of the nozzle or the paramedic treating a patient. In the medical field, the most important person is said to be the patient. This contrast leads to quarrels over who knows what is best for the patient. In public safety, all efforts are directed at supporting people to do their jobs properly and with adequate resources; the role of the public-safety captain is to ensure that this happens. There is sometimes an urge for the captain to perform some of the work for the firefighters and medics. When fire captains pick up the fire hose, they become firefighters and are no longer in charge. It is an important component of leadership to maintain some detachment from the action otherwise the leader becomes part of the action and unable to take in the larger setting.

In order to communicate, particularly with any distance from subordinates, the leader must *identify*, *interpret*, and *translate* information and events. HROs engage complex, time-compressed situations that are in constant flux. People are immersed in action, which leaves it to the leader to identify evolving threats, interpret the situation to better understand what is happening, and then translate that information to various organizations and professionals using language and words the other people will understand.

When working at a distance from the action it is important for the leader to communicate "commander's intent" which consists of purpose, objectives, and conditions that define the end state. This also means identifying objectives for decision-making and the problem space, acknowledging that some objectives may conflict at specific times. For example, according to William J. Corr (LAFD, retired), firefighters relieve smoke and heat in a house fire by cutting a hole in the roof. A firefighter once climbed to the roof using an attached fence; with him was Captain Corr. The battalion chief arrived and demanded to know why they were on the roof without a ladder, when department policy was to have a ladder on the roof at all times for emergencies. Captain Corr responded, "Isn't it also the department's policy to put out the fire?" (personal communication).

Communication in these settings must be objective, articulate, and succinct. Objective is the most difficult for people to learn because they believe their judgment of information is necessary for others to make good decisions. Be aware of words used to evaluate or persuade. The second most difficult thing to teach (after being objective), and most frustrating for the student, is to be concrete: students do not see, nor can they recognize, its importance until they are in a crisis. In an emergency, thinking moves to the concrete, and we lose our abstract thought. Concrete descriptions reduce ambiguity.

Bottom-Up and Top-Down Leadership

During critical moments in an emergency, a subordinate may observe decisions that seem counterproductive—not because the leader who makes these decision is unprofessional but because the leader lacks important information. It is the duty of the subordinate to bring this disconfirming information forward. In time-compressed states, however, or with a resistive leader, the subordinate may have to lead through persuasion by keeping within "commander's intent."

Karl Weick discusses the "group writ small" (personal communication), which is a critical concept, as it describes the dynamics of a bottom-up approach and supports the idea that safety and reliability are a self-organizing response to a particular situation in a local context. The combination of empowering the expert people who are closest to a problem and shifting leadership to those who have the answers to the problem at hand is central to success (Meshkati and Khashe 2015).

Renaud Vidal (2015) describes several models of leadership as "stances." The "gardener's stance" accepts that the leader cannot change the weather or the needs of the plants in the garden; the leader instead guides the growth of the garden and ensures that the plants receive what they need to grow. Vidal urges caution with the "engineer's stance" of leadership, which is "when lessons learned by organizations translate into the refinement of procedures, protocols, and proliferation of rules" (2015, 110). Creating rules to manage uncertainty typifies the engineer's stance.

Leadership in Ambiguity

Successful leaders seek out diverse perspectives and discrepancies (Barton et al. 2015). Leaders will engage diverse participants from inside and outside the organization to provide multiple perspectives and innovative suggestions that will contribute to "learning-by-doing" (Carroll 1995, 2015). Such leaders shuffle power and influence to those who can make sense of an ambiguous situation.

In the US Navy, only the captain of the ship can say no. A "bias for action" to make the system work developed from this situation so that people could work to say yes; if not successful, they then send the problem up the command ladder. In this manner, junior officers have the opportunity to solve problems and then are mentored in other solutions or problem-solving techniques (van Stralen and Mercer 2015). A deeper understanding of the "only the captain can say no" situation may be achieved by looking at how the captain sees a larger picture of events (Mercer, personal communication). In this manner, everyone on board a ship learns how to solve problems. If they can't solve a problem, then they move it up the command chain. Doing so also prevents people from blocking information and problems from moving upward.

John Carroll describes a CNO (chief nuclear officer of a nuclear power plant) who reversed the firings of two contract workers who had voiced safety concerns. The CNO saw the larger picture and, by acting *into* ambiguity, increased not only safety within the program but also transformed leadership in the ranks of management. Robert Bea, professor of civil engineering at UC Berkeley, has described the importance of corporate leadership; when the leaders who have originally developed a program retire, "the pipes start leaking again" (Bea, personal communication).

Assorted Methods of Leading

The following are independent leadership points we have accrued from various HROs. From discussions with members of the Joint Special Operations Command, for example, we have identified several key points:

- Relationships within an organization are important.
- Friction *will* occur when people have independent objectives and purposes.
- Maintain *interoperability* for mission success toward a common purpose.
- Be sure to "own your own error": if you do not identify an error you have made, somebody else will; when somebody else must call out the error, trust within the system will be reduced.

In the firefighting context, a veteran firefighter often gives a piece of advice to a rookie and then appears to leave. (In fact, the veteran firefighter often stands off a short distance and watches the rookie struggle—not for amusement, but to see how the rookie solves problems.) At a given moment, the veteran then steps in and, without passing any judgment, provides whatever additional assistance is necessary. This is how rookies learn that they must work on their own but that help is always nearby; they also learn that the help is always watching.

In the context of Bloom's taxonomy, HROs work in the affective domain of the taxonomy. Because people respond to the environment in ways that make sense to them, it is important for leaders to give meaning and context to information and events. Leaders also model attitudes and select attitudes necessary for use in an HRO. When one of the authors (Daved van Stralen) first started in a pediatric ICU, for example, he was concerned about how to combat the phrase "I know this is what Dr. van Stralen taught you, but let me tell you how it really works." Jim Holbrook, his educator guide at the time, told him to teach in the affective domain, particularly to focus on how the information helps the student. In effect, teach only what works. People now tell him precisely what he originally said about what works for given circumstances the next day (and even thirty years later). He finds that they fill in the space between what he taught—the cognitive domain—through their own study.

Van Stralen also recounts how his fire station commander valued everyone in his command and in the department. He asked why several firefighters had not moved up to fire engineer before their retirement; they had put in the years and had World War II veteran credits. The commander told him that they were successful; they had lived through the Depression and had fought in the war. Now each of them could provide a roof over his family's heads and food on the stove. Van Stralen used the same concept in a nursing home, where many people were dismissive of CNAs (certified nursing attendants). He told them that these CNAs were likely the most successful members in their families; they had completed some schooling and had jobs. Tone comes from the top. Leaders set the tone for the organization. When van Stralen and others created the pediatric intensive care unit, they had three simple rules that they used and modeled for the attitudes they sought in the staff: (1) do not criticize; (2) support the bedside caregiver; (3) you have a duty to the larger community.

Van Stralen's experience with developing safety, reliability, and independence among pediatric residents during their pediatric ICU rotations led to a series of four standard lectures:

- First day—complex patients are sorted into three elements: (1) What problem would kill the patient? (2) What problem would keep the patient in the ICU? (3) What problems would resolve from solving (1) and (2) along with routine treatment and time?
- Second day—discuss decision-making, problem-solving, and affective processes.
- Third day—discuss stress and unrecognized fear.
- Fourth day—learn to take a break. We can rest even in the busiest times, and the residents learned to trust the bedside staff. (Residents watch a 25 minute music video.)

The two attending intensivists also routinely walked through unit to identify the signs of stress in staff. In this way, the program grew over three years from a small, eight-bed unit that had no critically ill patients to the second-largest ICU in the in the state of California, with half the expected patient mortality.

In the context of the armed forces, General George S. Patton (US Army) once said, "Never tell a good man how to do something. Tell him what to do and he will surprise you with his ingenuity." While Patton is not unanimously recognized as a great leader, his quote does have meaning.

In the naval context, Rear Admiral Mercer (retired) was noted for his leadership methods on the USS *Carl Vinson*. During his routine and unscheduled walks around the carrier flight deck looking for debris, he would walk with the sailors. At some point during the walk, a sailor would have to talk to the ship's captain walking next to him or her. In this way, the captain maintained a connection with the crew, and they felt connected with him. He also described having three "cake celebrations" a day on the ship. He found that the presence of the captain at the celebrations was more important than almost any other reward or anything else he could do for the crew. The captain has a larger view of events on the ship. At that distance, the captain is more likely to resolve ambiguous information and assist in decision-making than others.

In another military context, foreign object debris (FOD) can be lethal on an aircraft carrier flight deck. One story we have heard is of a mechanic who lost a tool and quickly announced the loss; thus causing a delay in recovering aircraft, which is a dangerous situation if the planes are low on fuel. The crew eventually found the tool in a different location, and the mechanic was thanked for stopping operations. If the tool had been in the wrong place, it could have led to the loss of an aircraft and the death of the pilots.

Florence Nightingale: Leadership Foundation for the Science of Nursing

From her efforts to distinguish nursing as a distinct profession, Florence Nightingale originated the science of nursing. Out of concern that "petty management" would undermine the constructs that would delineate nursing as a profession, Nightingale insisted that nursing education should include personal and systems-management skills (Nightingale 1992 [1859]).

Nightingale knew "the most devoted friend or nurse cannot be always there. Nor is it desirable that she should" (1992 [1859]). This placed nursing as a discipline at risk, for "all the results of good nursing, as detailed in these notes, may be spoiled or utterly [negated] by one defect, viz.: in petty management, or in other words, by not knowing how to manage that what you do when you are there, shall be done when you are not there." Nightingale understood that the nurse must manage the patient in the absence of the nurse, and this must be taught before the absence occurs.

It was clear to Nightingale that petty management would not build a sustainable culture of care or provide resilience to ensure that all patients, every time, would receive optimal care, regardless of the variation in each patient's case or individuals' needs. Nightingale warned of managerial complacency arising from the inability of managers to assess skills and properly assign responsibilities and tasks. Her fear was of an organizational culture that gave the impression that "the house is in charge of itself." To that end, she provided the following managerial strategies "to be in charge" that closely correlate to the development of a High Reliability Organization.

To be "in charge" is:

- to carry out the proper measures yourself and to ensure that everyone else does as well;
- to see that no one either willfully or ignorantly obstructs or prevents such measures;

- to not do everything yourself or to appoint a number of people to each duty, but to ensure that each is capable and does his or her appointed duty;
- to not develop the egotistical belief that that no one can understand or carry on his or her assignments or responsibilities without your presence.

Rather, to be in charge means to strive to develop a system with rules that everyone can understand in order to do their work and, in case of the leader's absence or illness, know that all will go on as usual.
    —Patricia E. Sokol, RN, JD

Team Formation

This section describes convergent teams in the VUCA-T environment. Team organization and structure develop through interactions between team members, the problem, and the environment. Discussions of "team" are often conducted under the rubrics of team development, teamwork, and team organization, among others. These approaches imply that the team exists and would benefit from improved structure and refined processes. Other team discussions for structured or predictable environments can be found elsewhere in the healthcare or organizational literature. This chapter will discuss the convergent team, a team formed by a shared objective that is directed at the unexpected discrepancy or disruption.

When faced with an unexpected event, people naturally converge around the situation and join together to solve the problem. This system works well in natural settings, but when the problem is within VUCA-T environments, any actions the team participants take risk creating victims. We must avoid creating victims or the need to rescue the rescuer.

The confusion of a rapidly emergent event with novel properties challenges the most experienced of people. These events will attract others who are nearby, all of whom will make sense of the situation differently. For reliability in these situations, people must come together, engage as a team, and begin enactment toward resolution and a better end-state. This temporarily organized team is created and becomes operational between the beginning of the event and the arrival of a formal team, which is the start of collective enactment toward the unexpected.

Discussions of teamwork commonly focus on performance, purpose, team structure, hierarchy, and the roles of team members as work groups. What these discussions miss are the minutes immediately following a discrepancy or disruption when the emergency creates its own environment. In those moments, some routines must shift and some must be maintained, while information must be collected and interpreted; at the same time, action must commence. These minutes between discovery and the arrival of a more formal team can be stressful and chaotic or calm and controlled. These are the moments, not observable in simulations, when a group forms into a team for the creation of reliability. This early action by the convergent team creates structures that facilitate sensemaking (Maitlis and Christianson 2014).

In an environment with a team atmosphere, someone's initial engagement actions will be noticed as a discrepancy and will initiate team behavior. The first people are entering the problem environment and forming a team while making sense of events. In fact, sensemaking, actions, and team formation are deeply entwined, because they read one another and the situation. Those who are nervous or anxious can be calmed by more experienced experts, who will keep the team focused and performing. On the other hand, the team can begin to fall apart not only from this anxiety and nervousness but also from attempts to meet the system's expectations for performance and outcome or from acting toward idealized normative behaviors rather than working the problem.

Self-Organization

We design systems for people that include instructions, commands, and a hierarchy, all of which give us teams and workgroups. These structures are external to the team. Self-organizing systems, in contrast, develop through interactions internal to the system, without intervention by *external directing* influences. The key is the absence of external directing influences. Those who respond to an emergency and are focused on the problem will also self-organize through interactions internal to the group and in response to the problem. The physical environment is a sensemaking resource for storing and distributing sense.

This is not to say that people will not follow directions but that they will follow the directions as they make sense in this evolving situation. Unfortunately, signals from the event tend to be nuanced, subtle, or ambiguous, which leads people to follow different and possibly conflicting rules. Self-organization is beneficial in these situations: if people watch one another (as in heedful interrelating), then the actions they take in response to the problem and to one another can coalesce into a smoothly functioning team (Weick and Roberts 1993).

Self-organization builds from the amplifying nature of positive feedback. While negative feedback stabilizes a system in order to avoid undesirable fluctuations, maintain homeostasis, and identify safe boundaries, positive feedback promotes growth and pattern formation, which is a characteristic of self-organization. Such feedback is beneficial for a "refractory" problem, but if too much growth occurs, then inhibition (a form of negative feedback) occurs. An emergent property of self-organization is that growth should occur where it is needed and inhibition should occur after too much growth. This is not to say that we lose the safety value of negative feedback. Because self-organization is a response to local conditions, negative feedback and its concomitant safety information will be communicated through the small group. Group members respond not only to the environment but to one another. Information from the environment can then be shared more rapidly. Positive and negative feedback with the environment and between group members like this creates a stable pattern for problem-solving and group cohesiveness.

Teamwork then becomes an emergent property that is unique to the specific problem but recurring for each new emergency. The emergency creates its own environment, no matter how unstable it appears. Self-organizing teams respond by creating their own stabilizing environments. This stabilizing structure also facilitates sensemaking (Maitlis and Christianson 2014).

This situation describes another emergent property of self-organized teams: team cognition. Team cognition describes the organization of knowledge that is important for the problem, how that knowledge is represented, and how it is distributed throughout the team (DeChurch and Mesmer-Magnus 2010). This knowledge can be task-related knowledge (which describes duties necessary for problem-solving) or team-related knowledge of how to interact with team members and rely on the interdependence with team members.

Distributed Sensemaking

Sensemaking in this emergent model is a distributed process of shared understanding. People hold different pieces of information and bring in different types of knowledge; through interaction with one another, they collectively construct new meaning (Maitlis and Christianson 2014). As different signals become salient during the evolution of the problem, team members' understandings of the situation will shift, and their behaviors will change in response; this situation then develops into collective problem-solving and collective enactment toward the end-state.

In larger-scale emergencies, smaller convergent self-organizing teams become nodes linked to similar nodal teams. Node linkages occur through *information flow* and *authority migration*, both of which create a scale-free network that grows in response to the size of the crisis.

Hierarchy

In a self-organizing team, the hierarchy is not imposed from outside by status but is internally based on people's pertinent knowledge needs and roles at that time. In this sense, the phrase "task ambiguity" describes situations in which the task must be performed, but it can be performed by any of the professionals involved. For example, a physician or nurse can establish an intravenous line, depending on the difficulty and who has the available time. Except for those procedures a physician cannot delegate, most tasks can be performed by multiple specialties on the team.

A medical emergency requires multiple types of emergency responders to make sense of the evolving situation and coordinate their actions. Certain roles must be filled, but they can generally be filled by anyone who has the ability to perform a necessary task. These role structures may be a critical component to maintaining sensemaking (Maitlis and Christianson 2014). The collapse of role structures can lead to the collapse of sensemaking (Weick 1993).

Shared Objectives

When people have a shared objective, each member identifies what is required for the objective and works toward that goal. If they see that someone needs help, then they help that person, even if it means doing more work or slowing their own work. Doing so allows them to work from their strengths while watching out for one another. A French fighter pilot once described this behavior within an operational mission. If pilots cannot complete their own missions, then the mission becomes helping the other pilots reach their missions (personal communication to the authors).

> Identified, shared objectives are essential when acting within an environment with undetectable structure. Outsiders, or sojourners, have trouble working without structure and may create structure to help make sense of activities. You then see teams and team captains wearing a vest that says "Pit Crew" and standing in a certain spot so people know who they are and what they do. Teams don't need captains for "team by objective."
>
> In unstructured environments, it should be "team by shared objective." Note that the captain in "team by shared objective" uses less hierarchical authority, reserving perceptions for sensemaking of the larger setting. When a fire captain picks up a fire hose, for example, he is no longer captain; he becomes a firefighter. I used to joke to my staff at the hospital that I wasn't allowed on the linoleum during resuscitations; I had

to stand off to the side, on the carpet. I found that once I stood on the linoleum, the residents thought I was leading the resuscitation.

—Daved van Stralen

The Success of Teams

The past ten to fifteen years have seen developing appreciation that success in high-risk but uncommon surgical procedures may be derived from teamwork and institutional volume for the procedure, related with the number and frequency of procedures. Studies of survival following the performance of the Norwood procedure (the initial corrective surgery for hypoplastic left-heart syndrome) have demonstrated better outcomes related to institutional volume compared to individual surgeon case volumes (Checchia et al. 2005; Hornik et al. 2012; Pasquali et al. 2012; Pieper et al. 2014). This situation appears to hold true for congenital surgery in general (Anderson et al. 2016; Kansy et al. 2016). Kansy et al. also found a higher risk of complications in high-volume centers, but the mortality associated with the risk was lower. This inverse correlation has been identified with adverse events during pediatric cardiac catheterization (Jayarm et al. 2017) but not with extra-corporeal membrane oxygenation, or ECMO (Gupta and Rettiganti 2015).

> "Now I know what you mean by affective knowledge," an emergency medicine physician once said to me at a meeting. He said he'd been intubating an infant's airway and "realized how bad I'd look if I missed it. That pressure made it more difficult to intubate. My emotion began to get in the way." He told me how his team had helped him and the duty he'd felt toward them to succeed. We also talked about the criticisms we'd heard about paramedics intubating children and how they would view failure, since many of them had successfully intubated children in the past. In the EMS field, a lot of people talk about the number of procedures that are necessary to maintain procedural skills; many people believe that paramedics can't reach the necessary number. The emergency medicine physician I was talking to wondered how many failures in paramedic intubation may have occurred because of the pressure that physicians and the system in general place on EMTs.
>
> —Daved van Stralen

We included earlier in this book the observation by Martin Eisner, a surgeon practicing trauma surgery early in the history of the field, that surgeons at trauma centers may decide not to operate on a patient when a surgeon at a non-trauma medical center could do the job. Experienced and knowledgeable ICU nurses can capably observe a patient rather than the surgeon performing exploratory surgery (Eisner, personal communication). As the emergency medicine physician in the vignette above discovered, teams provide not only technical support but also affective support. Teams can create success where there would have been failure.

Conclusions

(1). In High Reliability, leadership shows when the emergency is present and the leader is not.

(2). Good leadership is invisible and occurs long before it is needed.

(3). In High Reliability, we develop "leader-leaders" rather than "leader-followers."

(4). Leadership before the extreme event utilizes elements of transformational, indirect, and motivational leadership.

(5). Practical wisdom emphasizes judgment by the individual for particular situations; such wisdom is modeled for less experienced people.

(6). Authority for decision-making as *line authority* derives from the need to control the operations of an organization; for *functional authority*, the purpose of authority is to control local events.

(7). In a "team by shared objective," each member identifies what is necessary for the objective and works toward that goal.

(8). Convergent teams begin as disaggregated elements and create an identity from the shared knowledge base; they anticipate the capabilities, limits, and needs of the other unknown participants.

CHAPTER 13

MODELS OF LEADERSHIP

We will discuss several models of leadership in this chapter. In HROs, it may be hard to isolate leadership from its context or situation. There is the abstract part of leadership—the concepts and thoughts of being a leader. Then there is the concrete part of leadership—giving direction in turmoil, helping when people falter, and providing a physical presence when possible. At times the leader must be authoritative or democratic, while at other times the leader must be autocratic or take full control. This is leadership in real time, done under uncertainty and ambiguity, in time-compressed states, and facing immediate peril. The leader cannot suddenly shift to these states and adopt a heroic leader stance. Leadership is created in the downtimes of the routine.

This style of leadership is difficult to observe, since numerous individual interactions add up to a concerted action. It is not a fair proxy to watch a leader of a large system who works apart from the event, such as an incident commander at a public-safety emergency or the medical director of a healthcare organization. These leaders may have learned while immersed in the crisis but now are removed and away from immediate danger. They now call upon their experience and practical wisdom while they observe the situation as a complete whole, ensuring command and authority, providing logistic support, monitoring tactics, and updating strategy.

Transformational-Transactional

Since the beginning of this century, a substantial body of research has accumulated on transformational-transactional leadership theory. James Burns (1978) first introduced the concepts of transformational and transactional leadership in his treatment of political leadership. Transformational leaders offer a purpose that transcends short-term goals and focuses on higher-order intrinsic needs. Transactional leaders, in contrast, focus on the proper exchange of resources. While transformational leadership results in followers identifying with the needs of the leader, transactional leaders give their followers something they want in exchange for something the leader wants (Kuhnert and Lewis 1987).

Bernard Bass (1985) based his theory of transformational leadership on Burns's (1978) conceptualization, with several modifications or elaborations. First, Bass did not agree with Burns's assessment that the transformational and transactional leadership styles represent opposite ends of a single continuum. Bass argued that transformational and transactional leadership are separate concepts and further argued that the best leaders are both transformational and transactional. Second, Bass elaborated considerably on the behaviors that manifest transformational and transactional leadership (Judge and Piccolo 2004).

The four dimensions of transformational leadership are charisma or idealized influence, inspirational motivation, intellectual stimulation, and individualized consideration.

(1). *Charisma,* or *idealized influence,* is the degree to which the leader behaves in admirable ways that causes followers to identify with the leader. Charismatic leaders display conviction, take stands, and appeal to followers on an emotional level.

(2). *Inspirational motivation* is the degree to which the leader articulates a vision that is appealing and inspiring to followers. Leaders with inspirational motivation challenge followers to have high standards, communicate optimism about future goal attainment, and provide meaning for the task at hand.

(3). *Intellectual stimulation* is the degree to which the leader challenges assumptions, takes risks, and solicits followers' ideas. Leaders with this trait stimulate and encourage creativity in their followers.

(4). *Individualized consideration* is the degree to which the leader attends to each follower's needs, acts as a mentor or coach to the follower, and listens to the follower's concerns and needs.

The three dimensions of transactional leadership are contingent reward, management by exception (active), and management by exception (passive). *Contingent reward* is the degree to which the leader sets up constructive transactions or exchanges with followers: the leader clarifies expectations and establishes the rewards for meeting these expectations. *Management by exception,* in general, is the degree to which the leader takes corrective action on the basis of results of leader-follower transactions. The difference between *management by exception (active)* and *management by exception (passive)* lies in the timing of the leader's intervention:

- Active leaders monitor follower behavior, anticipate problems, and take corrective actions before the behavior creates serious difficulties.
- Passive leaders wait until the behavior has created problems before taking action.

Transformational leadership has an impact on follower motivation and performance. Leaders transform and motivate their followers through their idealized influence (sometimes referred to as charisma), intellectual stimulation, and individual consideration. In addition, this type of leader encourages followers to come up with new and unique ways to challenge the status quo and to alter the environment to support being successful. In his book *Leadership and Performance beyond Expectations*, Bass (1985) developed the concept of transformational leadership further. Such a leadership style:

- is a model of integrity and fairness;
- sets clear goals;
- has high expectations;
- encourages others;
- provides support and recognition;
- stirs people's emotions;
- gets people to look beyond their self-interest; and
- inspires people to reach for the improbable.

The *transformational leadership* approach is based on the leader's personality, traits, and ability to make a change through example and by embodying a vision. Transformation is not based on a "give and take" relationship or on punishment-reward. The leader articulates an energizing vision and challenging goals. A transforming leader is idealized, in the sense that he or she is a moral example of working toward the benefit of the team, organization, and/or community.

The *transactional leadership* approach is based on processes and clear structures of what is required of subordinates; compliance is achieved through contingent reward and contingent penalization rather than via processes and example, as in transformational leadership. The central difference is the use of extrinsic motivators such as pay against intrinsic motivators such as pride and vision. Transactional leaders are generally passive and work within the existing system.

Indirect Leadership

Culture is social knowledge—the social response to the environment—and is passed down through stories. Howard Gardner's approach is also how culture changes from the indirect leader. The leader "owns" the story or narrative. There must be a relationship between the stories that leaders tell and the traits they embody. Every story has a purpose and a principle. In the preface to *Leading Minds: An Anatomy of Leadership* (written with Emma Laskin), Gardner states:

> A leader is an individual (or, rarely, a set of individuals) who significantly affects the thoughts, feelings, and/or behaviors of a significant number of individuals…I have called attention to an unrecognized phenomenon: indirect leadership. In this variety of leading, individuals exert impact through the works that they create…It is important that a leader be a good story-teller, but equally crucial that the leader embody that story in his or her life. When a leader tells stories to experts, the stories can be quite sophisticated; but when the leader is dealing with a diverse, heterogeneous group, the story must be sufficiently elemental to be understood by the untutored, or "unschooled," mind. (Gardner and Laskin 2011, xiii.)

Because the ability to adapt based on the situation is an integral part of HROs, they are constantly changing, growing, and organizing; Gardner's description of indirect leadership is particularly appropriate in context with the lessons learned from HROs.

Stories

Studies of leadership generally address *power, policies, public,* and *personality* (Gardner and Laskin 2011). Indirect leadership is not derived from models of leadership but from studying effective leaders who have changed society. These leaders have exerted their leadership through the works they create and the stories they tell. Indirect leaders influence people across both space and time, in contrast to direct leaders, who address the public face-to-face.

Leaders *relate* the story; they do not *tell* the story. In this manner, the leader embodies the story, thus lending authenticity to both leader and story. Gardner realized that presenting a story is but one way to communicate: leaders also convey the meaning of stories to the lives they live in the examples they set. Stories are important in human affairs and have distinct purposes for tacit knowledge, identity, values, and leadership. Gardner taught that the most effective lessons are often couched in good stories, particularly the relationship between the stories leaders tell and the traits they embody. Stories carry social knowledge. Some stories tell about the group and carry its identity to individual people, while other stories carry the knowledge held by the group itself, which is a form of tacit knowledge.

Stories for identity. These stories are conveyed through narrative in such a way that newcomers adopt the story as their own. They learn stories about the group that everybody must know; they also begin to shape their own stories into their new culture.

Stories for tacit knowledge. Knowledge can be *tacit* or *explicit.* As noted earlier, tacit knowledge is subconsciously understood and applied, difficult to articulate, developed from direct experience and action, and usually shared through highly interactive conversation, storytelling, and shared experience. Explicit knowledge, in contrast, can be more precisely and formally articulated. Although more abstract, it can be more easily codified, documented, transferred, or shared. Language is the most direct form of tacit knowledge; one must articulate information in the language rules of a culture. Part of the knowledge of language includes knowledge of discourse forms: how and when to tell a story. Anecdotes are stories that carry values and tacit social knowledge. Unfortunately, in health-care we tend to depreciate the anecdote despite its use in case reports. Stories provide a bridge between the tacit and the explicit, which allows tacit social knowledge to be demonstrated and learned without the need to make formal presentations of ethics or to specify in detail the proper behavior. Stories convey the speaker's moral attitude toward events in the social memory.

Stories with pedagogical function. Just as cultural stories guide people through the stages of life, organizational stories guide members from novice to manager and above. During enculturation, at each step of advancement, people will encounter many psychological challenges particular to the organization and its environment. Stories may serve as a guide for successful passage. Stories are the narrative for learning. Sometimes we say that we should tell a story, but in time-constrained events we may want to describe a scene. A German film director once described the differences between a story and a scene: a story has a beginning, middle, and end, while a scene takes us from A to B and contains only one or two story arcs. Rather than telling a story during an emergency, we can describe a scene with two salient story or incident arcs. Stories are powerful for leadership and enculturation; the one who controls the narrative is the one who leads.

The Questions We Ask, and the Answers We Accept

Einstein influenced many scientists by the conclusions he drew, but more so in the way in which he posed questions to formulate, approach, and solve problems. The very best instructor pilots rarely instruct; they simply embody the characteristics of the "best" pilots, demonstrating by example and deed rather than from a traditional model of instruction. Because such people embrace and live by HRO practices, their students come to accept a higher standard of performance as being what is expected. They embody HRO characteristics and raise the bar, albeit not through direct instruction. When an HRO experiences loss of structure, it may be best to lead through the questions we ask and in the answers we accept.

This model represents the questions you ask and the answers you accept: ask questions directed to move people, identify discrepancy, or appreciate complexity and ambiguity. People must develop alternative explanations for events and circumstances. When they offer plans, they must have descriptions to identify (1) the benefits of their suggested action, (2) any undesired consequences, and (3) how to interpret the absence of a response. This forms a "decision space" within which people can act freely, which describes the effect of acting too soon or too late and the effect of using too much or too little.

> Captain Bill Corr of the Los Angeles City Fire Department changed the culture of a fire station by asking firefighters to describe or explain what they were doing, and he would complement them on their skill, expertise, and ingenuity. Over time he began to talk to the firefighters, not to offer suggestions but to ask if they had considered anything else since they'd last spoken. Within a few months, the culture of the fire station had changed.
> —Daved van Stralen

Errors and mistakes should be investigated from the point of view that someone did the right thing and did what you would have done. This will change your perspective to that person's view, and you will see events quite differently. Everyone acts in a manner that makes sense to him or her. If you can see this, then you can learn where and what you need to teach. Error in these cases is gold, since it helps you identify vulnerabilities to your system. As Christopher A. Hart, chair of the NTSB has said, "Once you find out who did it, then you begin your investigation" (personal communication).

When the environment contains information, the leader must change the environment (part of the engagement with the emergency) while recognizing that the environment changes the leader. This is a dynamic interaction. Leaders must develop a relationship with their subordinates to know when to nurture them in times of stress or to guide them in situations of complexity and ambiguity. A relationship also builds a reservoir of goodwill one can use when it is necessary to be direct (if not blunt) in order to transform subordinates experiencing difficult circumstances or having undefined problems. While leaders provide direction, they must do this for the purpose of internalizing direction, as in the concept of "leader's intent."

To develop thinking skills for High Reliability problems, the leader asks questions: not to add pressure but to encourage decision-making and the development of adaptive, divergent responses. Information flow will then improve as the subordinates learn descriptive techniques that are objective, articulate, and succinct. To change culture to High Reliability, leaders "own" the narrative and use stories to demonstrate principles, decision-making, and problem-solving. Questions from the leader reframe the problem; questions from other people reappraise the situation.

The Motivational Interviewing Approach for Transformation

The following discussion is modified from Rollnick, Miller, and Butler (2008). People resist change: not from denial or inertia but from internal conflict between current beliefs and behaviors and new beliefs and behaviors. Demonstrating the discrepancy between what people have and what they would like and instilling self-efficacy can motivate people to change, but doing so requires an empathetic, nonjudgmental relationship with the leader. This style is referred to as a motivational interview (MI) approach to leadership.

The MI approach attempts to increase people's awareness of potential problems caused by specific beliefs and behaviors, any consequences experienced from those beliefs and behaviors, and any risks faced as a result of the belief and behavior in question. The approach is practical in its focus by developing strategies in a collaborative approach—more through persuasion than coercion—and is supportive rather than argumentative. It is designed to strengthen personal motivation for and commitment to a specific goal and to explore people's own reasons for change. MI is a formal approach that physicians use to change behavior (originally for addictive behaviors) and has been described in numerous articles on the subject since 1981.

MI facilitates and engages intrinsic motivation *within* people that is not imposed by a leader; it is a goal-oriented, person-centered, supportive style developed to elicit change in behavior by exploring and resolving ambivalence. The approach, which is nonjudgmental, nonconfrontational, and nonadversarial, is generally used for specific situations rather than for a broad approach to change. The five general principles of MI are:

(1). *Express empathy* through reflective listening.
(2). *Develop discrepancy* between people's goals or values and their current beliefs and behaviors.
(3). *Avoid arguments* and direct confrontation.
(4). *Adjust to resistance* rather than opposing it directly.
(5). *Support self-efficacy.*

Leaders establish interaction skills at the outset, such as the ability to provide affirmations. While working in adverse environments, people experience uncertainty and stress, both of which impair thinking. Their leaders encourage self-efficacy and engagement. They engage people in talking about the issues, concerns, and hopes, then focus by narrowing the conversation to habits or patterns to be changed by evoking the sense of importance of this change and the confidence to change. *This evokes from people what they already have and activates their own motivation and resources for change.* The use of MI follows a pattern of ambivalence, drivers for change, motivational interviewing, discrepancy development, and self-efficacy support, described below.

- Ambivalence: there are reasons to change and reasons not to change.
- Drivers for change: present change as problems to solve.
- Motivational interviewing: activate people's own motivations.
- Discrepancy development: determine the consequences of behavior conflict with knowledge and values.
- Self-efficacy support: instill belief that people can influence outcomes.

These principles are described in the following sections.

MI Principle 1: Ambivalence

The main problem encountered is not resistance or denial; it is ambivalence. The interpretation of ambivalence as resistance or denial creates friction. People's motivations to change are conflicted between desire, ability, and reasons. Ambivalence is a response to the tension between two pressures, where people may not know which way they want to go or do not feel they have the confidence or ability to change. Ambivalence about change has two components: (1) people tend to build pressure about making decisions when others tell them to change; (2) people are frustrated for not changing; this pressure contributes to becoming stuck in a chronically ambivalent state.

MI Principle 2: Drivers for Change

Motivation is situation specific. *Motivation for change* is malleable, particularly when formed in the context of relationships. Motivation is used for *specific situations* rather than being a broad approach to changing people. We can identify drivers for change as what we identify as local problems that subordinates and novices can solve with minimal guidance; by doing so, they learn engagement and decision-making in real time. "Drivers" are the problems that people can solve and, by solving the problems, they will change themselves. This process is transformational; our job is to assist in motivation to make this transformation. In MI, this is a problem-solving exercise to show that things can begin to happen. Use the resources people already have—they have been successful to get where they are now. We want to identify the things they may have brought with them that are currently impeding further or greater success. Doing so will increase our understanding of the situation and will identify their skills that they can draw on for change.

You should develop your own drivers for change that are specific to your domain and authority. Identify how to decompose the larger problem to smaller, more easily attainable objectives to match the ability of individuals or the group. Identify the risks of not acting or acting with insufficient force. Most people fear making decisions because of the belief that they will do more harm than good. "First, do no harm," the medical maxim, may harm more people than it helps; sometimes, doing nothing can be harmful.

Search for drivers that educate while being solved, develop insight into the mechanisms of your program, and instill tacit knowledge of the environment and operations. While solving small problems, people change themselves. Success is achievable. The release of the neurotransmitter dopamine for problem-solving gives satisfaction and pleasure. Small wins create self-efficacy and drive self-learning. The search for drivers is also a method of information flow (i.e., communication) of what works and what did not and where to focus resources; the process will grow into collaborative problem-solving. As an example, stress impairs cognition along with loss of abstract thought and makes initial acts difficult. Decomposing the problem to a small, easily managed problem that one can think about in concrete terms will facilitate engagement. A more critical thing to do is to create a problem driver that people cannot walk away from.

MI Principle 3: Motivational Interviewing

Motivational interviewing is a particular kind of conversation about change that activates people's own motivation for change. This kind of interviewing activates change within people, it avoids arguments during the interview, and the interviewer can be vigilant for blocks to interviewing. Motivation builds on what people already have, and a motivational interview will evoke from them their existing capabilities. From these findings we can help activate their motivation and resources for change. Use attribution theory over persuasion theory by telling them what they are, not what they need to be. They are successful: that is how they got to where they are today. Now, what do they have that hurts their success?

We want to understand their motivation to change, help them express the problem to be solved, and reduce the sense of threat, particularly the threat of change. We are working in an environment that can be confusing, bewildering, and, at times, adverse. We should acknowledge this.

Motivational interviewers must use certain leadership skills. The interviewer must proceed with a strong sense of purpose, have clear strategies and skills for pursuing that purpose, and maintain a sense of timing to intervene in specific ways at incisive moments. Interviewers should maintain being in control as the leader but avoid the expected complementary role of demanding adherence or compliance from their subordinates. As a guide, we help people learn to problem-solve with imperfect information and in time-compressed states. We want to understand their motivation to change, discuss problem-solving, and reduce threat, since we are working in an adverse environment. Doing so requires a level of interpersonal finesse that translates to effectiveness. Such interpersonal effectiveness can overcome adversity, motivate employees, and maintain effective relationships throughout the organization. When absent, these same characteristics may lead to labor disputes, legal action, poor morale, and generally ineffective organizational performance.

Motivational interviewing is a process of *eliciting* information, *providing* information, and then *eliciting* further information. By establishing the pattern of response, you are effectively guaranteeing that people will have a higher probability of communicating critical information in the future. You draw from people what they need and want to know and give them the meaning of the new information you provide. Work with their intrinsic motivations and values. Listen to their reasons to change and their reasons not to change. Provide simple information in digestible chunks; do not overload them. Consider the broader priorities of their organizations. As they change, their change talk advances. They:

- express the desire to change (*want*, *like to*, or *wish*);
- say they have the ability to change (*can* or *could*);
- state specific reasons for a certain change;

- use imperative language (*need*), which indicates that they are beginning to feel the necessity for change;
- end with talk of commitment.

Our purpose as leaders is to guide people through this change talk. Expressing too strong of a feeling that one is right can breed defensiveness and lead to counterproductive arguments. Resistance from a subordinate is a signal to change strategies; adjust to their resistance rather than opposing it directly. Support their self-efficacy and optimism. Some subordinates have problems that stem from psychological problems, not from a lack of skills; for such people, know when to refer them to counseling.

The use of persuasion, some forms of agreement, and some types of questioning can block the motivational interview. The use of logic, argument, and lecturing assume that people have not reasoned through the problem adequately. What is most likely true, though, is that they have not reasoned out the consequences of their beliefs or actions. When we agree, approve, or praise something, we may appear to be sanctioning or implying agreement with their statements. Questioning or probing can give the message that the right answer can be found if one asks enough questions.

> "When you listen, you learn. When all you do is
> talk, you cannot listen and you will not learn."
> —SPENCE BYRUM

For reflective listening, we do not have to agree with people or ask questions. In fact, intensive questioning interferes with the spontaneous flow of communication and diverts the conversation to our interests rather than those of the interviewee. Other traps we can fall into include withdrawing, becoming distracted (or introducing distractions), humoring people, or changing the subject. The use of humor, particularly in a sensitive or emotional moment, diverts communication and implies that people's beliefs are not important.

We will ask, listen, and inform. We will ask to understand their problems. We will listen to understand their meaning correctly. We will inform them to convey the knowledge that they need.

MI Principle 4: Discrepancy Development
Seeing discrepancies between one's current behaviors and beliefs and the desired outcomes will enhance motivation for change. For this principle, you should

develop team awareness of consequences. Assist in examining people's behavior and beliefs, differentiating adaptive from nonadaptive or maladaptive beliefs and behaviors. Some people have behaviors and beliefs that are commonly held as "normal" but that will have serious downstream effects in the HRO environment.

Identify any discrepancies within people's patterns. First you can highlight these discrepancies by presenting the negative consequences of a specific behavior. Help characterize and separate the belief or behavior that has contributed to the current consequences. Separate the behavior from the person: criticize the behavior, not the person. Help the team focus on how their current behavior differs from an effective behavior. Follow the belief or behavior to its logical end, the point at which it is more likely to result in undesired consequences. We often stop this process prematurely and do not see the actual or negative consequences. In real time, others may step in to capture the error, thus shielding people from the consequences of their error.

> In our pediatric ICU, the surgeons transferred several children for care in our service one time. The pediatric residents complained of "dumping"—that is, transferring the patients to our service for an easily treated condition but leaving our team with all the paperwork for hospital discharge. I followed that train of thought but with a different case, an infant on a surgical specialty service in which the resident had not bothered to consult the pediatric team for an easily treated problem—diet orders. The PICU team agreed that such a consultation or transfer was akin to dumping and that the surgical resident could easily write feeding orders. I then reported the outcome: excess feeding volume and overly frequent feeding. The infant aspirated food-gastric contents into the lung and died. We then discussed that a "dump" is something easily handled *only* because of our knowledge. An "acute abdomen" to pediatricians is an urgent problem, while to a surgeon it is routine and could be considered a "dump."
> —Daved van Stralen

The "Columbo" approach (Kanfer and Schefft 1988) is particularly useful with those who prefer to be in control, such as other leaders. Though you express understanding when using this approach, you appear unable to find a solution and continuously ask questions to clarify the problem. This stance of uncertainty or confusion can motivate people to offer solutions (Van Bilsen 1991).

Support the change once people begin to understand how the consequences of their current behavior conflict with significant personal, organizational, and

HRO values. Amplify this discordance until they can articulate consistent concerns and commitment to change and present their arguments for change. Keep the following in mind while doing so: (1) developing awareness of consequences helps people examine their own behavior; (2) showing a discrepancy between present behavior and important goals motivates change; (3) those who are being interviewed should present their own arguments for change.

MI Principle 5: Self-Efficacy Support

This principle refers to the strength of one's beliefs in one's own ability to complete tasks and reach goals. This is the single-most important skill we can instill in an HRO program. Without self-efficacy, people will not solve undefined problems and will fail to engage, which will lead to "diffusion of responsibility." Self-efficacy is entwined with the internal locus of control. For subordinates who lack a well-developed sense of self-efficacy, it may be difficult for them to believe that they can solve problems in real time. They may also have a misplaced or false sense of self-efficacy. It can be helpful to share stories about others in similar situations who have succeeded. Other employees can serve as role models (*social modeling*, as noted above) and offer encouragement.

Leaders must elicit and support optimism and the feasibility of managing problems in real time. They should recognize and acknowledge people's strengths, bring those strengths into the open, and support subordinates in believing that they can manage a series of problems on their own. Conveying four principal sources of information—enactive, vicarious, persuasive, and somatic—can instill self-efficacy (Bandura 1986).

Rationalizations or denial reduce the discomfort from perceived discrepancies between the desire to work and feelings about accomplishing the job. Self-efficacy is a critical component of working in an HRO environment; it is crucial that you as the leader also believe in your subordinates' capacity to independently manage problems.

A well-developed sense of self-efficacy will not develop in an organization with a disciplinary or punitive environment for error and mistakes. People have difficulty believing they can change or that change will be allowed. Improving self-efficacy requires supporting optimism and the feasibility of change. Because self-efficacy is a critical behavioral component in an HRO, it is crucial that you believe in your subordinates' capacity to engage and manage a series of problems in real time. Your subordinates must ultimately come to believe that engagement is their responsibility and that long-term success begins with a single step forward.

Reasons for Self-Efficacy

Self-efficacy leads to motivated, persistent, goal-directed, resilient, and clear thinkers under pressure. It can determine whether people experience self-hindering versus self-aiding thought patterns. It can predict how well people respond to threatening circumstances and supports resilience when people are faced with adversity and setbacks. As Albert Bandura (2009, 179) has said, "Unless people believe that they can produce desired effects and forestall undesired ones by their actions, they have little incentive to act or to persevere in the face of difficulties."

Self-Efficacy versus Self-Confidence

Self-confidence and self-efficacy are not identical conceptually. Self-confidence is a generalized sense of competence: a personal trait that is not generally subject to change. Self-efficacy is personal belief or self-judgment about one's task-specific capabilities, which is a social cognition that can change given appropriate conditions. The two are related to some extent. A highly confident person who is a leader would also likely report a high level of self-efficacy for leadership tasks. According to self-efficacy theory, self-confidence does not directly contribute to leader success. It is people's *beliefs* regarding their capabilities to successfully perform leadership tasks that is the key causal factor.

Using *enactive mastery experiences* that are structured through graduated attainments is an effective method for achieving self-efficacy. The path to high attainment is strewn with failure and setbacks. Success is achieved by learning from mistakes. Resilient efficacy requires experience in overcoming obstacles through perseverant effort. Train how to manage failure, and *make the training informative rather than demoralizing*. Only experiencing easy successes causes the expectation of quick results but will easily be discouraged by failure.

Social modeling develops personal and collective efficacy. Competent models convey knowledge, skills, and strategies for managing task demands and models the attitudes from Bloom's affective domain of learning. The leader's example in pursuing challenges models and fosters interest for engagement. When seeing colleagues at similar levels, people tend to persevere, which then raises their beliefs in their own abilities. *Social persuasion* increases people's chances of success. People who are persuaded to believe in themselves will exert more effort than those who are not. For leaders to act as credible persuaders, they must be knowledgeable and "practice what they preach" by modeling when they don't think they are being observed. Leaders, as effective efficacy builders, do more than convey faith in others; they arrange situations for others in ways that will bring success. Avoid prematurely placing your subordinates in situations where they are likely to fail. Measure their success by self-improvement rather than by triumphs over other people. Having pep talks without enabling guidance and telling narrative stories without a principle achieve little.

> When developing the pediatric ICU, we observed a strong hesitance to engage severe problems. People had never made decisions on their own that others would later rely on or that would have serious consequences. I asked people to identify if the action was reversible or irreversible; if it wasn't reversible, then they'd call me for assistance. If they could reverse it, then they could make the decision. This setup was not sufficient for decision-making, however, which led me to never make the final decision. When I asked for a decision and someone declined to answer, I provided more information, continuing this until they decided. At some point, they'd have to decide between two values that, unknown to them, were inconsequential. The most critical step was for them to decide. Simultaneously, I also identified knowledge gaps.
> —Daved van Stralen

We can ensure the achievement of self-efficacy. How do you know people have changed? What do you look for? How do people know that they were effective or effected change or reached a solution? How do people know they were right? The answers to these questions may be specific to the leader, individual people, or culture. Education can also increase the sense of self-efficacy, with credible, accessible, and accurate information. Teach from the affective domain of learning in Bloom's hierarchy. Understand the neurophysiology of change: that fear and stress have biological roots. Fear is not a weakness; it is neurochemicals released in the brain that can be suppressed.

A leader can take a process that initially feels overwhelming and break it down into small, achievable steps by decomposing or reducing the problem into elements. Solving problems, *particularly by making decisions that are acted on without review*, increases self-efficacy and trust in the system.

(1). If a wrong decision has been made, then provide sufficient information to change the decision; continue this iteration until a decision is reached that is reasonable.

(2). When a choice does not matter, let people choose.

(3). Do not criticize outcomes or results.

In these steps, belief in the possibility of change is an important motivator, subordinates are responsible for choosing and carrying out changes, and a range of alternative approaches is available.

Practical Wisdom: Aristotle's Prudence

It is not enough to give people information or instruction. People will evaluate such material from their knowledge, beliefs, and experience. The leader must also have values toward the good of the organization and place information and instruction within the context of a particular situation. This is practical wisdom.

Leadership represents practical wisdom rather than a body of knowledge and acts as interpretation, individual and collective, through shared narratives. In routine practical endeavors, we encounter the necessity of situational reasoning—those events where abstract concepts and principles do not neatly align with evolving events and where we encounter the full spectrum of processes yet can only call on categorized knowledge. It is in such cases, where we determine the best course of action in a given case, where we see the importance of practical wisdom or prudence, the first of the four cardinal virtues described by Aristotle.

In Aristotle's words, *phronesis* (prudence) is an intellectual virtue or characteristic that is "bound up with action, accompanied by reason, and concerned with things good and bad for a human being" (*Nicomachean Ethics* 1140b5-7). Those with prudent judgment consider the good of the community, which makes this one of Aristotle's four cardinal virtues (the others are justice, temperance, and fortitude).

The risk to organizations or to individuals is greatest from the unexpected or surprises, for it is here where the environment carries information particular to the event. The time compression of events limits communication between people and leaders, leaving less experienced or knowledgeable people to interact and risking the creation of a cascading series of mistakes from which they will not be able to recover. In this environment, the central problem is (1) the complexity from nonlinear interactions between causative principles and responders, (2) time compression as events change faster than one can identify or initiate controlling responses, and (3) developing stress reactions that impair cognitive function.

We will review leadership through the framework of a specific type of knowledge, practical wisdom: Aristotle's phronesis. Aristotle described three types of knowledge in *Nicomachean Ethics*, as discussed earlier in this book: episteme, techne, and phronesis.

- Episteme, or universal truth, is rational, context-independent, objective (explicit) knowledge that focuses on universal applicability independent of time or space; it is similar to "knowledge" as we recognize it today.
- Techne, or roughly technique, technology, and art, is the know-how or practical skill required to be able to create; it is instrumentally rational, context-dependent, practical (tacit) knowledge that is similar to "technology."
- Phronesis, or prudence or practical wisdom, is situational (i.e., having to do with contextual circumstances, context-dependent information, and the particulars of a situation). It is adaptive and pragmatic toward the greater good. Tacit knowledge is acquired from *practical experience* to make prudent decisions and to take action specific to each situation, guided by values and ethics (an intellectual virtue). Phronesis is the ability to determine and undertake the best action in a specific situation to serve the common good. The three elements of phronesis are: (1) the person (as actor; possesses character); (2) the particular (situation and context); (3) values (a vision of the good of the community, which makes it a virtue). Values include (3a) the highest good, or flourishing; (3b) values can be situational; (3c) values must be analyzed for a situation.

Wisdom (as an intellectual virtue) is sometimes translated as both *sophia* and *phronesis*, with sophia more closely related to "theoretical wisdom," a combination of the ability to discern reality and knowledge (episteme) or science; sophia refers to reasoning about universal truths. Phronesis adjusts knowledge to the peculiarity of local circumstances, similarly to the goals of other performance models, and sees the particular as a higher level of knowledge.

Dreyfus and Dreyfus (1986) studied the acquisition of expert performance among chess players, fighter pilots, and jazz-improvisation musicians. Contrary to what one might expect, they found that increasing expertise does not come from having a greater grasp of the abstract (episteme) but from having the ability to apply knowledge to particular situations (phronesis). The integration of general and situational knowledge in expert practice is a characteristic of mastery. As Patricia Benner has written in *From Novice to Expert: Excellence and Power in Clinical Nursing Practice,*

> Phronesis is the particular situation, the proficiency level in the Dreyfus model. Today, many industries and organizations use competency as their preferred measure...The competent level is supported and reinforced institutionally, and many nurses may stay at this level because it is perceived

as the ideal by their supervisors. The standardization and routinization of procedures, geared to manage the high turnover in nursing, most often reflect the competent level of performance. Most inservice education is aimed at the competent level of achievement; few inservice offerings are aimed at the proficient or expert level of performance. (1984, 30.)

The skills, rules, and knowledge (SRK) framework developed by Jens Rasmussen (1983) places emphasis on knowledge for the novel. The significance of local or special knowledge is the foundation of SRK, particularly in extreme cases where the particular is novel or unexpected. Rasmussen (1987) studied error in human-technological systems as an ecological model (called ecological interface design, or EID). James Reason, creator of the swiss cheese model of error containment discussed earlier in this book, classified human error on Rasmussen's framework. As Rasmussen and Vicente have stated, "Operators are maintained in [complex technological] systems because they are flexible, can learn and do adapt to the peculiarities of the system, and thus they are expected to plug the holes in the designer's imagination" (Rasmussen 1980, 97).

Having the wisdom to make judgments in everyday life with deliberation and emotion, and to make a right action, is wisdom embedded in practice. Having practical wisdom is to make the best judgment for the common good in a particular context.

The Priority of the Particular

We can evaluate the specific, the context, the essence of the situation, and the effect these elements have on knowledge and belief. The specific is the analysis of values—"the things good or bad for a human being" (*Nicomachean Ethics* 1140b6-7)—as a point of departure for managed action. We focus on what is variable, on that which cannot be encapsulated by universal rules, and on specific cases. This requires an interaction between the general and the concrete; it requires consideration, judgment, and choice. Rules can help only in specific situations; in the complex and dynamic world, we need "here and now" judgment that depends on the context. Context is important to pursue practical wisdom. Context is a relationship between things and situation. We can only understand meaning by knowing the relationship with our surroundings. Knowledge is a resource that we create within this context. Context-dependent knowledge and information arise when the environment contains information that is independent or influences our object or event. Context gives meaning to ambiguous information.

The essence of something is best described by the saying "the devil is in the details." The kind of consciousness that enables one to sense truth in individual details is the starting point of creativity. This consciousness contains the "why," which comes from the environment. We use our ability to intuitively fathom the true nature and meaning of people, things, and events. The ability to quickly sense what lies behind phenomena and accurately project an image of the future is based on this intuition; this intuition refers to the ability to recognize constantly changing situations correctly and to quickly sense what lies behind phenomena to envision the future and decide on the best action to be taken. We can recognize the situation correctly and grasp the essence. One can envision the future and decide on the best action to be taken to realize that future. *One must be able to see at both the micro and the macro levels simultaneously.*

We appreciate the effect of the particular regarding knowledge and belief. Knowledge and belief are found on a spectrum of value and degree of justified belief. We face limits of knowledge as we move toward belief; there is a seduction of belief as we move toward knowledge. We are not all at the same place at the same time.

The particular can be evidence for what is reasonable to believe based on evidence and not chance. The situation or particular fits a pattern of knowledge, coherent to what is already known, and guides the type of evidence that is accepted. Perception is empirical, in that it is our personal experience. How we think and reason is rational, but it is a rationality bounded by our perception and the limits of cognition (Simon 1957). The authority of the information we accept is subjective, since it is judged by each of us individually.

Disbelief during a crisis, the unexpected, or a surprise has importance. Those who, during an event, adhere to beliefs that are grounded in their (limited) knowledge will then resist revising their beliefs during a novel event. Disbelief helps avoid aversion to engagement; otherwise we risk falling back on aversive behaviors.

Because tacit knowledge is subjective and context specific, it is also phronesis knowledge, or practical wisdom. Phronesis is problem-solving and action. In Rasmussen's (1983) SRK framework, the routine and predictable are not particular. It is the particular that requires knowledge and thinking. This is practical wisdom, or prudence. The known and expected are more like episteme, while the skill-based is techne. Phronesis goes beyond the cognitive aspect of problem-solving. People use character values and place value on information within its context; this is tacit knowledge.

Why Phronesis Matters

Practical wisdom relies on dynamic interaction between perception, experience, and character. It offers an insightful vision of what is proximately and ultimately good for people, organizations, and business. Practical wisdom illuminates the thinking and actions of senior managers for novices. Among the most challenging things managers face are not questions of accumulating facts but questions of judgment. Business is essentially a human activity in which judgments are made with messy, incomplete, and incoherent data. As Warren Bennis and James O'Toole have written, "statistical and methodological wizardry blinds rather than illuminates" (2005, 98).

True executive abilities are matters of "feeling, judgment, sense, proportion, balance, appropriateness" (Barnard 1938, 235). To emphasize the need for synthesis and judgment, and for having a sense of proportion and appropriateness, is to emphasize the need for earlier and more widespread development of practical wisdom in managers. The concept of "a creative response" refers to "the ability to perceive new opportunities that cannot be proved at the moment at which action has to be taken, and on the other hand, will prove adequate to break down the resistance that the social environment offers to change" (Schumpeter 1947, cited by Duggan 2003, 46). To be disposed in one's character to creatively respond to the unexpected, and to willfully press forward to make the most of opportunity, is therefore part of what it means to be wise in a management sense.

Knowledge-creating companies (Halverson 2004) have the ability to make a judgment on "goodness," which refers to

- the ability to share contexts with others in order to create the shared space of knowledge;
- the ability to grasp the essence of particular situations/things;
- the ability to reconstruct the particulars into universals and vice versa using language/concepts/narratives;
- the ability to use any necessary political means well to realize concepts for the common good;
- the ability to foster phronesis in others to build a resilient organization.

This model highlights three features of practical wisdom: (1) the way in which wisdom is developed over time through reflective attention to the meaning of experiences; (2) the way in which wisdom requires cognitive schemas but also and essentially involves character and vision; (3) the way in which wisdom results from its enabling elements operating as a whole and in concert rather than individually or sequentially.

Phronesis as Leadership

Management is often viewed as "a way of life" rather than a tool to make money. In individuals, it is influenced from their leaders by modeling. Leaders stimulate people to act on their own in an interface with their environment. Leadership in a knowledge-creating company is not a matter of fixed administrative control. With flexible, distributed leadership, leading is determined by context and accepts deference to expertise, local knowledge, and context. Practical wisdom is the capacity to choose appropriate goals and successfully devise means to reach them (Halverson 2004).

Leaders use a sense of the details to "see" or "feel" the problems of their organizations *as being solvable within local constraints.* They develop successful plans to address identified problems in decision-making. Leaders make a synthesis of contextual knowledge from experience with universal knowledge from training. The tenets of educational theory (Halverson 2004) help leaders in organizations with collective phronesis create organizational structures. The structure then shapes the problems they identify and the solutions they offer. The organization develops shared practice and detects and processes problems toward a solution.

HRO Leadership

The authors suggest that a basic social process occurs within dangerous contexts they have termed "organizing ambiguity." From this process we may identify *framing, heedful interrelating,* and *adjusting,* described below. After analyzing firefighter near-miss records, Baran and Scott (2010) identified eight leadership categories: situational awareness, direction setting, communication, knowledge, role acting, agility, role modeling, and trust. They also identified several higher-order categories.

Framing involves effectively gauging the level of risk present in the environment. Firefighting teams place the ambiguity of their situations into an initial context, or frame, which is a means to focus their attention so that they can enact what is important and what is not important about an event. Leaders must draw on lessons learned from prior equivocal experiences—past successes and failures—to contextualize the type of situation they have encountered. Not only do they use their collective experience for framing, but framing is also influenced by organizational structures such as policies, procedures, and formal reporting relationships.

Heedful interrelating describes how a group comes to a joint conclusion about what is plausible in the environment, which is an interactive process of collective sensemaking. They are actively trying to understand the situation with the serious realization that each change in evaluation also changes the rules. They always question assumptions, including the communications they receive. They do not want to assume that they have heard a communication correctly. "Freelancing" hinders heedful interrelating by being heedless of the situation, which brings a serious risk of harm to others.

Adjusting describes having a flexible posture toward change that firefighters continually maintain. They not only maintain awareness of their surroundings but also continually revise their conclusions, which is a form of collective mindfulness.

Elements of Leadership

While various models of leadership have been put forth, there is not a specific model of HRO leadership. The following material comes from experience or from what we have learned from discussions with known leaders of High Reliability organizations.

- Resist efforts to categorize the leadership traits we have described.
  - It is important to create categories for definitions, descriptions, measurement, and research.
  - We lose knowledge and information when we categorize.

- Recognize the constraints and benefits of Bertrand Russell's concept of knowledge by description versus knowledge by acquaintance.
  - In knowledge by description, observers who are not engaged in leadership may miss the subtle and nuanced part of communication and will not recognize the rapid feedback that occurs in leadership.
  - In knowledge by acquaintance, leaders may function at such a high level of tacit knowledge that they neither recognize nor can describe their thoughts, actions, and purposes.

This lack of specific models makes it difficult for the leadership literature to be accurate in its descriptions or to be prescriptive for the purposes of teaching and learning. Another important point is to use "information flow," rather than communication:

Information is objective; communication is subjective and a behavior. Descriptions must be objective, articulate, and succinct.

- *Objective* descriptions are the most difficult, as people do not realize when they insert opinion, interpretation, or persuasion.

(One of the authors (Daved van Stralen) learned from family conferences about withdrawal support for children in the pediatric ICU that one cannot be totally objective, as the first words that are said always have the greatest influence. The choice of those words is subjective.)

- *Articulate* means that the words must come together in some form of structure that makes sense.

    A US marshal described to the authors how he teaches the importance of articulate description by telling his students that, once they have articulated the problem, they have identified half the solution. For example, he said that a white male found in an expensive car in Watts at two in the morning is probably lost, looking for drugs, or looking for prostitutes. This gives you probable cause to pull the man over.

- *Succinct*, from a Roman gladiator's method of girding for combat, means enough without being too much.

Pragmatic, Operant Leadership

To a great extent, leadership for an HRO is pragmatic; it must get the job done.

- It is adaptive and resists simple solutions and binary decisions.
- As a cultural entity, HROs are a social response to dynamic, unstable environments.
- An HRO leader can create a culture of High Reliability by (1) reframing the environment, (2) changing people's perceptions of the environment, and (3) reorganizing the problems to be solved.

Because the HRO is closely connected to the environment, it can almost be described as operant leadership. The environment operates *on* the leader, while the leader *changes* the environment. The leader adapts to the environment while at the same time changing the environment; this is a form of operant learning in real time.

Developmental Leadership

We can observe principles of leadership in the natural setting of child development and parental interactions. As we find in HRO, the parent prepares the child for life in an adverse environment, titrating reality as the child's neurological development occurs. We can identify four stages in this process: create a relationship, provide nurturing, assist in transformation, and develop direction.

Relationship. The social smile develops about two weeks into life; this is the smile adults respond to by smiling back, thus creating a *relationship* with the infant. One sign of neurologic injury is failure to develop a social smile, and those adults with a poor response can have difficulties bonding with the infant. Recall what is it like when your subordinate does not, or cannot, smile. When you have a relationship with your subordinates, you can read them and know better what to do during stressful performances.

Nurture. Your mother is effectively your first leader. She *nurtures* you physically during breastfeeding, which releases oxytocin, the trust or social hormone, in both mother and infant. Oxytocin makes you feel good, contributes to social memory, and causes you to trust others. Oxytocin is also released through touch, such as in hugging or hand-holding. We can nurture employees for their personal growth and development but also, in a crisis, we must know when they need a break or support.

Transformation. While admittedly sexist, your father, bearer of testosterone, introduces you to the world, including its hazards and pain, which involves decision-making in new situations. The child is *transformed* into an adult and, ideally, becomes a better person for it.

Direction. The last part of an adolescent's brain to develop is the prefrontal cortex, where the executive functions reside. This process starts at about seventeen years of age and is complete by about twenty-five (in some people, it may never become fully complete). In the prefrontal cortex, you gain control of emotions; think of the future; begin to make adaptive, rather than binary, decisions; and, most critically, you develop *direction*. Until this stage of development, your parents provide your direction for you.

As elements of leadership, *develop* a relationship with your subordinates to the level you can read them and their mood individually and collectively. *Nurture* them when they are overextended, and get them the resources they need to do their jobs. *Transform* your subordinates: challenge them, make them better, and increase their personal attributes. Help them identify resources and attributes that will then exceed demands and expectations of the problem or situation. Give your subordinates *direction* so they know where *you* are headed, and guide them in developing their own direction. If they cannot reach their objectives, then you decompose their objectives for them.

Conclusions

(1). Indirect leadership is effective and occurs by the changing of social knowledge through stories and narrative that the leader "owns."

(2). Motivational leadership, modified here from motivational interviewing in healthcare, identifies discrepancies to develop "drivers for change" and to support the creation of self-efficacy.

(3). People are less likely to be resistant to change or in denial than to be ambivalent; that is, they feel pressure to change but are also frustrated for not changing.

(4). Practical wisdom (phronesis or prudence), Aristotle's first cardinal virtue, adjusts knowledge to the peculiarity of local circumstances; it creates judgment by those who use situational values applied to the particular in specific contexts.

(5). HRO leadership is a social process that supports framing the situation and heedful interrelating toward collective sensemaking.

(6). Elements of leadership include building a relationship with subordinates, nurturing their growth, transforming their performance, and providing direction.

CHAPTER 14

CULTURE

> "Culture is the acquired knowledge people use to
> interpret experience and generate behavior."
> —JAMES P. SPRADLEY, ANTHROPOLOGIST (1984)

Culture gives meaning about the world and guidance for accepted behaviors and beliefs within a defined group. The immediate environment in which the group operates and the technology it uses will heavily influence an organization's culture. This helps explain the actions and beliefs of the members of an organization.

Culture as Function

An extreme event creates its own environment, much like a large wildland fire creates its own environment. Continuing culture across the liminal threshold into the VUCA-T environment (volatile, uncertain, complex, ambiguous, and threatening; see "The Environment" in chapter 2, "What Problem Does HRO Solve?") risks the transgression of limits across that threshold. We lose our cosmology to this new reality and experience the limits of our logic, rationality, cognition, strategic intent, and "followership." More than having sensitivity to operations, we pass the limits of strategic intent and strategic leadership. The result is deadly. This is the problem of the wrong culture or a misguided interpretation of the culture of HRO (Tempest et al. 2007).

Culture gives guidance and meaning to sensemaking and for leadership. Weick (1993) described the collapse of sensemaking, role structures, and leadership during the 1949 Mann Gulch Fire and how these elements contributed to disorganized action. Such abrupt breaches in the environment involve the entire group or organization. The loss of internal logic in the environment, what Weick calls "cosmology episodes," does not necessarily lead to disaster. Cultures exist that give frame and reference. HRO describes one such culture.

> During the Mann Gulch Fire in Montana a "blow up" caused the deaths of 13 smokejumpers. One firefighter lit an "escape fire" in which he entered the burnt area for protection from the blow up. A blow up describes a sudden acceleration in spread or intensity fire that prevents direct control and is often accompanied by violent air convection currents. It has characteristics of a fire storm. The Mann Gulch Fire deaths changed the culture of US wildland firefighting and directly led to changes in training and safety for wildland firefighting. It also became the story Weick (1993) used the fire to describe how sudden loss of orientation and structure can collapse sensemaking. Don Berwick (1999 and 2010) presented the escape fire used in the Mann Gulch Fire as a metaphor to bring safety to healthcare and support culture change.

Dramatic as a large fire is, the loss of cosmology can appear more slowly to challenge people, isolating them from those who do not recognize the change or from veterans who do not experience it in the same way. In addition to threat from the environment is the threat to cognitive functions and the ability to control behavior. This challenge can overwhelm some members of the organization, and the effects then can spread to others, creating a parallel loss of sensemaking and additional challenges to leadership. The filtering of perceptions and low-key leadership during an event with increasing tempo, combined with severe negative emotions, damages team coordination in such situations. This situation contributed to the crash of an Air France jet, flying from Rio de Janeiro to Paris, into the Atlantic Ocean (Berthod and Müller-Seitz 2017).

The belief that we can change the culture as needed—for example, that at the threshold of lost cosmology we "become High Reliability"—is a mistake. As the plane crash into the Atlantic Ocean demonstrates, catastrophes can develop from apparently routine operations as the environment changes and as different people respond differently to similar signs and signals. An embodied HRO culture adapts to crises evolving from the mundane and prepares for the sudden collapse of sensemaking. In this chapter we will define and describe culture as various sociological and anthropological constructs before we discuss the culture that enables operations in the VUCA-T environment. For these reasons, we must view HRO as an organizational culture adapted for the VUCA-T environment. From such a view, we can study how HRO as a culture can help us operate in the VUCA-T environment (a liminal environment) and understand the nature of the human-environment and human-human interactions that create this culture.

"The Extensions of Men"

Edward T. Hall said that we evolve by biology (genetics) but can evolve much faster by our "extensions." He described technology and culture as "extensions of man" that improve or specialize various functions. Language is another extension; it "extends experience in time and space while writing extends language" (1966, 3).

As Hall wrote in *The Silent Language*,

> Today man has developed extensions for practically everything he used to do with his body. The evolution of weapons begins with the teeth and the fist and ends with the atom bomb. Clothes and houses are extensions for man's biological temperature-control mechanisms. Furniture takes the place of squatting and sitting on the ground. Power tools, glasses, TV, telephones, and books which carry the voice across both time and space are examples of material extensions. Money is a way of extending and storing labor. Our transformation networks now do what we used to do with our feet and backs. In fact, all man-made material things can be treated as extensions of what man once did with his body or some specialized part of his body. (1959, 55.)

Culture, in Hall's view, is one of many types of extension humanity has created. Weapons, clothing, shelter, and so on have all extended us into otherwise adverse and hostile environments. Marshall McLuhan, who focused on the media extension of this idea and was in frequent correspondence with Hall, feared that these extensions would innervate or numb us emotionally. In 1964 McLuhan wrote in *Understanding Media: The Extensions of Man*, "Examination of the origin and development of the individual extensions of man should be preceded by a look at some general aspects of the media, or extensions of man, beginning with the never-explained numbness that each extension brings about in the individual and society" (1994, 6).

In less rigorous discussions we have used culture for broader, less technical, purposes. We start a program and the organization's culture changes, thus giving support for calling the program a success. Anthropologists and sociologists have a stricter definition ("description" may be a better term) and have produced several models that can inform our discussion of HRO as a social system. Culture has specified elements, generally accepted to be behaviors, beliefs (including attitudes, values, and a spiritual component), and some artifact or structure of significance. Cultures function within and in response to specific environments. We will describe HRO with the elements of culture and will then place "HRO culture" in the context of culture as social knowledge (J. Spradley), as social and technological response to the environment (Steward), and as contextual knowledge (Hall). We conclude with the development of safety culture out of the development of nuclear weapons and nuclear propulsion and a description of HRO as a culture.

Culture as the Extension of Man (Humanity)

McLuhan, agreeing that technology is an extension of man, had a different twist to language. Language as the *form* of communication (the medium), rather than the message itself, is the extension of man and should be the target of academic study. The technology of the message influences the way we think.

Both men, frequent correspondents, agreed that the patterns and structures we use to make sense and understand the world enable us to assess problems more realistically and accurately. McLuhan believed that the perception of reality depends on the structure of information, and he searched for those ground rules. Hall described how we are not aware of the rules in our culture—the rules that guide perception and behavior. He sought to unveil the "hidden dimensions" of these rules. These dimensions structure our experience and are molded by deep, common, unstated experiences shared within a culture (Song 2005; Hall 1966).

The rules of language and communication in a culture, particularly an HRO culture, are hidden both to outsiders and to the members of the HRO. Language, communication, and the means of communication create, and are created by, culture. Hall observed that these dimensions are hidden to participants. Observers search for these rules in HROs, seeking to make visible the invisible, yet these rules are most visible only when they are most useful—in the midst of an emergency. Any observations made at that moment would be confused in the mind of the observer by the observer's own efforts to keep safe. We must be wary of attractive but contrived good rules made by distant observers.

Culture adapts to the environment. Culture can adapt to adverse or hostile environments to produce High Reliability and the HRO. The study of the High Reliability organization as a culture, using the tools of anthropology and the observer as participant, is difficult to do because the rules that are vital for adaptability may be an accessory and appear unnecessary in a stable environment, only becoming critical in the VUCA-T environment. Well-designed studies in an HRO, though, can make these invisible rules visible.

Elements of Culture

What drive and strategies for survival led humans to occupy, as a single species, almost every environment on earth, many of them hostile to human beings? How was this accomplished? What did it take? Rather than taking on the definition of culture, a nebulous target, we will describe what are commonly accepted as descriptions of culture in this section. The following sections will discuss a few relevant theories of culture: culture as social knowledge, cultural ecology, and high-context cultures.

A culture is a way of life of a group of people. It consists of social knowledge, beliefs, behaviors, norms, symbols, and rituals, which are passed along to each generation by communication, modeling, and imitation. A culture occurs in an environment and makes use of a specific technology the culture is organized around; behaviors occur in response to the environment and for the use of the technology. Beliefs develop when behaviors are repeated. Over time, behaviors and beliefs extend to normative qualities, attitudes, and values. The descriptive elements of culture include:

- the environment
- behaviors
- beliefs
  - attitudes
  - values
- artifacts
  - technology
  - policies

The *environment*, and the human response to the environment, influences the culture but not in a deterministic manner. That is, different cultures can develop within an identical environment. High Reliability is concerned with VUCA-T environments (volatile, uncertain, complex, ambiguous, and threatening) with a fundamental problem set of uncertainty, time compression, and threat. The fact that threat comes in many forms does not mean that the core elements and principles of HRO change. Only the manifestation of High Reliability changes, while the core principles remain the same.

The *behaviors and norms* of a culture are directed toward engagement and collaboration. Members understand that they can watch the safety of three or four other people better than they can watch their own safety. For this reason, they can focus on the problem, observe their colleagues, and not worry about their own safety. Members respond positively to criticism. This behavior allows for entry into a hostile environment.

Ritual plays a key part in socialization and the embodiment of important beliefs and concepts. Ritual induces an emotional component that increases motivation, embodiment, and a sense of membership. Ritual also acts as a rule to ensure thoroughness. For example, a novice may be instructed to follow a procedure in detail; if the novice follows the procedure as a ritual, then the novice can perform more complex processes with less need for detailed education.

Beliefs, attitudes, and *values* embody a culture, characterizing the culture and making it unique. Each problem an HRO encounters is the same, only different. There is no standard or general situation for which an HRO can reliably plan with sufficient detail. Attitudes, therefore, become important initiators of behavior. Attitudes do not predict behavior to the same level as a belief or value, but they do influence behavior. The military and public-safety services internalize specific attitudes necessary for performance in adverse or hostile environments. The civilian sector has a more difficult time with this internalization, because initial training is less controlled, and changing attitudes would appear as brainwashing (though it is not).

Repeating specific behaviors creates beliefs and attitudes, both of which are important during initiation into the culture. Positive feedback (reinforcement) encourages behavioral change and thus leads to change in belief systems. In a closed social system, such as the military or public safety, negative punishment is sometimes used. In this approach, a recruit receives some form of acceptable punishment, such as strict demands for detailed skill performance, with the demands (the negative aspect) reduced or removed as the desired behaviors appear and become stable.

A value is an arbitrary conception of what is *desirable* in human experience. During socialization, all children are exposed to a constant barrage of evaluations—the arbitrary "rating system" of their culture. Nearly everything they learn is labeled in terms of its desirability. The value attached to each bit of information may result from the pain of a hot stove, the look of disapproval from a parent, the smile of appreciation from a teacher, or some specific verbal instruction. When parents tell a child, "You should go to college and get a good education," they are expressing a value.

Socialization may be ineffective for some people, but for the vast majority of people in any society, conformity results from the internalization of values. As we learn through imitation, identification, and instruction, we internalize values. As an embodiment of culture, values provide security and contribute to a sense of personal and social identity. For this reason, people in every society cling tenaciously to the values they have acquired and feel threatened when confronted with others who live according to different conceptions of what is desirable.

US Marine Corps Recruit Training, Part 1: Cultural Initiation

Perhaps those who say changing culture is hard, if not impossible, do not know how to change culture or they are not willing to change themselves to change culture. The US Marine Corps must indoctrinate recruits into the Corps. Primary methods for culture change were creation of internal locus of control, control of emotions, and task performance.

As discussed earlier in this book, in a study of US Marine Corps recruit attrition, Raymond Novaco and his group found the major determinant of attrition to be organizational factors and social environment (Novaco et al. 1979), with the social environment of the training units to be a key determinant (Sarason et al. 1981a). Their evidence suggested that drill instructors' beliefs, expectations, and attitudes all play significant roles in influencing rates of attrition (Sarason et al. 1981). Addressing these areas contributed to a change in culture.

The development of the recruits' capabilities for effective performance under stress conditions lowered the attrition rate at no cost to the quality of performance. The drill instructor played a significant part in this dynamic (Novaco et al. 1979). Low-attrition drill instructors encouraged the belief that successful outcomes result from skill and effort, while high-attrition drill instructors were more likely to shape the belief that powerful others, luck, fate, or chance controlled outcomes. Drill instructors could change the recruits' perception of their responsibility for their own behavior, which represents a change in their "locus of control" (Sarason and Novaco 1982). The locus of control became more internal in the lower-attrition units, while it became more external in high-attrition units.

Drill instructors with low-attrition units used reward contingencies favorable toward the internalization of locus of control, thus developing among recruits a belief that success will result from their own efforts. The internalization of locus was true even for those recruits who'd originally had an external locus of control. High-attrition drill instructors induced an expectation among recruits that rewards are controlled by forces outside of one's control (Cook et al. 1980). This finding was true even for those recruits who'd had negative or failed experiences in life, such as failure, rejection, and emotional disruption.

Sarason and Novaco (1982) found that "recruits who have had negative or failure experiences in life can develop a belief that success results from their own efforts if they are trained in units whose reward contingencies are favorable to the formation of internal locus of control expectancies." These recruits tended to initially have an external locus of control. After placement in low-attrition platoons, they became more internally oriented.

The authors developed televised material for initial training to emphasize two key themes: (1) self-control of emotions and (2) the importance of task-performance effectiveness (Sarason and Novaco 1982). Abnormal or undesired feelings such as fear, anger, disappointment, and worry are normal. The authors intertwined the "regulation of emotion" theme with the "task performance" theme. For a demanding training task, the recruit must learn to control self-defeating emotional states and preoccupying thoughts that may engender those emotions. They must learn to "process information efficiently, exercise good judgment, attend to detail under duress, learn from mistakes, and develop the skill of teamwork." Viewing the thirty-minute film increased the recruits' self-efficacy across training tasks. They expressed more self-confidence in their ability to endure stress, control emotions, and live up to a drill instructor's expectations.

US Marine Corps Recruit Training, Part 2: Drill Instructor Characteristics

Drill instructors are the ones who bring recruits into the culture of the Marine Corps. The instructors' beliefs, expectations, and attitudes strongly influence rates of recruit attrition (Sarason et al. 1981). Low-attrition drill instructors believed that their attitudes influenced platoon attrition rates. The drill instructor sets the tone of the training situation and significantly influences the recruits' appraisals and expectations (Sarason and Novaco 1982).

Several traits identified successful drill instructor candidates (Sarason and Novaco 1982): more job involved, more competitive, and higher in internal control expectations, while also being significantly less impatient, lower in proneness to anger, and lower in physiological arousal. They have greater empathy for recruits.

Other Characterizations of Culture

We use two methods to characterize culture to help understand HRO as a culture. First, a cultural framework (Hofstede 1980) characterizes cultural value systems in "universal" patterns that include individualism and collectivism as values.

Second, we use Trompenaars and Hampden-Turner's (1997) seven dimensions to characterize people in a culture. The authors found that each culture has its own way of thinking, its own values and beliefs, and different preferences, all of which are placed along the seven dimensions. Culture may be the single-most important determinate of whether an organization becomes an HRO or not. Culture frames every aspect of an organization's actions, and an HRO "raises the bar" for everyone in the group. A good culture is as important to an HRO as oxygen is to a human being.

Cultural Framework

As noted above, a cultural framework (Hofstede 1980) characterizes cultural value systems in universal patterns, as described below.

Power distance (PD or PDI). This refers to the extent to which less powerful members expect and accept unequal power distribution. High-PD cultures usually have centralized, top-down control, while low power distance implies greater equality and empowerment.

Self: individualism vs. collectivism. In an individual environment, individuals and their rights are more important than those of the groups they may belong to. In a collective environment, people are born into strong extended families or tribal communities, and these loyalties are paramount.

Gender: masculinity versus femininity. This aspect focuses on the degree to which traditional gender roles are assigned in a culture. For example, men might be considered aggressive and competitive, while women would be expected to be gentler and concerned with home and family.

Predictability: uncertainty avoidance. This element defines the extent to which a culture values predictability. Avoidant cultures have strong traditions and rituals and tend toward formal, bureaucratic structures and rules.

Time: long-term versus short-term. Time orientation is the cultural trait that focuses on the extent the group invests for the future, is persevering, and is patient in waiting for results.

The Seven Dimensions of Culture

As noted above, Trompenaars and Hampden-Turner (1997) defined seven dimensions to characterize people in a culture:

(1). Universalism vs. particularism: What is more important, rules or relationships?

(2). Individualism vs. collectivism (communitarianism): Do we function in a group or as individuals?

(3). Neutral vs. emotional: Do we display our emotions?

(4). Specific vs. diffuse: How separate do we keep our private and working lives?

(5). Achievement vs. ascription: Do we have to prove ourselves to receive status, or is status given to us?

(6). Sequential vs. synchronic: Do we do things one at a time or several things at once?

(7). Internal vs. external control: Do we control our environment, or are we controlled by it?

Culture as Social Knowledge

Knowledge acquired locally and shared with others enables people to live in hostile environments. The use of knowledge as facts, concepts, and beliefs supports adaptive behaviors. Using communication to share this knowledge through language, communication, and mutual rules increases safety and binds a group socially. Hall (1959) describes cultures through communication, and the degree context, or the environment, contains information. James Spradley (1984) describes cultures through acquired knowledge.

Communication style can differentiate cultures along a spectrum from high- to low-context cultures. In short, we can look at information in its context as well as the use of verbal or nonverbal elements in language and social rules (Hall 1959). In a high-context culture, information contains contextual elements, language has more nonverbal elements, and social interactions follow implicit rules. The style of communication for these high-context cultures relies on close relationships and knowledge internalized over time. In a low-context culture, nothing is taken for granted. Information is codified independently of context, with greater reliance on descriptions using words and rules. Such cultures have greater focus in language for direct, explicit verbal communications. Explicit rules for social interaction allow for a flexible, decentralized social structure. This style of communication for low-context cultures is independent of relationships and relies on well-defined constructs with explicit, open, and clear messages.

Rather than defining culture through social interactions or behavior, James P. Spradley (1984) placed the greatest importance on the culture's acquired knowledge: what people learn and share. He wanted to discover the *insider's view* of not only the acquired knowledge but of how people use this knowledge to interpret the world, generate social behavior, design their own actions, construct their own behavior, and interpret the behavior of others. As people learn their culture, they acquire new ways to interpret experience.

Culture as knowledge is learned and shared. Culture is also arbitrary and adaptive, both of which are traits that give culture flexibility to invent technologies or strategies when stressed or in the face of change. Diverse and distinct cultures worldwide have been created by cultures' ability to change within necessary timeframes as well as from the human mind's resourcefulness at acquiring new knowledge, building from traditional knowledge, and adapting to the knowledge of locality.

As Fabio Y. Lee Perez states in "Survival Tactics of Indigenous People" in reference to the December 2004 Indian Ocean tsunami:

> Another tsunami survivor is the Moken, the "sea gypsies" of the Andaman Sea. They survived the tsunami because they knew it was coming. The Mokens are nomads, who constantly move from island to island, living most of the year in boats. The Moken believe that ocean waves are created by the spirits of the sea, according to Saleh Kalathalay (a Moken man interviewed by CBS). In response to why the tsunami came, he said, "The big wave had not eaten anyone for a long time, and it wanted to taste them again." The Moken [have] a legend that is passed from generation to generation about the Laboon, the "wave that eats people." It is believed that the angry spirits of the ancestor brought the tsunami. The myth tells that, before the giant wave comes, the sea recedes. Then the waters flood the earth, destroy it, and make it clean again. On these islands the cicadas are usually loud, but suddenly went silent before the tsunami hit. Saleh Kalathalay noticed the silence and warned everyone about the tsunami. The Moken started to flee toward higher ground long before the first wave struck and were saved. (Fabio Y. Lee Perez 2005.)

According to Subir Bhaumik's 2005 *BBC News* article "Tsunami Folklore 'Saved Islanders'" on the same topic,

> Traditional knowledge handed down from generation to generation helped to save ancient tribes on India's Andaman and Nicobar Islands from the worst of the tsunami, anthropologists say. But other isolated communities who moved to the islands from South East Asia centuries ago fared far worse than the indigenous peoples, evidence suggests.
>
> The aboriginal tribes—some of the oldest and most isolated in the world—have oral traditions apparently developed from previous

earthquakes that may have allowed them to escape to higher ground before the massive tsunami struck the island chain off Indonesia.

The Onge tribe, for example, have lived on Little Andaman for between 30,000 and 50,000 years and, though they are on the verge of extinction, almost all of the 100 or so people left seem to have survived the 26 December quake and the devastating waves which followed. Their folklore talks of "huge shaking of ground followed by high wall of water," according to Manish Chandi, an environmental protection worker who has studied the tribes and spoke to some Onges after the disaster.

"When the earthquakes struck, the Onges moved to higher ground deep inside their forest and escaped the fury of the waves that entered the settlements," he told the BBC News website after talking to some of the inhabitants who knew some Hindi as well as their own ancient languages.

He said another aboriginal people—the Jarawa on South and Middle Andaman—also fled to higher ground before the waves.

"There's clear evidence that the aboriginals know about tsunamis and they know how to deal with them," he said.

But research on the more southern Nicobar part of the archipelago suggests that tribes who were not indigenous to the islands fared far less well.

Thousands of Nicobarese, who some say migrated from South East Asia 500 or 600 years ago, are dead or missing. Many of their islands suffered more in the huge waves—in some cases being washed off the horizon entirely.

And even those who survived face more dangers along with their aboriginal fellow island dwellers—partly because of the renewed interest in them from outside. (Bhaumik 2005.)

We can consider culture to be a social response to the environment that continues through generations or as a belief system that determines human nature. People are what they learn, and what they learn may be to survive in a harsh environment or to live socially with the least friction. The limiting factor on the abilities of human beings is survival in adverse environments on one hand and survival against onerous social pressures (a passive existence) on the other. Human nature, being what it is, does surmount adverse physical or social environments. HRO describes a culture that not only survives adverse physical or social environments but also changes, if not improves, those environments.

Social Knowledge

This kind of knowledge is not the same as *mutual knowledge* or *common knowledge*, as used in epistemic logic. Mutual knowledge is knowledge that all people have, but they are not aware if others also have the same knowledge, while common knowledge is shared, mutual knowledge in which everyone knows that everyone else also knows that knowledge. Common knowledge underwrites much in social life. Social knowledge, for our use, is that knowledge transmitted from elder to novice; it is dependent on what has been taught and is commonly known and shared among the cultural group. Novices willingly accommodate these learned behaviors and internalize beliefs toward their embodiment of cultural ideals. For HROs, this type of knowledge produces members who act appropriately when the stress of a crisis impairs their cognitive processes and disrupts rationality.

Language

Language also sets a culture apart, by using clichés as a form of abbreviated knowledge, using jargon from technical knowledge, or using slang for exclusivity. Language is representational and full of symbolic references. Language can refer to spoken word or tone, body language, or gestures but must be adaptable to adverse environments and malleable enough to describe something that one has never seen before. Language operates in environments where environmental "noise" corrupts communication; due to separation and distance, the language is also *caused* by communication. A structure in the language must support honest communication and must contain some form of redundancy for reliability. Message feedback for calibration reduces the effect of noise (Weick, personal communication).

Stories as Values and Social Knowledge

Anecdotes are stories that carry values and tacit social knowledge. Stories can be adapted to the individual and to the particular situation, thus giving multiple uses for a single story. (Unfortunately, despite the use of anecdotes in case reports, the healthcare field typically dismisses or depreciates the use of anecdotes.) Stories provide a bridge between the tacit and the explicit, which allows tacit social knowledge to be demonstrated and learned without the need to make formal presentations of ethics or specify in detail the proper behavior. Stories convey the speaker's moral attitude toward events in the collective social memory.

Stories as Myth

Mythology has several functions within culture. Joseph Campbell (1976) identified four functions in his book *The Masks of God: Creative Mythology*—the metaphysical, cosmological, sociological, and pedagogical functions.

The *metaphysical* function awakens a sense of awe before the mystery of being; the absolute mystery of life cannot be captured directly in words or images but requires symbols and metaphors. The *cosmological* function explains the shape of the universe; in this function, stories operate as a form of science by offering explanations for the physical phenomena that we encounter in an organization's environment. The *sociological* function validates and supports the existing social order. Members of an organization must conform to an existing social order; in an HRO, this conformity to the social order communicates important tacit information that is not available in the world outside the organization. Campbell often refers to these "conformity" myths as the "right-hand path" to reflect the brain's left hemisphere's abilities for logic, order, and linearity. Together with these myths, however, he observed the existence of the "left-hand path," which refers to mythic patterns such as the "hero's journey." These patterns are revolutionary in character, in that they demand from people a surpassing of social norms and sometimes even of morality. Finally, the *pedagogical* function guides people through the stages of life. During enculturation, we encounter many psychological challenges; stories may serve as a guide for our successful passage through these challenges.

Stories are the narrative for learning. Sometimes we say that we should tell a story, but during time-constrained events, we may want to describe a scene instead. As noted earlier, a German film director once described the differences between a story and a scene as the former having a beginning, middle, and end, while the latter takes us from A to B and contains only two story arcs. Rather than telling a story during an emergency, we can describe a scene using its two most salient story or incident arcs.

Stories are powerful for leadership and enculturation. Who controls the narrative is the one who leads.

> The greatest barrier to adopting HRO principles and practices is a cultural hierarchy where autonomy is the core value. Physicians, the very people we need desperately to champion a cultural change, frequently complain that the applicability of HRO principles to their practice is "cookbook medicine." Many physicians claim that tools such as checklists detract from their autonomy and lack a personal touch. Knowing what we know today about human error, these objections are not only dangerous but

absurd. Very simply put, if you had the opportunity to choose between an OR that could statistically ensure greater safety by using HRO principles and one that did not, which one would you choose? From an ethical perspective, healthcare demands that we "get it right" the first time. It is our moral obligation to significantly decrease the chance for human error.
　　—Spence Byrum

The meaning we bring to our stories is crucial, since these narratives develop and transmit social norms. People can assimilate their own loss into their own existing self-narrative, thereby contributing to their resilience. Experienced and veteran HRO operators tell stories *with* meaning to demonstrate a principle or truth (Calhoun and Tedeschi 2014).

Cultural Ecology

The field of cultural ecology analyzes the relationship between culture and environment. That is, how does the physical environment affect culture? Do people like fish because they live near the sea or because they like fish? Julian Steward (1955) believed that the physical environment determined culture and technology rather than biology determining behavior. Instead of undergoing deterministic, unilinear evolution, a culture could evolve along several lines through the interactions between people, technology, and the environment. Social organization is not a strict interaction with the environment but a type of ecological adaptation.

Steward recognized that the ecology of humans has distinct biological and cultural aspects. Cultural responses include technology and the organization of economic, political, and social systems. Compared to biology, culture is an extremely flexible and rapid adaptive mechanism. Behavioral responses can be developed and taught within the lifetime of an individual (Henry 1995).

Cultures categorize knowledge about the environment for the purposes of adapting to that environment. One culture may classify energy by how it is used, another by how it is produced, and another by the difficulty of containing or controlling it. As a cultural construction, the way in which the reality of that particular culture is biased by the culture's worldview. This experience depends on how that culture looks at reality. In some environments, stability may cause this reality to drift and appear arbitrary or idiosyncratic; in other environments that are either unstable or where the culture interacts closely with that environment, people constantly test their beliefs against reality to adapt behaviors or to correct beliefs as necessary and as experience demonstrates.

Social knowledge is associated with, if not intertwined with, technology. In his *Theory of Culture Change: The Methodology of Multilinear Evolution* (1955), Steward represented cultural ecology as the "ways in which culture change is induced by adaptation to the environment" (1955, 5). Human adaptation to the environment comes from social knowledge inherited from the past and the technologies and practices that allow people to live in that environment. Environment influences human adaptation but does not determine adaptation.

His approach was groundbreaking. Steward's (1955) primary arguments were that (1) cultures in similar environments may have similar adaptations; (2) all adaptations are short-lived and are constantly adjusting to changing environments; and (3) changes in culture can elaborate on an existing culture or can result in the creation of entirely new ones.

Steward was the first to combine four approaches to study the interaction between culture and environment: (1) an explanation of culture in terms of the environment where it existed, rather than just a geographic association with economy; (2) the relationship between culture and environment as a process, not just a correlation; (3) a consideration of small-scale environment, rather than culture-area-size regions; and (4) the connection of ecology and multilinear cultural evolution ("parallel and different" versus "unilinear" and less versus more evolved).

High- and Low-Context Culture

Edward T. Hall, an American anthropologist who worked for the US Army during World War II and for the US State Department afterward, studied cultural differences and the problems that developed with diplomats and the military due to ignorance of these differences. He identified two types of culture that he could describe by their means of communication and whether information was dependent on or independent of context: high-context versus low-context cultures, respectively.

Hall's 1976 book *Beyond Culture* first discussed high-context culture, in which communication is primarily through the use of contextual elements (i.e., body language, tone of voice, or someone's status). Information is not explicitly stated in such cultures, which is in direct contrast to low-context cultures, where information is communicated primarily through language, and the rules are explicitly spelled out. (No culture is completely high-context or low-context, since all societies contain at least some parts that are both high- and low-context.)

A military officer in the medical corps of the Royal Thai Air Force once invited me to a luncheon with his fellow officers. We sat down and were served what in the United States we would call a family-style meal, with the serving dishes placed in the middle of the table. There we no serving utensils, so I waited to see how the food would be served. Each guest at the table used his chopsticks to put food from the communal dishes on his plate, so I did the same.

My host leaned over and, in a soft voice, politely told me that it was impolite to use the end of the chopsticks that go in the mouth to serve oneself from the community dish. He must have seen the consternation in my face, since he took his chopsticks and slowly showed me how to flip them around in the same hand and to use one end for serving and one end for eating. I looked more closely and saw that each of the other guests was indeed using this flipping motion.

In a similar experience in the Nepal Himalaya, a poor Sherpa family invited a group of us for dinner at their home in Nepal. They did this because, after we had finished a climbing trek, our sirdar, our guide for the climb, had found this family and had suggested that we give the remainder of our food to them. They served us boiled potatoes to dip into a mixture of chili and star anise. As honored guests, we were to start eating first. We each took a small boiled potato, dipped it in the community sauce, and ate.

Our sirdar whispered in our ear that we were to peel the potato, as that part of the potato is unclean. Even though they were boiled, he said that they don't eat what comes in contact with the ground. We were to perform this act solely with the right hand. I am left-handed, which made this quite awkward.

—Daved van Stralen

Hall later proposed a cultural framework in which he stated that all cultures can be situated in relation to one another through the styles in which they communicate. People communicate through space, time, and context.

Defining High-Context Culture

Besides context, Hall found a difference in how different cultures consider time and space. Hall's first major publication relates to the three dimensions of time, space, and context. *Time* refers to how members of different cultures orient themselves toward time and the way in which they perceive time (monochronic versus polychronic). *Space* refers to differing cultural frameworks for defining and organizing space, with frameworks internalized in everyone at an unconscious level.

Context refers to the nature of how meaning is constructed differently across cultures using different ratios of context and information.

To Hall, high-context cultures: (1) primarily use nonverbal methods to relay meaningful information in conversations, such as with facial expressions, eye movement, and tone of voice; (2) the situation, people, and nonverbal elements are more important than the actual words that are communicated; (3) people are comfortable standing close to one another; and (4) the preferred way of solving problems and learning is in groups.

High-context cultures can be difficult to enter if you are an outsider, because you don't carry the context information internally and because you cannot instantly create close relationships. Low-context cultures, in contrast, are relatively easy to enter if you are an outsider, because the environment contains much of the information you need to participate, you *can* form relationships fairly quickly, and because what is important is accomplishing a task rather than feeling your way into a relationship.

Hall (2000, 37) argues that "the level of context determines everything about the nature of the communication and is the foundation on which all subsequent behavior rests." Information in context produces meaning. Context is a form of preprogramming within the receiver that allows people to avoid information overload, which increases their capacity to cope with higher amounts of complex information. High-context communication allows for the transmission of a coherent message with minimal information. In contrast, low-context transmissions are more explicit and require more information for a coherent message to be delivered. Context, information, and meaning are central terms to Hall's concept. There is no meaning without a combination of information and context.

Context, Information, and Meaning

Hall's conceptual idea of *context* can be understood with the classification of context by Harrington and Rogers (1988), who proposed context as conventionalized use or as a vantage point; that is, "a transparent vantage point around which individuals orient meaning" (p. 7). Defined as a vantage point, context describes preprogrammed cues for activation with information from the environment. This is in contrast to the culture-specific cues found in low-context cultures; to establish meaning in such cultures, the cues only require minor activation through information. The nature of context in this understanding is usually, but not exclusively, nonverbal implicit content.

In *information theory*, a message carries information, to the degree that it conveys something not already known by the receivers. According to Shannon and

Weaver (1949), information is a phenomenon that reduces uncertainty and fosters entropy. This definition does not define information in terms of Hall's concept, however. Hall refers to a higher degree of complexity of information than does the information theorist: "The information human beings are required to process, because they have evolved themselves, their cultures, their theories, their technologies, and their languages, is of a different sort of complexity than physical phenomena" (Hall 1992, 212). The nature of information in this understanding is usually (but not exclusively) verbal, providing explicit content.

Meaning is the result of the synthesis of context and information. Beyond information theory, according to Radford (1994), is the notion that meaning has a subjective aspect beyond the idea of information processing. As Hall remarks, "In a context model the same information together with altered context yields different meaning" (Hall 1973, 19). Consequently, meaning can be understood as the result of a cognitive combination of context and information (Kittler, Rygi, and Mackinnon 2011).

Time and Space

High- and low-context cultures appreciate *time* in a different manner. High-context cultures see time as polychronic, a system where several things can happen or be done at once, while low-context cultures see time as monochronic, more like a ribbon or road. Each system has its own logical operators, as we described in the section on temporal logic (see chapter 3, "The Logic of Practice and the Logic of Operations.").

A monochronic time system means that things are done one at a time, and time is segmented into precise, small units. Under this system, time is scheduled, arranged, and managed. Time is tangible and is viewed as a commodity to be scheduled, arranged, and managed. Monochronic time more closely represents time-dependence as a single vector, which is the system of time used in academic research. Time-dependence describes the evolutionary value of a variable or parameter, with the value differing along the time vector. Time-dependence can also refer to the timing of events, where something may happen or an action should be performed at a given time.

A polychronic time system takes a wider view of time, in which time is perceived in large, fluid sections, as in multitasking. Polychronic cultures are much less focused on the preciseness of accounting for each and every moment. Polychronic cultures are more focused on tradition and relationships than on tasks—a clear difference from their monochronic counterparts. In this sense, polychronic time has variable time density, or the number of instants or events that can occur in sequence. Polychronic time better describes what we mean by time compression.

Space is a form of communication. In Hall's 1992 book *An Anthropology of Everyday Life: An Autobiography*, the author recounts how, during World War II, he found that subordinates in the US Army were to stand three feet from their superior officers when talking to them. At this distance, it is normal to raise your voice to be heard, but raising your voice is also a means to communicate anger. As a result, the two people would be caught in a cycle of raising their voices and becoming angry, all because they were standing too far apart. Their anger increased because the voices were raised, and the voices were raised because of anger. Hall offered the solution of standing six inches closer, which solved the problem.

All animals have a distance from other animals at which they no longer feel safe. This holds true from reptiles to large mammals. For humans, the distance depends on the culture: high-context cultures stand closer together than low-context cultures, where people tend to keep a greater distance from one another. We contact people across a distance—or "orientation," as Hall describes it—that can be surprisingly specific.

Hall described four spaces or zones known as realms of *personal territory*: intimate, personal, social, and in public. The distances for each space are not only dependent on culture but also on individual factors and location, such as an open versus closed public space, an office workspace, or a home. *Intimate space* is a distance of about two feet, where only very close people can enter. In this case, you're probably less than a foot away and you might even be touching the other person. *Personal (friend) space*, from two to four feet, is reserved for talking to friends or family. *Social space*, from four to twelve feet, used during meetings or shopping, is the kind of space you're probably in if you're talking to a colleague or a customer at work. *Public space* is for collective contact with strange people; it characterizes how close we sit or stand to someone such as a public figure or public speaker. At an event such as listening to a professor give a lecture, you are probably about twelve to twenty-five feet away from the speaker.

Safety Culture: A Different Kind of Safety

"Safety culture" developed in the period after 1945 from US nuclear weapons research and the development of the nation's nuclear navy. Nuclear weapons research produced a different type of radiation injury from previous experience, in which lower radiation dosages caused damage over greater periods of time. Radiation injury in weapons research occurred in seconds, with health effects appearing over the next twenty-four hours. Out of concern of the effects of a reactor accident in an enclosed ship, Admiral Hyman G. Rickover (USN) enforced specific procedures to manage safety in nuclear power and the US nuclear-propulsion program.

Fissile Material

A *criticality accident* or *critical excursion* occurs when a mass of fissile material (the critical mass) accidently comes together in a way that is sufficient to sustain a fission chain reaction. A *fission* chain reaction is the radioactive decay of the nucleus into smaller parts; a *fusion* chain reaction is the combination of two or more atomic nuclei. In either case, the difference in mass from before the event to after is the amount of energy that is released. Controlled reactions occur in a nuclear reactor; uncontrolled, *explosive* criticality is used in a nuclear bomb. Uncontrolled criticality of a lesser amount of radioactive material is the typical case of the accidents that cause acute radiation syndrome, or ARS.

Radiation from gamma rays, x-rays, and beta particles (high-speed electrons or positrons) are ionizing because of their ability to dissipate energy in matter by causing the ionization of atoms. Ionizing radiation ejects an electron from the atom with such force that the atom remains ionized until it binds with an oppositely charged particle. The ability to produce ion pairs is responsible for the biological effects of the radiation and distinguishes this type of radiation from ultraviolet light or infrared light. Ultraviolet light does not have the necessary energy to ionize atoms, though it can cause chemical reactions. The lower energy of infrared light is only sufficient to cause heat by increasing the vibrational movements of atoms. The energy spectrum of radiation, then, is one of ionization (ionizing radiation), chemical reactivity (ultraviolet light), visibility (visible light), and thermal effects (infrared light).

Ionizing radiation required a different kind of safety. Normally we consider safety as protection from an identifiable direct threat, yet with ionizing radiation the energy is (1) invisible, (2) the damage is delayed, and (3) the disease is untreatable (supportive care is the only option). One can have a fatal, untreatable exposure to ionizing radiation *without knowing that the event happened*. In the early period of nuclear weapons work, it was not even known how much exposure could cause injury (Hempelmann et al. 1952).

Before the use of more dangerous fissile material, radiation injuries developed over time from the use of radium or overdosage of x-rays in clinical or industrial settings. Chronic radiation syndrome injuries include anemia, cataracts, bone fractures, and cancers after a latent period; more acute injures include skin burns. Following the recognition of the dangers of x-rays and radium, most chronic radiation injuries by the 1940s developed from medical treatments, diagnostic procedures, or technical work (Uhlmann 1942).

ARS injuries caused by the exposure of the whole body to penetrating radiation include acute degenerative changes in the bowel, the blood vessels, and the blood and blood-forming organs; the condition is characterized clinically by nausea, vomiting, diarrhea, prostration, hemorrhagic diathesis, and epilation (hair loss). Death, if it occurs, happens in days to weeks. The experience of the atomic bomb victims in Hiroshima and Nagasaki contributed little to knowledge of ARS, as trained medical examination and laboratory evaluation were significantly delayed. ARS death takes place in days to weeks (Warren and Bowers 1950).

The first experience researchers had with ACS came from Japan as well as a few laboratory accidents that occurred there and elsewhere. Working with nuclear material, researchers found that the injury from acute exposure of a high level produces a different injury pattern than chronic exposure of lower levels. The fundamental damage happens to the cell, with higher-metabolic cells, such as stomach-lining and hair cells, having a greater response. Because of the novelty and rarity of the injuries, scientists did not know how much radiation exposure would cause injury. Calculations had to be made from the type of material, distance of the victim from the material, exposure time, and the presence of any protective clothing or material. The calculation of radiation doses based on the fissile material and type of radiation created further uncertainties in the computation of radiation dose period of nuclear weapons work; it was not even known how much exposure could cause injury (Hempelmann et al. 1952).

By 1948, in recognition that radiation injuries were untreatable, the safety-management field began a focus on *prevention* (Morgan 1948). After several criticality accidents killed two people and injured eight at Los Alamos National Laboratory (Hempelmann et al. 1952) in New Mexico, the laboratory began to correlate physical and biological data. By 1954 California was using the concept of permissible dose to provide legal protection to workers. Safety management for nuclear power had begun.

Safety Culture in Nuclear Power

Admiral Hyman G. Rickover (USN) reduced nuclear power generation to a contained, small space. He realized that the navy could not have even the slightest incident, or the navy's nuclear propulsion system would end. Admiral Rickover established certain core values in naval reactors that remain very visible today: people, formality, and discipline; technical excellence and competence; and responsibility.

According to Rear Admiral Mercer, "Safety is the responsibility of everyone at every level in the organization. Safety is embedded across all organizations in the program, from equipment suppliers, contractors, laboratories, shipyards, training facilities, and the fleet to our headquarters. Put another way, safety is mainstreamed. It is not a responsibility unique to a segregated safety department that then attempts to impose its oversight on the rest of the organization. Admiral Rickover was told of each accident" when it occurred (personal communication). From this unique safety-management problem developed the idea of safety culture and the better definition of safety. Rickover did not call it a culture, but it became one.

A catastrophic failure of the Chernobyl nuclear power plant in 1986 led to the introduction of the term "safety culture." The term was first used in a report by the International Nuclear Safety Advisory Group (INSAG) called the "Summary Report on the Post-Accident Review Meeting on the Chernobyl Accident" (1988) as "that assembly of characteristics and attitudes in organizations and individuals which establishes that, as an overriding priority, nuclear plant safety issues receive the attention warranted by their significance." The phrase "safety culture" in the Chernobyl investigation filled the gap between technology and error. Though called culture and though culture elements were used, safety culture was never described fully as a culture in the anthropologic or social science sense (Carroll 2015).

Conference participants repeatedly called for a "nuclear safety culture" that would envelop all reactor operations. The INSAG 4 report (INSAG 1991) traced the then current safety culture to national laws related to nuclear safety. These laws had established the proper chain of responsibility in both operating and regulatory regimes. The report found that safety culture had been instilled through the attitudes and practices of management (note the recurrence of attitudes toward creating a culture).

Safety when in the presence of nuclear radiation strives for zero injuries. Keep in mind that "safety" as used in High Reliability organizations describes the efforts taken to enable entry into a dangerous, or VUCA-T environment, or to operate high-risk processes. Nuclear safety does meet these two safety goals of HROs but with the addition of *zero* consequential accidents.

Safety Culture in Healthcare and Public Health

Great Britain's Health and Safety Commission (HSC) developed one of the most commonly used definitions of safety culture (Health and Safety Commission 1993) : "The product of individual and group values, attitudes, perceptions, competencies, and patterns of behaviour that determine the commitment to, and the style and proficiency of, an organisation's health and safety management." A "culture of safety," according to the United States' Agency for Healthcare Research Quality (AHRQ), encompasses these key features:

(1). acknowledgment of the high-risk nature of an organization's activities and the determination to achieve consistently safe operations;

(2). a blame-free environment where people are able to report errors or near misses without fear of reprimand or punishment;

(3). encouragement of collaboration across ranks and disciplines to seek solutions to patient safety problems;

(4). organizational commitment of resources to address safety concerns.

Safety as a culture in healthcare must include providers' attitudes toward patients, not only attitudes to colleagues and to error. Showing neutrality toward all patients regardless of how they acquired a disease, providing dignity to all people, and identifying one's bias toward certain classes of people or diseases are all part of HRO and must become recognized for their part in safety culture.

Safety Culture and Prejudice

According to Faher E. Koteira of the American Board of Internal Medicine (in a personal comment to one of the authors), "I've noticed some residents draw back when they meet certain patients, for example those with HIV. They express a judgment about the patient and how he or she acquired the disease. I want them to see the patient as a person, as human, with a disease, and we treat the disease—not as someone who may have acquired the disease through his or her choice of action."

Two female residents tell me that they're admitting a drunk female adolescent. One adds, "She's in the emergency department and has been seen by the emergency physician, residents, and a social worker." Several questions come to my mind because of what may be a harrowing, dangerous situation: What is she drunk on? How old is she? Has this happened before? I know that some men get young girls drunk for sex, to carry drugs, or to hide contraband in their purses (they tell them the cops won't look in a girl's purse). If she's been drinking a mint-flavored drink, it may hide the smell of marijuana; if sweet, she may be a novice drinker; and if vodka, then she's been drinking for a while, or someone wants to hide the smell of alcohol.

I learn that she is fifteen years old, and it is indeed vodka. One resident immediately finds in the records that she had been admitted a year earlier, also drunk on vodka. I then ask for her Tanner stage (the level of physical sexual development) and breast size; my fear is that she is cognitively an early to middle adolescent with a mature woman's body. The residents could not answer this question. We examine the young woman, who is almost fully developed physically, with larger than average breast size (possibly juvenile macromastia).

The residents sit down with me, and I can only say one thing: "This young lady is likely being sexually abused and has been for over a year. Of all the patients we'll admit tonight, whether ICU or any other critical area, she's the one who's most likely to be dead in five years, acquire a lethal infection such as HIV or hepatitis B, or experience multiple unwanted pregnancies. And she was evaluated by multiple healthcare professionals, each one calling her a delinquent, drunk, adolescent girl. She's in the one place she should feel safe, yet we fix her up and send her back into her world. It must be hell for her." This situation does not meet the definition of safety culture or of a patient-safety problem. It does meet the criteria for High Reliability Organizing.

—Daved van Stralen

Safety culture developed in response to invisible energy causing untreatable, lethal injury that appeared days later. A similar pattern occurs in certain infectious diseases, particularly communicable diseases, as well as cardiovascular diseases and cancers. AHRQ's key features of a culture of safety readily apply to many public-health diseases: (1) acknowledgment of the high-risk nature of *human* activities and the determination to *promote safe behaviors*; (2) the existence of a blame-free environment where *patients* are able to report *exposures and symptoms* (errors) without fear of *prejudice or loss of dignity*; (3) the encouragement of collaboration across disciplines to seek solutions to *public-health problems*; and (4) community and government identification of resources to address *public-health concerns*.

My patients who have risk factors for stroke or cardiovascular disease may not change their lifestyle, undergo medical evaluation, or not follow through on treatment. Their disease develops over years, is unnoticed while it develops, then presents as a debilitating disease. This is much like acute radiation syndrome. The only difference is the timeframe.

—Dr. Faher E. Koteira, American Board of Internal Medicine

Conversely, the methods the public-health field uses can also improve safety culture. While a full development of this topic is beyond the scope of this book, we will present a brief description of the Haddon matrix for error. William Haddon argued that we can treat injuries in an ecosystem much like we treat arthropod-borne parasitic disease. Malaria is caused by *Plasamodium*, a species of protozoan that is carried to humans by an infected female *Anopheles* mosquito. Thus, a host (in this case a human) is infected by an agent (*Plasmodium*) carried to the human by a vector (the *Anopheles* mosquito). An infectious agent (*Plasmodium*) is involved. Knowing this epidemiology and the ecology of mosquitos allows for the use of public-health measures to reduce the spread of malaria.

Haddon applied this ecological model to injuries (Haddon 1970) using the same human-as-host concept. He described the "infectious" agent as energy and the vector as a carrier of that energy. A host (human) is injured by an agent (a form of energy) carried by a vector (automobile, chemical release, fire, and the like). With the addition of the phases pre-event, event, and post-event as distinct time elements (Haddon 1980), the science of epidemiology could now identify more effective interventions to prevent or reduce injuries. (See table 13.)

Phase	Human	Vehicle	Environment (Physical)	Environment (Social)
Pre-event				
Event				
Post-event				

Table 13—Haddon's ecological model

Novel situations or unexpected events place people in situations where the correctness of decisions and actions is not known until the response can be observed. This response could be inconsequential, but when consequential, the action becomes identified as a mistake or error (see chapter 10, "Sensemaking of Noise"). Actions are not mistakes; actions *become* mistaken (Paget 1988).

For the public-health model, error becomes the agent or pathogen, much as a protozoan is the pathogen for a vector-borne disease or energy for injuries. We can use public-health approaches (including epidemiology) to identify characteristics in the three phases of pre-event, event (or incident), and post-event (or recovery). We can also identify characteristics of the human host, such as knowledge and experience, personality, and ability to block fear responses and moderate threat responses. The vector or vehicle is broad but is generally covered by the three threats of uncontrolled energy, behavior, or physiology. The social environment is HRO.

When we consider error as an agent, we see that error must achieve a certain threshold of infectivity, the threshold of which is dependent on the virulence ("infectiousness") of the error and the vulnerability of the host (the organization or system). The host must be available for the infection—that is, enter an adverse or hostile (physical) environment and/or have unsafe behaviors or beliefs (social environment)—or a vector "brings" the agent to the organization, such as an unexpected event, discrepancy, or disruption in routine. The use of an error matrix, patterned after Haddon's energy-injury matrix, facilitates the use of local and regional ecology in error management and the utilization of epidemiologic techniques and public-health methodologies. Because of the widespread moral opprobrium to consequential errors, the use of a public-health philosophy for sexually transmitted diseases may prove fruitful. (The clinical term "sexually transmitted disease" was a shift from the more moralistic "venereal disease.")

We can see the influence of using an ecological approach in Rasmussen's ecological interface design, where Rasmussen and Vicente (1989) identified the workplace as an ecosystem that includes perceptions (i.e., from the interface) and behaviors (from skills, rules, and knowledge). They identified signs and signals as perceptions and a framework for performance, known as the skills, rules, knowledge (SRK) framework. James Reason (1990) then adapted this framework as a model of error management.

HRO Culture

HROs anticipate problems and contain them when they occur. Doing so involves the elements of culture: communication, social knowledge, behaviors, beliefs, attitudes, and values. We can see HRO culture through various interpretations, including Hall's communication and high-context culture, James Spradey's (1984) social knowledge, or Karl Weick's (1995) shared sensemaking.

A few traits HROs share are counterintuitive or commonly considered wrong.

- *HROs use anecdotal evidence*—because events are rare and their elements often overlap, HROs often use anecdotes for education; because of the high-context culture of an HRO, the meaning and significance of these anecdotes may be lost to outsiders.
- *Threat is to be engaged*—this engagement may take the form of sounding an alarm or entwining yourself into a situation.
- *The environment contains information*—HROs have many of the characteristics of high-context cultures.

The physical danger and limitations experienced in the enactment of highly reliable practices are equally as influential as the cognitive and linguistic components associated with collective mindfulness (R. T. Spradley 2012). HROs, as developed and described in this book, emerged from operations in which harm was immediate and deadly. This new form could also support not only routine operations but any situation where action must be taken but information is uncertain and ambiguous, not necessarily just because of a threat. Time compression drives the need to act immediately.

Having a defined set of attitudes (Weick and Sutcliffe's five principles) supports the behaviors, while having a defined set of values (van Stralen and Mercer's five values with Weick's modification) guides thinking and beliefs. The most critical factors are to exhibit the behavior for directly engaging threat, to collaborate with others at some point, and to have the ability to engage as solo actions. Doing so requires modulation of the fear response and the use of short-feedback decision-making to operate close to the edge of danger.

Shared HRO Culture

Gary Provansal (a deputy fire chief) and I once toured a petrochemical plant in Europe, where we studied the use of HRO. At lunch our host asked us, "What do you do?" Through the language barrier and his accent, I thought he had asked me what my hobbies were. I then proceeded to tell him how the principles of HRO had helped me during a trekking trip to a peak in the Himalayas with novice mountaineers. He was surprised and said, "You really 'do' HRO!" At that point, he described the problems he'd had with establishing safety in the plant and the lack of support he was getting from administration, management, and line workers. Nothing new there—we've all encountered these problems—but this opening about shared HRO culture led to more discussions. At the end of the conversation, I told him that Gary and I had more in common with him, through HRO, than he had with his countrymen, region, and fellow employees. HRO creates a culture that we share to a greater extent than we do our national cultures.

—Daved van Stralen

452

The goal of HRO culture is to create knowledge in real time through interaction with the environment, but doing so requires authority migration and information flow. That is, information must freely and aggressively flow, since we do not know who needs information or who has it. Authority must migrate, thus enabling those nearest the problem to make timely decisions. This is not to say that people should engage in random activity: people also must have the judgment to know if they are the right people to be making the decisions or if they must pass the information and authority to someone else. It is important to note that in certain situations, someone who is farther from the event will be in a better position to decide.

Summary: Change and Barriers to Change

Most individuals and organizations have been organizing reliably, or else they would not currently be operating. Within each organization are teams who perform better than others, but a more critical element is the team who engages High Reliability situations. This team may not be the most experienced, but they were the most experienced *at that time*; the more experienced teams were simply occupied. That High Reliability situation then provides learning for the organization and becomes a move toward greater reliability.

The discussion, then, should focus not on whether an organization is an HRO but whether it possesses any teams who are excellent at handling High Reliability situations. Such teams become nodes, and the HRO can then self-organize within the organization. In addition, the use of loop decision-making (such as Boyd's OODA loop); the recognition of a few, basic biases and heuristics; the implementation of complete support (without criticism) for those who make decisions and act; and the holding of realistic expectations are a few of the small number of changes that allow HROs to self-organize.

HRO principles seem to activate an unusual resistance. Some of this resistance may come from an early loss of lives; following such loss, the organization new to HRO values may compare itself as a young organization (when it was a novice to the process) to organizations that have functioned as HROs for decades. Such organizations may focus on their past failures.

The use of scientific processes, or the misconception of scientific processes, has often impeded the acceptance of HRO. The knowledge gained in well-controlled, safe environments can inform and improve HRO processes but cannot replace them. HRO processes are scientific; they are simply a broader science than experimental empiricism. HROs use experiential empiricism—the empiricism of perceived experience. Cognitive dissonance risks placing greater emphasis on strongly held beliefs over beliefs that come from experience and the reality of cascading failures. Situations in which someone says, "I can't believe my eyes" do happen, as when a subordinate describes a situation and the supervisor responds, "That can't happen."

We hope, with this book, that we have introduced you to the sciences that support High Reliability Operations. We hope you will engage High Reliability situations as the most qualified person available at that time. Thank you.

Conclusions

(1). Culture allows the extension of humans into austere, adverse, and even hazardous environments.

(2). Culture consists of behaviors, beliefs (including attitudes and values), and a type of artifact or technology.

(3). Culture is social knowledge, particularly knowledge that is acquired through continual interaction with the environment and shared socially through generations.

(4). In high-context cultures, information is dependent on context; the environment carries, or gives meaning to, information.

(5). Safety culture, developed within nuclear weapons research and US naval nuclear propulsion, reduces or prevents system failure.

(6). High Reliability culture supports the engagement of extreme events with information flow and authority migration.

For updates and additional information please visit www.hrobook.com.

REFERENCES

Aristotle. 2011. *Nicomachean Ethics* Trans. Bartlett, Robert C., Susan D. Collins. Chicago, Illinois: The University of Chicago Press.

Agarwal, Naresh K. 2012. "Making Sense of Sense-Making: Tracing the History and Development of Dervin's Sense-Making Methodology." *International Perspectives on the History of Information Science and Technology: Proceedings of the ASIS&T 2012 Pre-Conference on the History of ASIS&T and Information Science and Technology.* https://s3.amazonaws.com/academia.edu.documents/37347262/Agarwal-ASIST-History-preconf-2012-author-formatted-6Jan2013_1.pdf?AWSAccess KeyId=AKIAIWOWYYGZ2Y53UL3A&Expires=1507298811&Signature=Yyw CfzVPGogOEsqpohYe8rRQbyM%3D&response-content-disposition=inline %3B%20filename%3DMaking_sense_of_sense-making_tracing_the.pdf

Ahmadjian, Christina L., and James R. Lincoln. 2001. "Keiretsu, Governance, and Learning: Case Studies in Change from the Japanese Automotive Industry." *Organization Science* 12 (6): 683–701.

Anderson, Brett R., Adam J. Ciarleglio, David J. Cohen, Wyman W. Lai, Matthew Neidell, Matthew Hall, Sherry A. Glied, and Emile A. Bacha. 2016. "The Norwood Operation: Relative Effects of Surgeon and Institutional Volumes on Outcomes and Resource Utilization." *Cardiology in the Young* 26 (4): 683–92.

Anon, Report NTSB. 1979. "Aircraft Accident Report 79-7." *United Airlines flight* 173 McDonnel-Douglas DC-8-61 Portland, OR December 28, 1978. http://libraryonline.erau.edu/online-full-text/ntsb/aircraft-accident-reports/AAR79-07.pdf Accessed Nov 17, 2017.

Arnsten, Amy F. 2009. "Stress Signaling Pathways That Impair Prefrontal Cortex Structure and Function." *Nature Reviews Neuroscience* 10 (6): 410–22.

Ashforth, Blake E., and Ronald H. Humphrey. 1995. "Emotion in the Workplace: A Reappraisal." *Human Relations* 48 (2): 97–125.

Avolio, Bruce J., William L. Gardner, Fred O. Walumbwa, Fred Luthans, & Douglas R. May. 2004. Unlocking the mask: A look at the process by which authentic leaders impact follower attitudes and behaviors. *The leadership quarterly, 15*(6), 801-823.

Banaji, Mahzarin R., and Larisa Heiphetz. 2010. "Attitudes." In *Handbook of Social Psychology*, edited by S. T. Fiske, D. T. Gilbert, and G. Lindzey, 353–93. Hoboken, NJ: John Wiley.

Bandura, Albert. 1982. Self-efficacy mechanism in human agency. *American Psychologist, 37*(2), 122-147.

———. 1986. *Social Foundations of Thought and Action: A Social Cognitive Theory.* Englewood Cliffs, N.J.: Prentice-Hall.

———. 2009. "Cultivate self-efficacy for personal an organizational effectiveness." In *Handbook of Principles of Organization Behavior: Indispensable knowledge for evidence-based management.* edited by Edwin A. Locke, 179-200. New York, New York: John Wiley & Sons.

Banzett, Robert B., Sarah H., Pedersen, Richard M., Schwartzstein, and Robert W. Lansing. 2008. "The Affective Dimension of Laboratory Dyspnea: Air Hunger Is More Unpleasant Than Work/Effort." *American Journal of Respiratory and Critical Care Medicine* 177 (12): 1384–90.

Baran, Benjamin E., and Marisa Adelman. 2010. "Preparing for the Unthinkable: Leadership Development for Organizational Crises." *Industrial and Organizational Psychology* 3 (01): 45–7.

Baran, Benjamin E., and Cliff W. Scott. 2010. "Organizing Ambiguity: A Grounded Theory of Leadership and Sensemaking within Dangerous Contexts." *Military Psychology* 22 (S1): S42.

Barnard, A. 2016. "Why Good People Make and often Repeat Bad Decisions … and How to Reduce Avoidable Decision Mistakes." *TOCICO White Paper Series.*

Barnard, C. 1938. *The Functions of the Executive.* Cambridge, MA: Harvard University Press.

Barnett, James A. 2003. "A History of Research on Yeasts: The Fermentation Pathway." *Yeast* 20: 509–43.

Bartholomew, Kathleen. 2006. *Ending nurse-to-nurse hostility: Why nurses eat their young and each other.* Marblehead, MA: HC Pro, Inc.

Bartlett, Robert C., and Susan D. Collins. 2011. *Aristotle's* Nicomachean Ethics*: A New Translation.* Chicago: University of Chicago Press.

Barton, Michelle A., Kathleen M. Sutcliffe, Timothy J. Vogus, and Theodore DeWitt. 2015. "Performing under Uncertainty: Contextualized Engagement in Wildland Firefighting." *Journal of Contingencies and Crisis Management* 23 (2): 74–83.

Bass, Bernard M. 1985. *Leadership and Performance beyond Expectations.* New York, NY: Free Press; Collier Macmillan.

Bea, Robert. 2008. "Managing the Unpredictable." *Mechanical Engineering* 130 (3): 27–31.

Bengtsson, Bo, and Nils Hertting. 2014. "Generalization by mechanism: Thin rationality and ideal-type analysis in case study research." *Philosophy of the social sciences* 44 (6): 707-732.

Benner, Patricia. 1984. *From Novice to Expert: Excellence and Power in Clinical Nursing Practice.* Menlo Park, CA: Addison-Wesley.

Bennis, Warren G., and James O'Toole. 2005. "How Business Schools Lost Their Way." *Harvard Business Review* 83 (5): 96–104.

Berenholtz, Sean M., Peter J. Pronovost, Pamela A. Lipsett, Deborah Hobson, Karen Earsing, Jason E. Farley, Shelley Milanovich, Elizabeth Garrett-Mayer, Bradford D. Winters, Haya R. Rubin, Todd Dorman, and Trish M. Perl. 2004. "Eliminating Catheter-Related Bloodstream Infections in the Intensive Care Unit." *Critical Care Medicine* 32 (10): 2014–20.

Berkun, Mitchell M. 1964. "Performance Decrement under Psychological Stress." *Human Factors* 6: 21–30.

Berkun, Mitchell M., Hilton M. Bialek, Richard P. Kern, and Kan Yagi. 1962. "Experimental Studies of Psychological Stress in Man." *Psychological Monographs: General and Applied* 76 (15): 1-39.

Berthod, Olivier, and Gordon Müller-Seitz. 2017. "Making Sense in Pitch Darkness: An Exploration of the Sociomateriality of Sensemaking in Crises." *Journal of Management Inquiry.* published on line: https://doi.org/10.1177/1056492616686425.

Berwick, Donald Mark.1999. *Escape fire.* Boston, MA: Institute for Healthcare Improvement.

Berwick, Donald M. *Escape fire: designs for the future of health care.* John Wiley & Sons, 2010.

Bhaumik, Subir. 2005. "Tsunami Folklore 'Saved Islanders.'" *BBC News,* 20 January. http://news.bbc.co.uk/2/hi/south_asia/4181855.stm.

Bierly, Paul E., and J. C. Spender. 1995. "Culture and High Reliability Organizations: The Case of the Nuclear Submarine." *Journal of Management* 21 (4): 639–56.

Bigley, Gregory A., and Karlene H. Roberts. 2001. "The Incident Command System: High-Reliability Organizing for Complex and Volatile Task Environments." *Academy of Management Journal* 44 (6): 1281–99.

Bloom, Benjamin S., Max D. Engelhart, Edward J. Furst, Walker H. Hill, and David R. Krathwohl. 1956."Taxonomy of Educational Objectives: The Classification of Educational Goals. Handbook I: Cognitive Domain. New York: David McKay Company." *Inc. (7th Edition 1972).*

Boole, George. 1854. *An Investigation of the Laws of Thought: On Which Are Found the Mathematical Theories of Logic and Probabilities.* London, UK: Cambridge Macmillan and Co. .

Bolton, Patrick, and Mathias Dewatripont. 2013. "Authority in Organizations." In *Handbook of Organizational Economics*, edited by Robert Gibbons and John Roberts, 342–72. Princeton, NJ: Princeton University Press.

Bonanno, George A. 2004. "Loss, Trauma, and Human Resilience: Have We Underestimated the Human Capacity to Thrive After Extremely Aversive Events?" *American Psychologist* 59: 20–8.

Bonanno, George A., and Charles L. Burton. 2013. "Regulatory Flexibility: An Individual Differences Perspective on Coping and Emotion Regulation." *Perspectives on Psychological Science* 8 (6): 591–612.

Bonanno, George A., and Anthony D. Mancini. 2012. "Beyond Resilience and PTSD: Mapping the Heterogeneity of Responses to Potential Trauma." *Psychological Trauma: Theory, Research, Practice, and Policy* 4 (1): 74–83.

Bonanno, George A., Maren Westphal, and Anthony D. Mancini. 2011. "Resilience to Loss and Potential Trauma." *Annual Review of Clinical Psychology* 7: 511–35.

Boonstra, Rudy. 2013. "The Ecology of Stress: A Marriage of Disciplines." *Functional Ecology* 27 (1): 7–10.

Brehmer, Berndt. 1992. "Dynamic Decision Making: Human Control of Complex Systems." *Acta Psychologica* 81 (3): 211–41.

Brown, John Seely, and Paul Duguid. 1991. "Organizational Learning and Communities-of-Practice: Toward a Unified View of Working, Learning, and Innovation." *Organization Science* 2 (1): 40–57.

———. 2001. "Knowledge and Organization: A Social-Practice Perspective." *Organization Science* 12 (2): 198–213.

Burke, Brian L., Andy Martens, and Erik H. Faucher. 2010. "Two Decades of Terror Management Theory: A Meta-Analysis of Mortality Salience Research." *Personality and Social Psychology Review* 14: 155–195.

Burns, James M. 1978. *Leadership: Transformational Leadership, Transactional Leadership.* New York: Harper and Row.

Calhoun, Lawrence G., and Richard G. Tedeschi. 2014. The Foundation of Posttraumatic Growth: An Expanded Framework, In *Handbook of Posttraumatic Growth: Research and Practice,* edited by Lawrence G. Calhoun and Richard G. Tedeschi, 1-23. New York, NY: Routledge.

Campbell, Joseph. 1976. *The Masks of God: Occidental Mythology.* Vol. 3. New York, NY: Penguin.

Carroll, John S. 1995. "Incident Reviews in High-Hazard Industries: Sense Making and Learning under Ambiguity and Accountability." *Organization and Environment* 9 (2): 175–97.

———. 2015. "Making Sense of Ambiguity through Dialogue and Collaborative Action." *Journal of Contingencies and Crisis Management* 23 (2): 59–65.

Catino, Maurizio, and Gerardo Patriotta. 2013. "Learning from Errors: Cognition, Emotions and Safety Culture in the Italian Air Force." *Organization Studies* 34 (4): 437–67.

Chassin, Mark. and Jerod Loeb. The Joint Commission. 2013. "High Reliability Health Care: Getting There from Here." *Milbank Quarterly* 91 (3): 459–90.

Checchia, Paul A., Jamie McCollegan, Noha Daher, Nikoleta Kolovos, Fiona Levy, and Barry Markovitz. 2005. "The Effect of Surgical Case Volume on Outcome After the Norwood Procedure." *Journal of Thoracic and Cardiovascular Surgery* 129 (4): 754–9.

Cohen, Marvin S., Jared T. Freeman, and Steve Wolf. 1996. "Meta-Recognition in Time-Stressed Decision Making: Recognizing, Critiquing, and Correcting." *Human Factors* 38 (2): 206–19.

Cole, Dana. 2000. *The Incident Command System: A 25-Year Evaluation by California Practitioners.* Emmitsurg, MD: National Fire Academy.

Cook, Thomas M., Raymond W. Novaco, and Irwin G. Sarason. 1980. *Generalized Expectancies, Life Experiences, and Adaptation to Marine Corps Recruit Training* (no. AR-002). Arlington, Virginia: Office of Naval Research.

———. 1982. "Military Recruit Training as an Environmental Context Affecting Expectancies for Control of Reinforcement." *Cognitive Therapy and Research* 6 (4): 409–27.

Cooper, Joel M. 2007. *Cognitive Dissonance: 50 Years of a Classical Theory.* Thousand Oaks, CA: Sage.

Coram, Robert. 2002. *Boyd: The Fighter Pilot Who Changed the Art of War.* New York, New York: Little, Brown.

Cozolino, Louis. 2006. *The Neuroscience of Human Relationships: Attachment and the Developing Social Brain.* New York: W. W. Norton.

Cozzolino, Philip J. 2006. "Death Contemplation, Growth, and Defense: Converging Evidence of Dual-Existential Systems?" *Psychological Inquiry* 17 (4): 278–87.

Cozzolino, Philip J., Laura E. R. Blackie, and Lawrence S. Meyers. 2014. "Self-Related Consequences of Death Fear and Death Denial." *Death Studies* 38 (6): 418–22.

Cozzolino, Philip J., A. D. Staples, L. S. Meyers, and J. Samboceti. 2004. "Greed, Death, and Values: From Terror Management to Transcendence Management Theory." *Personality and Social Psychology Bulletin* 30 (3): 278–92.

Crano, William D., and Radmila Prislin. 2006. "Attitudes and Persuasion." *Annual Review of Psychology* 57: 345–74.

Cromwell, Howard Casey, and Jaak Panksepp. 2011. "Rethinking the cognitive revolution from a neural perspective: how overuse/misuse of the term 'cognition' and the neglect of affective controls in behavioral neuroscience could be delaying progress in understanding the BrainMind." *Neuroscience & Biobehavioral Reviews* 35 (9): 2026-2035.

Daft, Richard L., and Karl E. Weick. 1984. "Toward a Model of Organizations as Interpretation Systems." *Academy of Management Review* 9 (2): 284–95.

Damasio, Antonio R. 1994. *Descartes' Error: Emotion, Reason, and the Human Brain.* New York, NY; Penguin Putnam.

Darwin, Charles. 1857. Darwin Correspondence Project, "Letter no. 2130," accessed on 18 November 2017, http://www.darwinproject.ac.uk/DCP-LETT-2130

DeBono, Edward. 2010. *Lateral Thinking: A Textbook of Creativity.* New York, New York: Penguin.

DeChurch, Leslie A., and Jessica R. Mesmer-Magnus. 2010. "The Cognitive Underpinnings of Effective Teamwork: A Meta-Analysis." *Journal of Applied Psychology* 95 (1): 32–53.

Dekker, Sidney W. A. 2009. "Just Culture: Who Gets to Draw the Line?" *Cognition, Technology and Work* 11 (3): 177–85.

Deming, W. Edwards. 2000. *Out of Crisis*. Cambridge, Massachusetts; MIT Press.

Dervin, Brenda. 1983. "An Overview of Sense-Making Research: Concepts, Methods and Results." Paper presented at the annual meeting of the International Communication Association, Dallas, Texas, May. http://communication.sbs.ohio-state.edu/sense-making/lit/1983_4.html.

Dickerson, Sally S., and Margaret E. Kemeny. 2004. "Acute Stressors and Cortisol Responses: A Theoretical Integration and Synthesis of Laboratory Research." *Psychological Bulletin* 130: 355–91.

Diekhof, Esther K., Katharina Geier, Peter Falkai, and Oliver Gruber. 2011. "Fear Is Only as Deep as the Mind Allows: A Coordinate-Based Meta-Analysis of Neuroimaging Studies on the Regulation of Negative Affect." *Neuroimage* 58 (1): 275–85.

Dieterly, Duncan L. 1980. "Problem Solving and Decisionmaking: An Integration." NASA Technical Memorandum 81191. Moffett Field, California: NASA Ames Research Center.

Dismukes, R. Key, and Ben Berman. 2010. "Checklists and Monitoring in the Cockpit: Why Crucial Defenses Sometimes Fail." NASA/TM 216396. Moffett Field, California: NASA Ames Research Center.

Dodge, Kenneth A. 1991. "The Structure and Function of Reactive and Proactive Aggression." In *The Development and Treatment of Childhood Aggression*, edited by D. J. Pepler and K. H. Rubin, 201–18. Hillsdale, NJ: Lawrence Erlbaum.

Dreyfus, Hubert L., and Stuart E. Dreyfus. 1986. "From Socrates to Expert Systems: The Limits of Calculative Rationality." In *Philosophy and Technology II*, edited by Carl Mitcham and Alois Huning, 111–30. Hingham, MA: Kluwer Academic Publishers.

Dreyfus, Stuart E. 2004. "The Five-Stage Model of Adult Skill Acquisition." *Bulletin of Science, Technology and Society* 24 (3): 177–81.

Dreyfus, Stuart E., and Hubert L. Dreyfus. 1980. *A Five-Stage Model of the Mental Activities Involved in Directed Skill Acquisition.* No. ORC-80-2. Berkeley: University of California Operations Research Center.

Duchenne, Guillaume-Benjamin. 1990. *The mechanism of human facial expression.* Cambridge, UK: Cambridge University Press. First published as *Mécanisme* de la Physionomie Humaine, 1862, Paris, France.

Duncko, Roman, Linda Johnson, Kathleen Merikangas, and Christian Grillon. 2009. "Working Memory Performance After Acute Exposure to the Cold Pressor Stress in Healthy Volunteers." *Neurobiology of Learning and Memory* 91: 377–81.

Dunn, Robert F. 2017. "Gear Up, Mishaps Down: The Evolution of Naval Aviation Safety, 1950–2000." Annapolis, MD: Naval Institute Press.

Edwards, Betty. 1999. *The New Drawing on the Right Side of the Brain.* New York: Penguin.

Einstein, Albert, Leopold Infeld. 1938. The Evolution of Physics: The Growth of Ideas from Early Concepts to Relativity and Quanta. Cambridge, UK: Cambridge University Press.

Ekman, Paul, Richard J. Davidson, and Wallace V. Friesen. 1990. "The Duchenne Smile: Emotional Expression and Brain Physiology: II." *Journal of Personality and Social Psychology* 58 (2): 342.

Elzinga, Berner M., and Karlin Roelofs. 2005. "Cortisol-Induced Impairments of Working Memory Require Acute Sympathetic Activation." *Behavioral Neuroscience* 119: 98–103.

Endsley, Mica R. 1995a. Toward a Theory of Situation Awareness in Dynamic Systems." *Human Factors: The Journal of the Human Factors and Ergonomics Society* 37 (1): 32–64. "

———. 1995b. "Measurement of Situational Awareness in Dynamic Systems." *Human Factors* 37: 65-84.

———. 2013. "Situation Awareness-Oriented Design." In *The Oxford Handbook of Cognitive Engineering*, edited by John D. Lee, Alex Kirlik, and M. J. Dainoff, 272–85. New York: Oxford University Press.

———. 2015. "Situation Awareness Misconceptions and Misunderstandings." *Journal of Cognitive Engineering and Decision Making* 9 (1): 4–32.

Etkin, Amit, Tobias Egner, and Raffael Kalisch. 2011. "Emotional Processing in Anterior Cingulate and Medial Prefrontal Cortex." *Trends in Cognitive Sciences* 15 (2): 85–93.

Etkin, Amit, Tobias Egner, Daniel M. Peraza, Eric R. Kandel, and Joy Hirsch. 2006. "Resolving Emotional Conflict: A Role for the Rostral Anterior Cingulate Cortex in Modulating Activity in the Amygdala." *Neuron* 51 (6): 871–82.

Fallows, James M. 1981. *National Defense.* New York: Random House.

Fama, Eugene F., and Michael C. Jensen. 1983. "Separation of Ownership and Control." *The Journal of Law and Economics* 26 (2): 301–25.

Flavell, John H. 1979. "Metacognition and Cognitive Monitoring: A New Area of Cognitive-Developmental Inquiry." *American Psychologist* 34: 906–11.

Flin, Rhona. 2010. "Rudeness at Work." *British Medical Journal* 340: c2480.

Foushee, H. Clayton, and Karen L. Manos. 1981. "Information transfer within the cockpit: Problems in intracockpit communications." In *Information transfer problems in the aviation system NASA TP1875*, edited by Charles E. Billings and Ed S, 63-71. Cheaney. Moffett Field, CA: Ames Research Center, NASA.

Foushee, H. Clayton. 1984. "Dyads and triads at 35,000 feet: Factors affecting group process and aircrew performance." *American Psychologist, 39* (8), 885-893.

Fox, Craig R., and Amos Tversky. 1995. "Ambiguity Aversion and Comparative Ignorance." *Quarterly Journal of Economics* 110 (3): 585–603.

Frasnelli, Elisa. 2013. "Brain and Behavioral Lateralization in Invertebrates." *Frontiers in Psychology* 4 (939): 1-10.

Gardner, Howard, with Emma Laskin. 2011. *Leading Minds: An Anatomy of Leadership.* New York: Basic Books.

Garson, James. 2016. "Modal Logic." In *The Stanford Encyclopedia of Philosophy* (Spring 2016 edition), edited by Edward N. Zalta. https://plato.stanford.edu/archives/spr2016/entries/logic-modal/.

Gawande, Atul. 2010. *The Checklist Manifesto: How to Get Things Right.* New York: Metropolitan Books.

Gibson, James J. 1966. *The Senses Considered as Perceptual Systems.* Boston: Houghton Mifflin.

Gibson, James J. 1972. "A Theory of Direct Visual Perception." In *The Psychology of Knowing,* edited by Joseph Royce, William Rozenboom, 215-227. New York: Gordon & Breach.

Gigerenzer, Gerd. 2008. "Why Heuristics Work." *Perspectives on Psychological Science* 3 (1): 20–9.

Gigerenzer, Gerd, and Daniel G. Goldstein. 1996. "Reasoning the Fast and Frugal Way: Models of Bounded Rationality." *Psychological Review* 103 (4): 650–69.

Gladwell, Malcolm. 2008. *Outliers: The Secret of Success.* New York: Little, Brown & Co.

Gregory, Richard. 1970. *The Intelligent Eye.* London: Weidenfeld and Nicolson.

Gregory, Richard L. 2015. *Eye and brain: The psychology of seeing.* Princeton, New Jersey: Princeton university press.

Goffman, Erving. 2005. "Role distance." In *Life as theater. A Dramaturgical Sourcebook* 2, edited by Dennis Brisset and Charles Edgley, 101-111. New Brunswick, NJ: Aldine Transaction.

Goranko, Valentin, and Antony Galton. 2015. "Temporal Logic." In *The Stanford Encyclopedia of Philosophy* (Winter 2015 edition), edited by Edward N. Zalta. https://plato.stanford.edu/archives/win2015/entries/logic-temporal/.

Gortney, William E. 2016. *Department of Defense Dictionary of Military and Associated Terms.* No. JP-1-02. Joint Chiefs of Staff Washington United States.

Green, Jessica L., Alan Hastings, Peter Arzberger, Francisco J. Ayala, Kathryn L. Cottingham, Kim Cuddington, Frank Davis, Jennifer A. Dunne, Marie- Josée Fortin, Leah Gerver, and Michael Neubert. 2005. "Complexity in Ecology and Conservation: Mathematical, Statistical, and Computational Challenges." *BioScience* 55 (6): 501–10.

Greenberg, Jeff, and Jamie Arndt. 2011. "Terror Management Theory." *Handbook of Theories of Social Psychology* 1: 398–415.

Gupta, Punkaj, and Mallikarjuna Rettiganti. 2015. "Association between Extracorporeal Membrane Oxygenation Center Volume and Mortality among Children with Heart Disease: Propensity and Risk Modeling." *Pediatric Critical Care Medicine* 16 (9): 868–74.

Haas, Jack. 1977. "Learning Real Feelings: A Study of High Steel Ironworkers' Reactions to Fear and Danger." *Sociology of Work and Occupations* 4 (2): 147–70.

Haddon Jr., William. 1970. "On the Escape of Tigers: An Ecologic Note." *American Journal of Public Health and the Nation's Health* 60 (12): 2229–34.

Hall, Edward T. 1959. *The Silent Language.* New York: Doubleday.

———. 1966. *The Hidden Dimension.* New York: Anchor Press.

———. 1973. *The Silent Culture.* New York: Anchor Press.

———. 1976/1989. *Beyond Culture.* New York: Anchor Press.

———. 1980. "Advances in the Epidemiology of Injuries as a Basis for Public Policy." *Public Health Reports* 95 (5): 411–21.

———. 1992. *An Anthropology of Everyday Life: An Autobiography.* New York, NY: Doubleday Books.

———. 2000. "Monochronic and Polychronic Time." *Intercultural Communication: A Reader* 9: 280–6.

Halverson, Richard. 2004. "Accessing, Documenting, and Communicating Practical Wisdom: The Phronesis of School Leadership Practice." *American Journal of Education* 111 (1): 90–121.

Hammond, Grant T. 2001. *The Mind of War: John Boyd and American Society.* Washington, DC: Smithsonian Institution.

Hampden-Turner, Charles, and Fons Tromepenaars. 1997. *Riding the Waves of Culture: Understanding Diversity in Global Business.* New York, NY: McGraw-Hill.

Hansen, Christine H., and Ranald D. Hansen. "Finding the face in the crowd: An anger superiority effect." *Journal of personality and social psychology* 54, no. 6 (1988): 917-24.

Harken, Dwight E. 1946. "Foreign Bodies in, and in Relation to, the Thoracic Blood Vessels and Heart: Techniques for Approaching and Removing Foreign Bodies from the Chambers of the Heart." *Surgery, Gynecology and Obstetrics* 83: 117-125.

Harmon-Jones, E. 1999. *Cognitive Dissonance: Progress on a Pivotal Theory in Social Psychology.* Washington, DC: American Psychological Association.

Harrington, Anne W., and Priscilla S. Rogers. 1988. "What Is 'Communication Context'?" Working paper #584, Division of Research, Graduate School of Business Administration, University of Michigan. https://deepblue.lib.umich.edu/bitstream/handle/2027.42/35683/b1411792.0001.001.txt?sequence=1&isAllowed=y.

Hartley, Eugene L., & Hartley, Ruth E. 1952. Leadership-followership. In *Fundamentals of social psychology* edited by Eugene L. Hartley & Ruth E. Hartley, 603-650. New York, NY, US: Alfred A. Knopf.

Health and Safety Commission 1993. *Organizing for safety: Third report of the human factors study group of ACSNI.* Sudbury, UK: HSE Books.

Heggie, Vanessa. 2013. "Experimental Physiology, Everest and Oxygen: From the Ghastly Kitchens to the Gasping Lung." *British Journal for the History of Science* 46 (01): 123–47.

Helmreich, Robert L. 1984. "Cockpit management attitudes." *Human factors* 26 (5): 583-589.

Helmreich, Robert L., H. Clayton Foushee, Robert Benson, and William Russini. 1986. "Cockpit resource management: exploring the attitude-performance linkage. "*Aviation, space, and environmental medicine* 57 (12, Sect I): 1198-1200.

Helmreich, Robert L., Ashleigh C. Merritt, and John A. Wilhelm. 1999. "The evolution of crew resource management training in commercial aviation." *The international journal of aviation psychology* 9 (1): 19-32.

Hempelmann, Louis H., Hermann Lisco, and Joseph G. Hoffman. 1952. "The Acute Radiation Syndrome: A Study of Nine Cases and a Review of the Problem." *Annals of Internal Medicine* 36 (2, part 1): 279–510.

Hendricks, Vincent, and John Symons. 2015. "Epistemic Logic." In *The Stanford Encyclopedia of Philosophy* (Fall 2015 edition), edited by Edward N. Zalta. https://plato.stanford.edu/archives/fall2015/entries/logic-epistemic/.

Henry, Donald O. 1995. "Introduction and Overview: Evolutionary Ecology and Archaeology." In *Prehistoric Cultural Ecology and Evolution: Insights from South Jordan*, 1-21. New York, New York: Springer US.

Hilborn, Ray, and Stephen C. Stearns. 1982. "On Inference in Ecology and Evolutionary Biology: The Problem of Multiple Causes." *Acta Biotheoretica* 31: 145–64.

Hofstede, Geert. 1980. "Motivation, Leadership, and Organization: Do American Theories Apply Abroad?" *Organizational Dynamics* 9 (1): 42–63.

Hollander, Edwin P. 1992. "The essential interdependence of leadership and followership." *Current Directions in Psychological Science* 1 (2): 71-75.

Hollander, Edwin P., and Wilse B. Webb. 1954. Leadership, Followership and Friendship. No. NSAM-NM-001-058-16-03. Pensacola, Florida: Naval School of Aviation Medicine.

———. 1955. Leadership, followership, and friendship: an analysis of peer nominations. *The Journal of Abnormal and Social Psychology.* 50 (2): 163-167.

Hornik, Christoph P., Xia He, Jeffrey P. Jacobs, Jennifer S. Li, Robert D. B. Jaquiss, Marshall L. Jacobs, Sean M. O'Brien, Karl Welke, Eric D. Peterson, and Sara K. Pasquali. 2012. "Relative Impact of Surgeon and Center Volume on Early Mortality After the Norwood Operation." *Annals of Thoracic Surgery* 93 (6): 1992–7.

Inozu, Bahadir, Dan Chauncey, Vickie Kamataris, and Charles Mount. 2011. *Performance Improvement for Healthcare: Leading Change with Lean, Six Sigma, and Constraints Management.* New York, NY: McGraw-Hill.

Inhelder, Barbel, Jean Piaget. 1958. *The Growth of Logical Thinking from Childhood to Adolescence.* New York: Basic Books.

International Atomic Energy Agency (IAEA). 1986. "Summary Report on the Post-Accident Review Meeting on the Chernobyl Accident." Report by the International Nuclear Safety Advisory Group (INSAG). Vienna: IAEA.

Ioannidis, John P. 2005. "Why Most Published Research Findings Are False." *PLOS Medicine,* 2 (8): e124.

———. 2005. Contradicted and Initially Stronger Effects in Highly Cited Clinical Research. *Journal of the American Medical Association* 294 (2): 218–28.

Janis, Irving L., and Leon Mann. 1977. *Decision Making: A Psychological Analysis of Conflict, Choice, and Commitment.* New York, NY: Free Press.

Jayaram, Natalie, John A. Spertus, Michael L. O'Byrne, Paul S. Chan, Kevin F. Kennedy, Lisa Bergersen, and Andrew C. Glatz. 2017. "Relationship between Hospital Procedure Volume and Complications Following Congenital Cardiac Catheterization: A Report from the Improving Pediatric and Adult Congenital Treatment (IMPACT) Registry." *American Heart Journal* 183: 118–28.

Jensen, Eva. 2006. "Good Sensemaking Is More Important Than Information for the Quality of Plans." In *Proceedings of the 11th International Command and Control Research and Technology Symposium, Cambridge, UK.*

Judge, Timothy A., and Ronald F. Piccolo. 2004. "Transformational and Transactional Leadership: A Meta-Analytic Test of Their Relative Validity." *Journal of Applied Psychology* 89 (5): 755-768.

Kahneman, Daniel. 2003. "A Perspective on Judgement and Choice." *American Psychologist* 58: 697–720.

———. 2011. *Thinking, Fast and Slow.* New York, NY: Macmillan Press.

Kahneman, Daniel, and Amos Tversky. 1973. "On the Psychology of Prediction." *Psychological Review* 80 (4): 237–51.

Kanfer, Frederick H., and Bruce K. Schefft. 1988. *Guiding the Process of Therapeutic Change.* Champaign, IL: Research Press.

Kansy, Andrzej, Tjark Ebels, Christian Schreiber, Zdzislaw Tobota, and Bohdan Maruszewski. 2014. "Association of Center Volume with Outcomes: Analysis of Verified Data of European Association for Cardio-Thoracic Surgery Congenital Database." *Annals of Thoracic Surgery* 98 (6): 2159–64.

Katz, Daniel. 1960. "The Functional Approach to the Study of Attitudes." *Public Opinion Quarterly* 24: 163–204.

Keil, Frank C. 2006. "Explanation and Understanding." *Annual Review of Psychology* 57: 227–54.

Kerber, Bill, and Brian J. Dreckshage. 2011. *Lean Supply Chain Management Essentials: A Framework for Materials Managers.* Boca Raton, FL: CRC Press.

Kevles, Bettyann 1992. "BOOK REVIEW: Pioneering Physician Is Vividly Recalled : DIARY OF WILLIAM HARVEY: The Imaginary Journal of the Physician Who Revolutionized Medicine by Jean Hamburger." *Los Angeles Times* October 27, 1992. http://articles.latimes.com/1992-10-27/news/vw-741_1_william-harvey.

Khemlani, Sangeet S., and Philip N. Johnson-Laird. 2012. "Hidden Conflicts: Explanations Make Inconsistencies Harder to Detect." *Acta Psychologica* 139: 486–91.

Kittler, Markus G., David Rygl, and Alex Mackinnon. 2011. Special review article: "Beyond Culture or Beyond Control? Reviewing the Use of Hall's High-/Low-Context Concept." *International Journal of Cross Cultural Management* 11 (1): 63–82.

Klein, Gary A. 1993. *A Recognition-Primed Decision (RPD) Model of Rapid Decision Making*. New York: Ablex.

———. 1999. *Sources of Power: How People Make Decisions*. Cambridge, MA: MIT Press.

———. 2014. "An Overview of Naturalistic Decision-Making Applications." In *Naturalistic Decision Making*, edited by Caroline E. Zsambok and Gary Klein, 49–60. New York, New York: Routledge Press.

Klein, Gary A., Roberta Calderwood, and Donald Macgregor. 1989. "Critical Decision Method for Eliciting Knowledge." *IEEE Transactions on Systems, Man, and Cybernetics* 19 (3): 462–72.

Klein, Gary, Brian Moon, and Robert R. Hoffman. 2006. "Making Sense of Sensemaking 2: A Macrocognitive Model." *IEEE Intelligent Systems* 21 (5): 88–92.

Kolling, Nils, Tim E. J. Behrens, Marco K. Wittmann, and Matthew F. S. Rushworth. 2016a. "Multiple Signals in Anterior Cingulate Cortex." *Current Opinion in Neurobiology* 37: 36–43.

Kolling, Nils, Marco K. Wittmann, Tim E. Behrens, Erie D. Boorman, Roger B. Mars, and Matthew F. Rushworth. 2016b. "Value, Search, Persistence and Model Updating in Anterior Cingulate Cortex." *Nature Neuroscience* 19 (10): 1280–5.

Koutsikou, Stella, Jonathan J. Crook, Emma V. Earl, J. Lianne Leith, Thomas C. Watson, Bridget M. Lumb, and Richard Apps. 2014. "Neural Substrates Underlying Fear-Evoked Freezing: The Periaqueductal Grey–Cerebellar Link." *Journal of Physiology* 592 (10): 2197–213.

Kraiger, Kurt, J. Kevin Ford, and Eduardo Salas. 1993. "Application of Cognitive, Skill-Based, and Affective Theories of Learning Outcomes to New Methods of Training Evaluation." *Journal of Applied Psychology* 78 (2): 311–28.

Krathwohl, David R., Benjamin S. Bloom, and Bertram Masia. 1964. *Taxonomy of Educational Objectives Handbook II: Affective domain*. New York, New York: David McKay Company.

Krulak, Charles C. 1999. "The Strategic Corporal: Leadership in the Three-Block War." *Marine Corps Gazette* 83 (1): 18-22.

Kuhnert, Karl W., and Philip Lewis. 1987. "Transactional and Transformational Leadership: A Constructive/Developmental Analysis." *Academy of Management Review* 12 (4): 648–57.

Kurtz, Cynthia F., and David J. Snowden. 2003. "The New Dynamics of Strategy: Sense-Making in a Complex and Complicated World." *IBM Systems Journal* 42 (3): 462–83.

Lahti, David C., Norman A. Johnson, Beverly C. Ajie, Sarah P. Otto, Andrew P. Hendry, Daniel T. Blumstein, Richard G. Coss, Kathleen Donohue, and Susan A. Foster. 2009. "Relaxed Selection in the Wild." *Trends in Ecology and Evolution* 24 (9): 487–96.

Langer, Ellen J. 1989. *Mindfulness.* Boston, MA: Addison-Wesley.

———. 2014. *Mindfulness 25th Anniversary Edition.* Cambridge, MA: Da Capo Press.

La Porte, Todd R., and Paula M. Consolini. 1991. "Working in Practice but Not in Theory: Theoretical Challenges of 'High Reliability Organizations.'" Berkeley: Institute of Governmental Studies, University of California.

La Porte, Todd R., Karlene Roberts, and Gene I. Rochlin. 1988. "Aircraft Carrier Operations at Sea: The Challenges of High Reliability Performance" (no. IGS/OTP-1-88). Berkeley: Institute of Governmental Studies, University of California.

Lave, Jean, and Etienne Wenger. 1991. *Situated Learning: Legitimate Peripheral Participation.* Cambridge, UK: Cambridge University Press.

Lazarus, Richard S. 2006. *Stress and emotion: A new synthesis.* New York, New York: Springer Publishing Company.

LeBlanc, Vicki R., Meghan M. McConnell, and Sandra D. Monteiro. 2015. "Predictable Chaos: A Review of the Effects of Emotions on Attention, Memory and Decision Making." *Advances in Health Sciences Education* 20 (1): 265–82.

LeDoux Joseph. E. 2000. "Emotion Circuits in the Brain." *Annual Review of Neuroscience* 23: 155–84.

———. 2013. "The Slippery Slope of Fear." *Trends in Cognitive Sciences* 17 (4): 155–6.

———. 2014. "Coming to Terms with Fear." *Proceedings of the National Academy of Sciences* 111 (8): 2871–8.

LeDoux, Joseph E., and Daniel S. Pine. 2016. "Using Neuroscience to Help Understand Fear and Anxiety: A Two-System Framework." *American Journal of Psychiatry* 173 (11): 1083–93.

Lee Perez, Fabio Y. 2005. "Survival Tactics of Indigenous People." Waves of Devastation. http://academic.evergreen.edu/g/grossmaz/LEEPERFY/.

Lenzen, Sigurd. 2014. "A Fresh View of Glycolysis and Glucokinase Regulation: History and Current Status." *Journal of Biological Chemistry* 289 (18): 12189–94.

LePore, Stephen J., and Tracey A. Revenson. "Resilience and Posttraumatic Growth: Recovery, Resistance, and Reconfiguration." In *Handbook of Posttraumatic Growth: Research and Practice*, edited by Lawrence G. Calhoun and Richard G. Tedeschi, 24–46. Routledge: New York.

Lipshitz, Ranaan, and Marvin S. Cohen. 2005. "Warrants for Prescription: Analytically and Empirically Based Approaches to Improving Decision Making." *Human Factors* 47 (1): 121–30.

Lupien, Sonia J., Christian J. Gillin, and Richard L. Hauger. 1999. "Working Memory Is More Sensitive Than Declarative Memory to the Acute Effects of Corticosteroids: A Dose-Response Study in Humans." *Behavioral Neuroscience* 113: 420–30.

MacDougall-Shackleton, Scott A. 2011. "The Levels of Analysis Revisited." *Philosophical Transactions of the Royal Society of London B: Biological Sciences* 366 (1574): 2076–85.

MacDuffie, John Paul, and Susan Helper. 1997. "Creating Lean Suppliers: Diffusing Lean Production through the Supply Chain." *California Management Review* 39 (4): 118–51.

Mack, John E., and Holly Hickler. 1981. *Vivienne: The Life and Suicide of an Adolescent Girl.* Boston: Little, Brown & Co.

MacLean, Paul D. 1990. *The Triune Brain in Evolution: Role in Paleocerebral Functions.* Springer Science and Business Media (Plenum): New York.

Magee, John F. 1964a. "Decision Trees for Decision Making." *Harvard Business Review* 42 (4): 35-48.

———. 1964b. "How to Use Decision Trees in Capital Investment." *Harvard Business Review* 42 (5): 79–96.

Magee, Roderick R. 1998. *Strategic Leadership Primer.* Carlisle, PA: Army War College.

Maitlis, Sally, and Marlys Christianson. 2014. "Sensemaking in Organizations: Taking Stock and Moving Forward." *Academy of Management Annals* 8 (1): 57–125.

Maitlis, Sally, and Scott Sonenshein. 2010. "Sensemaking in crisis and change: Inspiration and insights from Weick (1988)." *Journal of management studies* 47 (3): 551-580.

Maitlis, Sally, Timothy J. Vogus, and Thomas B. Lawrence. 2013. "Sensemaking and Emotion in Organizations." *Organizational Psychology Review* 3 (3): 222–47.

Mani, Anandi, Sendhill Mullainathan, Eldar Shafir, and Jiaying Zhao. 2013. "Poverty Impedes Cognitive Function." *Science* 341 (6149): 976–80.

March, James G. 1991. "Exploration and Exploitation in Organizational Learning." *Organization Science* 2 (1): 71–87.

Martin, Rod A., Patricia Puhlik-Doris, Gwen Larsen, Jeanette Gray, and Kelly Weir. 2003. "Individual Differences in Uses of Humor and Their Relation to Psychological Well-Being: Development of the Humor Styles Questionnaire." *Journal of Research in Personality* 37 (1): 48–75.

Marx, David. 2001. *Patient Safety and the "Just Culture": A Primer for Health Care Executives.* Presentation to Trustees of Columbia University in the City of New York, Columbia University. April 17, 2001.

McAuley, Mark T., Rose Anne Kenny, Thomas B. Kirkwood, Darren J. Wilkinson, Janette J. Jones, Veronica M. Miller. 2009. "A Mathematical Model of Aging-Related and Cortisol Induced Hippocampal Dysfunction." *BMC Neuroscience* 10: 26-40.

McConnell, Mark, and Daved van Stralen. 1997. "Emergency Medical Decision Making in the Tactical Environment." *Tactical Edge Journal* 15 (3): 32–9.

McGhee, Paul E. 2013. "On the Cognitive Origins of Incongruity Humor": Fantasy Assimilation versus Reality Assimilation." In *The Psychology of Humor: Theoretical Perspectives and Empirical Issues*, edited by Jeffrey H. Goldstein, 61–80. New York, NY: Academic Press.

McLuhan, Marshall. 1994. *Understanding Media: The Extensions of Man.* Cambridge, MA: MIT Press.

McNamara, Paul. 2014. "Deontic Logic." In *The Stanford Encyclopedia of Philosophy* (Winter 2014 edition), edited by Edward N. Zalta. https://plato.stanford. edu/archives/win2014/entries/logic-deontic/.

Meier, Brian P., Simon Schnall, Norbert Schwarz, and John Bargh. (2012). Embodiment in social psychology. *Topics in cognitive science*, 4 (4), 705-716.

Meshkati, Najmedin, and Yalda Khashe. 2015. "Operators' Improvisation in Complex Technological Systems: Successfully Tackling Ambiguity, Enhancing Resiliency and the Last Resort to Averting Disaster." *Journal of Contingencies and Crisis Management* 23 (2): 90–6.

Meyer, John C. 2000. "Humor as a Double-Edged Sword: Four Functions of Humor in Communication." *Communication Theory* 10 (3): 310–31.

Miller, Richard L., Philip Brickman, and Diana Bolen. 1975. "Attribution versus Persuasion as a Means for Modifying Behavior." *Journal of Personality and Social Psychology* 31 (3): 430-41.

Mischel, Walter. 1998. "Metacognition at the Hyphen of Social-Cognitive Psychology." *Personality and Social Psychology Review* 2 (2): 84–6.

Morgan, Karl Z. 1948. "Radiation Safety Measures in an Atomic Energy Plant." *Engineering Journal* 31 (3): 154–61.

Morris, David J. 2015. *The Evil Hours: A Biography of Post-Traumatic Stress Disorder.* New York: Houghton Mifflin Harcourt.

Natterson-Horowitz, Barbara, and Kathryn Bowers. 2013. *Zoobiquity: The Astonishing Connection between Human and Animal Health.* New York: Vintage.

Neamy, Robert. 2011. "From Firescope to NIMS." *Fire Rescue* magazine 6 (8): 103.

Neimeyer Robert. 2014. Re-Storying Loss: Fostering Growth in the Posttraumatic Narrative. In *Handbook of Posttraumatic Growth: Research and Practice*, edited by L. G. Calhoun and R. G. Tedeschi, 68–80. New York, New York: Routledge.

Nightingale, Florence. 1992 [1859]. *Notes on Nursing: What It Is, and What It Is Not.* London: Lippincott Williams and Wilkins.

Nonaka, Ikujiro. 1994. "A Dynamic Theory of Organizational Knowledge Creation." *Organization Science* 5 (1): 14–37.

Nordwig, Arnold. 1984. "Carl Neuberg: Fate of a Jewish Biochemist in the Third Reich." *Trends in Biochemical Sciences* 9 (11): 498–9.

Novaco, Raymond W. 1979. "The cognitive regulation of anger and stress." In *Cognitive-behavioral interventions: Theory, research, and procedures,* edited by Philip C. Kendall and Stephen D. Hollon, 241-285. New York New York: Academic Press

Novaco, Raymond W., Irwin G. Sarason, Thomas M. Cook, Gregory L. Robinson, and Francis J. Cunningham. 1979. "Psychological and Organizational Factors Related to Attrition and Performance in Marine Corps Recruit Training." Arlington, VA: Office of Naval Research.

Novaco, Raymond W., Irwin G. Sarason, Gregory L. Robinson, and Christiane Parry. 1983. "Attributes of Drill Instructor School Graduates: Stress-Related Factors." Arlington, VA: Office of Naval Research.

Novaco, Raymond W., Irwin G. Sarason, Gregory L. Robinson, and Francis J. Cunningham. 1982. *Longitudinal Analyses of Stress and Performance among Marine Corps Drill Instructors* (no. AR-ONR-007). Arlington, VA: Office of Naval Research.

Oesper, Peter. 1968. "Error and Trial: The Story of the Oxidative Reaction of Glycolysis." *Journal of Chemical Education* 45 (9): 607–10.

Öhman, Arne, Daniel Lundqvist, and Francisco Esteves. 2001. "The face in the crowd revisited: a threat advantage with schematic stimuli." *Journal of personality and social psychology* 80 (3): 381-96.

O'Leary, Mike, and Sheryl L. Chappell. 1996. "Confidential Incident Reporting Systems Create Vital Awareness of Safety Problems." *ICAO Journal* 51 (8): 11–13, 27.

Orr, George E. 1983. *Combat Operations C3I: Fundamentals and Interactions.* Maxwell Air Force Base, Montgomery, AL: Airpower Research Institute.

Orton, J. Douglas, and Karl E. Weick. 1990. "Loosely Coupled Systems: A Reconceptualization." *Academy of Management Review* 15 (2): 203–23.

Orwell, George. 2008. "Shooting elephant." In *Facing Unpleasant Facts: Narrative essays* compiled by George Packer, 29-37. Boston, MA: Mariner Books.

Paget, Marianne A. 1988. The unity of mistakes: A phenomenological interpretation of medical work. Philadelphia, PA: Temple University Press.

Park, Crystal L. 2010. "Making Sense of the Meaning Literature: An Integrative Review of Meaning Making and Its Effects on Adjustment to Stressful Life Events." *Psychological Bulletin* 136 (2): 257-301.

Parrott, Lael. 2002. "Complexity and the Limits of Ecological Engineering." *Transactions of the American Society of Agricultural Engineers* 45 (5): 1697-1702.

Parry, Richard. "*Episteme* and *Techne.*" In *The Stanford Encyclopedia of Philosophy* (Fall 2014 edition), edited by Edward N. Zalta. https://plato.stanford.edu/archives/fall2014/entries/episteme-techne/.

Pasquali, Sara K., Jeffrey P. Jacobs, Xia He, Christoph P. Hornik, Robert D. B. Jaquiss, Marshall L. Jacobs, Sean M. O'Brien, Eric D. Peterson, and Jennifer S. Li. 2012. "The Complex Relationship between Center Volume and Outcome in Patients Undergoing the Norwood Operation." *Annals of Thoracic Surgery* 93 (5): 1556–62.

Pastel, Teague A. 2008. *Marine Corps Leadership: Empowering or Limiting the Strategic Corporal?* Quantico, VA: US Marine Corps Command and Staff College.

Pauly, Daniel. 1995. "Anecdotes and the Shifting Baseline Syndrome of Fisheries." *Trends in Ecology and Evolution* 10 (10): 430.

Paus, Tomáš, Robert Jech, Christopher J. Thompson, Roch Comeau, Terry Peters, and Alan C. Evans. 1998. "Dose-Dependent Reduction of Cerebral Blood Flow During Rapid-Rate Transcranial Magnetic Stimulation of the Human Sensorimotor Cortex." *Journal of Neurophysiology* 79 (2): 1102–7.

Pea, Roy, and John S. Brown. 1991. Series Foreword to *Situated Learning: Legitimate Peripheral Participation*, edited by Jeane Lave and Etienne Wenger, 11–12. New York, NY: Cambridge University Press.

Perrow, Charles. 1981. "Normal Accident at Three Mile Island." *Society* 18 (5): 17–26.

———. 2011. *Normal Accidents: Living with High-Risk Technologies.* Princeton, NJ: Princeton University Press.

Petty, Richard E., Duane T. Wegener, and Leandre R. Fabrigar. 1997. "Attitudes and Attitude Change." *Annual Review of Psychology* 48: 609–47.

Phelps, Elizabeth A. 2006. "Emotion and Cognition: Insights from Studies of the Human Amygdala." *Annual Review of Psychology* 57: 27–53.

Pieper, Dawid, Tim Mathes, and Boulos Asfour. 2014. "A Systematic Review of the Impact of Volume of Surgery and Specialization in Norwood Procedure." *BMC Pediatrics* 14 (1): 198.

Pirolli, Peter, and Daniel M. Russell. "Introduction to this special issue on sense-making." (2011): 1-8.

Pliske, Rebecca M., Michael J McCloskey, and Gary Klein. 2001. "Decision Skills Training: Facilitating Learning from Experience." In *Linking Expertise and Naturalistic Decision Making*, edited by Eduardo Salas and Gary A. Klein, 37–53. New York, NY: Psychology Press.

Polanyi, Michael. 1966. *The Tacit Dimension*. New York, New York: Doubleday New York.

Posner, Michael I., Mary K. Rothbart, Brad Sheese, and Yiyuan Tang. 2007. "The Anterior Cingulate Gyrus and the Mechanism of Self-Regulation." *Cognitive, Affective, and Behavioral Neuroscience* 7 (4): 391–5.

Post, Richard H. 1971. "Possible Cases of Relaxed Selection in Civilized Populations." *Human Genetics* 13 (4): 253–84.

Proulx, Raphael. 2007. "Ecological Complexity for Unifying Ecological Theory across Scales: A Field Ecologist's Perspective." *Ecological Complexity* 4 (3): 85–92.

Radford, Gary P. 1994 (November). "Overcoming Dewey's 'False Psychology': Reclaiming Communication for Communication Studies." Paper presented at the *80th Annual Meeting of the Speech Communication Association*, New Orleans, Louisiana. November 19-22, 1994.

Rasmussen, Jens. 1980. What Can Be Learned from Human Error Reports? in Duncan, K.D., Gruneberg, M.M. and Wallis, D. (eds), *Changes in Working Life*, New York, NY: Wiley: 97–113.

———. 1983. "Skills, Rules, and Knowledge: Signals, Signs, and Symbols, and Other Distinctions in Human Performance Models." *IEEE Transactions on Systems, Man, and Cybernetics*, SMC-13 (3): 257–66.

———. 1987. *Cognitive Control of Human Activities and Errors: Implication for Ecological Interface Design*. Roskilde, Denmark: Risø National Laboratory

———. 1989. "Coping with Human Errors through System Design: Implications for Ecological Interface Design." *International Journal of Man-Machine Studies* 31: 517–34.

Reason, James. 1990. *Human Error.* New York, NY: Cambridge University Press.

———. 1997. *Managing the Risks of Organizational Accidents.* Aldershot, UK: Ashgate.

———. 1998. "Achieving a Safe Culture: Theory and Practice." *Work and Stress* 12 (3): 293–306.

———. 2000. "Human Error: Models and Management." *British Medical Journal* 320 (7237): 768–70.

Roberts, Karlene H. 1989. "New Challenges in Organizational Research: High Reliability Organizations." *Organization and Environment* 3 (2): 111–25.

———. 1990. "Managing High Reliability Organizations." *California Management Review* 32 (4): 101–13.

Roberts, Karlene H., and Denise M. Rousseau. 1989. "Research in Nearly Failure-Free, High Reliability Organizations: Having the Bubble." *IEEE Transactions on Engineering Management* 36 (2): 132–9.

Robinson, Gregory L., Raymond W. Novaco, and Irwin G. Sarason. 1981. *Cognitive Correlates of Outcome and Performance in Marine Corps Recruit Training.* Arlington, VA: Office of Naval Research.

Rogers, Lesley J. 2002. "Lateralization in Vertebrates: Its Early Evolution, General Pattern, and Development." *Advances in the Study of Behavior* 31: 107–61.

Roe, Emery., and Paul R. Schulman. 2015. "Comparing Emergency Response Infrastructure to Other Critical Infrastructures in the California Bay-Delta of the United States: A Research Note on Inter-Infrastructural Differences in Reliability Management." *Journal of Contingencies and Crisis Management* 23 (4): 193–200.

Rollnick, Stephen, William R. Miller, and Christopher C. Butler. 2008. *Motivational Interviewing in Health Care: Helping Patients Change Behavior.* New York: Guilford Press.

Ron, Neta, Raanan Lipshitz, and Micha Popper. 2006. "How Organizations Learn: Post-Flight Reviews in an F-16 Fighter Squadron." *Organization Studies* 27 (8): 1069–89.

Rule, Brendan G. 1974. "The Hostile and Instrumental Functions of Human Aggression." In *Determinants and Origins of Aggressive Behavior,* edited by J. de Wit and W. Hartup, 125–145. The Hague, Netherlands: Mouton.

Russell, Bertrand. 1910. "Knowledge by Acquaintance and Knowledge by Description." *Proceedings of the Aristotelian Society* (11, January): 108–28.

Russell, Daniel M., Mark J. Stefik, Peter Pirolli, and Stuart K. Card. 1993. "The Cost Structure of Sensemaking." In *Proceedings of the INTERACT '93 and CHI '93 Conference on Human Factors in Computing Systems,* 269–76. New York: ACM.

Ryan, Craig. 2015. *Sonic Wind: The Story of John Paul Stapp and How a Renegade Doctor Became the Fastest Man on Earth.* New York: Liverwright Publishing Corp.

Ryan, Sharon. "Wisdom." In The *Stanford Encyclopedia of Philosophy* (Winter 2014 edition), edited by Edward N. Zalta. https://plato.stanford.edu/archives/win2014/entries/wisdom/.

Sandberg, Jorgen, and Haridimos Tsoukas. 2011. "Grasping the Logic of Practice: Theorizing through Practicality Rationality." *Academy of Management Review* 36 (2): 338–60.

Sandi, Carmen, and M. T. Pinelo-Nava. 2007. "Stress and Memory: Behavioral Effects and Neurobiological Mechanisms." *Neural Plasticity* 78970. Pages 1-20. https://www.ncbi.nlm.nih.gov/pmc/articles/PMC1950232/

Sarason, Irwin G., and Raymond W. Novaco. 1982. *Stress and Coping in Recruit Training: Roles of the Recruit and the Drill Instructor* (no. AR-ONR-008). Arlington, VA: Office of Naval Research.

Sarason, Irwin G., Raymond W. Novaco, Gregory L. Robinson, and Thomas M. Cook. 1981. *Recruit Attrition and the Training Unit Environment.* Arlington, VA: Office of Naval Research.

Sarason, Irwin G., Raymond W. Novaco, and Barbara R. Sarason. 1981. *A Follow-Up Study of Marines Two and a Half Years After Recruit Training* (no. AR-006). Arlington, VA: Office of Naval Research.

Schachter, Stanley, and Jerome E. Singer. 1962. "Cognitive, Social, and Physiological Determinants of Emotional State." *Psychological Review* 69 (5): 378–99.

Schmidt, Harold S. 1995. *Contingency Communications Planning for the Force XXI Army.* Carlisle, PA: Army War College.

Schumpeter, Joseph A. 1947. "The Creative Response in Economic History." *Journal of Economic History* 7 (02): 149–59.

Schwartz, Shalom H. 1992. "Universals in the Content and Structure of Values: Theoretical Advances and Empirical Tests in 20 Countries." In *Advances in Experimental Social Psychology* 25: 1-65, edited by M. Zanna. San Diego: Academic Press.

———. 1994. "Are There Universal Aspects in the Structure and Contents of Human Values?" *Journal of Social Issues* 50 (4): 19–45.

Schwartz, Shalom H., Jan Cieciuch, Michele Vecchione, Eldad Davidov, Ronald Fischer, Constanze Beierlein, Alice Ramos, Markku Verkasalo, Jan Erik Lönnqvist, Kursad Demirutku, Ozlem Dirilen-Gumus, and Mark Konty. 2012. "Refining the Theory of Basic Individual Values." *Journal of Personality and Social Psychology* 103 (4): 663-88.

Shannon, Claude E., and Warren Weaver. 1949. *The Mathematical Theory of Communication.* University of Illinois Press: Urbana, IL.

Shenhav, Amitai., Matthew. M. Botvinick, and Jonathan D. Cohen. 2013. "The Expected Value of Control: An Integrative Theory of Anterior Cingulate Cortex Function." *Neuron* 79 (2): 217–40.

Sherman, Paul W. 1988. "The Levels of Analysis." *Animal Behaviour* 36 (2): 616–9.

Shin, Jaiwon. (2000). The NASA aviation safety program: overview. *Proceedings of ASME Turbo Expo 2000,* 8-11. Munich, Germany May 8-11, 2000.

Shubik, Martin. 1962. "Some Experimental Non-Zero Sum Games with Lack of Information about the Rules." *Management Science* 8 (2): 215–34.

Simon, Herbert. A. 1957. *Administrative Behavior: A Study of Decision-Making Processes in Administrative Organization (2nd ed.). New York: Macmillan.*

Simon, Herbert A. 1962. The architecture of complexity. *Proceedings of the American Philosophical Society.* 106 (6): 467-82.

Soliday, Edmond L., & Erickson, E. (1999). Commercial Aviation Safety Team (CAST). In *Annual International Air Safety Seminar* (Vol. 52, pp. 51-66). Flight Safety Foundation; 1998.

Song, Li. 2005. "Seeing the Invisible: Reflections on E. T. Hall and M. McLuhan." *Intercultural Communication Studies* 14 (2): 114.

Spradley, James P. 1984. "Culture and Ethnography." In *Conformity and Conflict: Readings in Cultural Anthropology*, 1st ed., edited by James P. Spradley and David W. McCurdy, 1–13. Boston, MA: Pearson.

Spradley, James P., and David W. McCurdy. 1984. In "Culture and the Contemporary World." *Conformity and Conflict: Readings in Cultural Anthropology*, 1st ed., edited by edited by James P. Spradley and David W. McCurdy, 1–13. Boston, MA: Pearson.

Spradley, Robert T. 2012. "The Constitution of Highly Reliable Practices: Materializing Communication as Constitutive of Organizing." PhD diss., Texas A&M University.

Stadler, Christian, Tazeeb Rajwani, and Florence Karaba. 2014. "Solutions to the Exploration/Exploitation Dilemma: Networks as a New Level of Analysis." *International Journal of Management Reviews* 16 (2): 172–93.

Stanovich, Keith E. 1999. *Who Is Rational? Studies of Individual Differences in Reasoning.* Mahwah, NJ: Psychology Press.

Stanovich, Keith E., and Richard F. West. 2000. "Advancing the Rationality Debate." *Behavioral and Brain Sciences* 23 (05): 701–17.

———. 2002. "Individual Differences in Reasoning: Implications for the Rationality Debate?" In *Heuristics and Biases: The Psychology of Intuitive Judgment*, edited by Thomas Gilovich, Dale Griffin, and Daniel Kahneman, pp. xvi and 421–40. New York: Cambridge University Press.

Stevens, Francis L., Robin A. Hurley, and Katherine H. Taber. 2011. "Anterior Cingulate Cortex: Unique Role in Cognition and Emotion." *Journal of Neuropsychiatry and Clinical Neurosciences* 23 (2): 121–5.

Steward, Julian H. 1955. *Theory of Culture Change: The Methodology of Multilinear Evolution*. Urbana: University of Illinois Press.

Steward, Julian H., and Frank M. Setzler. 1938. "Function and Configuration in Archaeology." *American Antiquity* 4 (1): 4–10.

Swap, Walter, Dorothy Leonard, Mimi Shields, and Lisa Abrams. 2001. "Using Mentoring and Storytelling to Transfer Knowledge in the Workplace." *Journal of Management Information Systems* 18 (1): 95–114.

Taleb, Nassim N. 2005. *Fooled by Randomness: The Hidden Role of Chance in Life and in the Markets* (vol. 1). New York, NY: Random House.

Tedeschi, Richard G., and Lawrence G. Calhoun. 2004. "Posttraumatic Growth: Conceptual Foundations and Empirical Evidence." *Psychological Inquiry* 15 (1): 1–18.

Tempest, Sue, Ken Starkey, and Christine Ennew. "In the Death Zone: A Study of Limits in the 1996 Mount Everest Disaster." *Human Relations* 60 (7): 1039–64.

Tetlock, Philip. 2005. *Expert Political Judgment: How Good Is It? How Can We Know?* Princeton, NJ: Princeton University Press.

Thomas, David H. 1973. "An Empirical Test for Steward's Model of Great Basin Settlement Patterns." *American Antiquity* 38 (2): 155–76.

Thompson, Fred. 1995. "Business Strategy and the Boyd Cycle." *Journal of Contingencies and Crisis Management* 3 (2): 81–90.

Tinbergen, Niko. 1963. "On Aims and Methods of Ethology." *Zeitschrift fur Tierpsychologie* [*Journal of comparative ethology*] 20 (4): 410–33.

Trout, John D. 2002. "Scientific Explanation and the Sense of Understanding." *Philosophy of Science* 69 (June): 212–33.

Tugade, Michele M., and Barbara L. Fredrickson. 2004. "Resilient Individuals Use Positive Emotions to Bounce Back from Negative Emotional Experiences." *Journal of Personality and Social Psychology* 86 (2): 320-33.

Tversky, Amos, and Daniel Kahneman. 1973. "Availability: A Heuristic for Judging Frequency and Probability." *Cognitive Psychology* 5 (2): 207–32.

———. 1981. "The Framing of Decisions and the Psychology of Choice." *Science* 211: 453–8.

Uhl-Bien, Mary, Ronald E. Riggio, Kevin B. Lowe, and Melissa K. Carsten. 2014. "Followership theory: A review and research agenda." *The Leadership Quarterly.* 25 (1): 83-104.

Uhlmann, Erich. 1942. "Significance and Management of Radiation Injuries." *Radiology,* 38 (4): 445–52.

US Department of Defense. 2010. *Department of Defense Dictionary of Military and Associated Terms.* http://www.dtic.mil/doctrine/new_pubs/jp1_02.pdf.

Vallortigara, Giorgio, and Lesley J. Rogers. 2005. "Survival with an Asymmetrical Brain: Advantages and Disadvantages of Cerebral Lateralization." *Behavioral and Brain Sciences* 28 (4): 575–88.

van Bilsen, Henck. 1991. "Motivational Interviewing: Perspectives from the Netherlands with Particular Emphasis on Heroin Dependent Clients." In *Motivational Interviewing: Preparing People to Change Addictive Behaviour,* edited by William Miller and Stephen Rollnick. New York: Guilford Press.

van Stralen, Daved. 2015. "Ambiguity." *Journal of Contingencies and Crisis Management* 23 (2): 47–53.

van Stralen, Daved, Shanna Kissel. 2016. Physiological Pediatrics: An all-encompassing refresher on pediatrics. *JEMS The journal of emergency medical services*, 41(7):46-57.

van Stralen, Daved, and T. A. Mercer. 2015. "Ambiguity in the Operator's Sense." *Journal of Contingencies and Crisis Management* 23 (2): 54–8.

van Wingen, Guido A., Elbert Geuze, Eric Vermetten, and Guillén Fernández. 2011. "Perceived Threat Predicts the Neural Sequelae of Combat Stress." *Molecular Psychiatry* 16 (6): 664–71.

Vicente, Kim J., and Jens Rasmussen. 1988. "On Applying the Skills, Rules, Knowledge Framework to Interface Design." *Proceedings of the Human Factors and Ergonomics Society Annual Meeting* 32 (5).

———. 1992. "Ecological Interface Design: Theoretical Foundations." *IEEE Transactions on Systems, Man, and Cybernetics* 22 (4): 589-606.

Vidal, Renaud. 2015. "Managing Uncertainty: The Engineer, the Craftsman and the Gardener." *Journal of Contingencies and Crisis Management* 23 (2): 106–16.

Warren, Shields, John Z Bowers. 1950. "The Acute Radiation Syndrome in Man." *Annals of Internal Medicine* 32 (2): 207–16.

Wason, Peter C., and Jonathan St. B. T. Evans. 1974. "Dual Processes in Reasoning?" *Cognition* 3 (2): 141–54.

Weick, Karl E. 1964. "Reduction of Cognitive Dissonance through Task Enhancement and Effort Expenditure." *Journal of Abnormal and Social Psychology* 68 (5): 533–9.

———. 1979. *The Social Psychology of Organizing (2nd ed.)*. New York: McGraw-Hill.

———. 1988. Enacted sensemaking in crisis situations. *Journal of Management Studies*, 25 (4): 305–317.

———. 1993. "The Collapse of Sensemaking in Organizations: The Mann Gulch Disaster." *Administrative Science Quarterly* 38: 628–52.

———. 1995. *Sensemaking in Organizations* (vol. 3). Thousand Oaks, California: Sage.

———. 1998. Introductory essay: "Improvisation as a Mindset for Organizational Analysis." *Organization Science* 9 (5): 543–55.

———. 2002. "Puzzles in Organizational Learning: An Exercise in Disciplined Imagination." *British Journal of Management* 13 (S2): S7–S15.

———. 2011. "Organizing for Transient Reliability: The Production of Dynamic Non-Events." *Journal of Contingencies and Crisis Management* 19 (1): 21–7.

Weick, Karl E., and Karlene H. Roberts. 1993. "Collective Mind in Organizations: Heedful Interrelating on Flight Decks." *Administrative Science Quarterly* 38: 357–81.

Weick, Karl E., and Kathleen M. Sutcliffe. 2008. "Information Overload Revisited." In *The Oxford Handbook of Organizational Decision Making*, edited by Gerard P. Hodgkinson and William H. Starbuck, 56–75. Oxford, UK: Oxford University Press.

———. 2011. *Managing the Unexpected: Resilient Performance in an Age of Uncertainty* (Vol. 8). John Wiley and Sons.

———. 2015. *Managing the Unexpected: Resilient Performance in a Complex World*, Jossey-Bass; 3rd edition

Weick, Karl E., Kathleen M. Sutcliffe, and David Obstfeld. 2005. "Organizing and the Process of Sensemaking." *Organization Science* 16 (4): 409–21.

Westphal, Maren, and George A. Bonanno. 2007. "Posttraumatic Growth and Resilience to Trauma: Different Sides of the Same Coin or Different Coins?" *Applied Psychology* 56 (3): 417–27.

Wickens, Christopher D. 2008. "Situation Awareness: Review of Mica Endsley's 1995 Articles on Situation Awareness Theory and Measurement." *Human Factors* 50: 397–403.

Wolfberg, Adrian. 2006. "Full-Spectrum Analysis: A New Way of Thinking for a New World." *Military Review* 86 (4): 35-42.

Yates, Frank J. 2001. "Outsider: Impressions of Naturalistic Decision Making." In *Linking Expertise and Naturalistic Decision Making*, edited by E. Salas and G. A. Klein, 9–34. New York, New York: Psychology Press.

Zald, David H., and Jose V. Pardo. 1997. "Emotion, Olfaction, and the Human Amygdala: Amygdala Activation During Aversive Olfactory Stimulation." *Proceedings of the National Academy of Sciences* 94 (8): 4119–24.

Zotev, Vadim, Frank Krueger, Raquel Phillips, Ruben P. Alvarez, W. Kyle Simmons, Patrick Bellgowan, Wayne Drevets, and Jerzy Bodurka. 2011. "Self-Regulation of Amygdala Activation Using Real-Time fMRI Neurofeedback." *PLOS One* 6 (9): e24522.

Zsambok, Caroline E. 2014. "Naturalistic Decision-Making: Where Are We Now?" In *Naturalistic Decision Making*, edited by Caroline E. Zsambok and Gary Klein, 3–16. New York, New York: Routledge Press.

ABOUT THE AUTHORS

Daved van STRALEN, MD, FAAP

Dr. Daved van Stralen, an assistant professor of pediatrics, has created multiple healthcare programs using an approach Karlene Roberts of the University of California has described as "High Reliability Organizing." He assisted in creating a pediatric intensive care unit (PICU) at Loma Linda University Children's Hospital using principles from his pre-EMS fire rescue ambulance experience; he then used this same approach to expand and improve the pediatric critical care transport service, which had various quality, safety, morale, and service problems. Both the PICU and the pediatric critical care transport team served a geographic area four times the size of Vermont; within three years, both became the second largest in California. Other programs he developed include the creation of the first *clinical, academic* emergency medical care bachelor's degree program in the United States; the implementation of changes in a regional EMS system to that of an academic medical model; the creation of a chronic intensive care program for ventilator management to assist a struggling pediatric nursing home, which was later reproduced in another pediatric subacute care facility; and the development of a home mechanical ventilator program using the HRO methods described in this book. He regularly collaborates with safety, risk, and reliability experts from the fields of wildland firefighting, business, and healthcare in the United States and Europe to identify the common approaches people use to ensure safety and reliability. Through his extensive travels in Europe studying HRO in multiple industries, he developed a relationship with France's Bouches-du-Rhône Fire Service (known as SDIS 13), which became the source for the US Forest Service–SDIS 13 HRO collaboration.

Dr. van Stralen is an assistant professor of pediatrics on staff at Loma Linda University Children's Hospital and the Children's Subacute Center at Community Hospital of San Bernardino (both in California) and is president of Strategic Reliability, LLC. He has served as medical director for the Riverside County (California) Emergency Medical Services Agency (where he introduced HRO to a government regulatory agency and regional EMS) and medical director for the San Bernardino County Fire Department, which covers a twenty-thousand-square-mile area. He worked in South Los Angeles as an ambulance man and fire department rescue ambulance driver for the Los Angeles City Fire Department in the 1970s. By one estimation, he is the first career paramedic to attend medical school. He has a bachelor of arts degree in social ecology and a bachelor of science in biological science from the University of California, Irvine, and an MD from the UC Irvine College of Medicine, where he completed his pediatric residency. He completed a pediatric critical care fellowship at Children's Medical Center and Parkland Memorial Hospital in Dallas, Texas.

His publications include primary research, research abstracts, invited book chapters, and invited educational articles on the topics of business, medicine, emergency medical care, and public safety. A list of his publications is available on request.

This book has applicability to numerous fields (including healthcare) as well as various professional associations. Some of the associations Dr. van Stralen has given lectures for include the Society of Critical Care Medicine, the National Association of EMS Physicians, EMS Today, the American Medical Director's Association, and the American Society of Healthcare Risk Management. He is available for presentations to medical conferences and meetings for quality of care, risk management, patient safety, and quality improvement.

Spencer L. BYRUM

Spencer L. Byrum is the chief executive officer of HRS Consulting, Inc., a premier human performance improvement company that was specifically created and designed to enhance individual and team decision-making in high-risk industries. Mr. Byrum's specialty is taking lessons learned in aviation and other high-risk fields and developing innovative process improvements and training for professions in which people need to make critical decisions in stressful, demanding environments.

Mr. Byrum is a former US Coast Guard rescue pilot, head of standardization and training, and an internationally known expert on the subject of human performance in demanding, time-critical environments. He has developed and delivered training to all US combat air forces, the Air National Guard, and the Air Force Reserve; multiple NATO forces; various domestic and international commercial airlines; several commercial heavy-construction crews; a number of undergraduate and graduate university programs; the Federal Aviation Administration (FAA); and NASA Dryden test pilots, project engineers, and project managers.

Since becoming integrally involved in healthcare almost twenty years ago, Mr. Byrum has worked with over six hundred healthcare facilities, ranging from major tertiary care centers to ambulatory surgery centers to critical access hospitals. He has developed tools for the quantitative and qualitative assessment of the processes associated with healthcare-associated infections (HAIs), surgical site infections (SSIs), histories and physicals (H&Ps), informed consent, surgical time out, surgical site marking, surgical counts, medication errors, and other processes that some of the largest healthcare institutions and companies in the United States have implemented. Mr. Byrum has developed and delivered medical training for over a hundred thousand participants on the introduction of High Reliability Organization (HRO) processes for staff and physicians; the introduction of "time out"; the elimination of retained surgical items, OR burns, and "look-alike, sound-alike" medications; the use of patient scheduling optimization; and the role of the surgeon in surgical counts. Hundreds of facilities across the United States, Canada, and Europe have utilized these processes. He has developed a web-based "safety culture" survey tool that has assessed over three-quarters of a million responses to questions about organizational safety and culture. HRS Consulting's "intro to HROs" and the "role of the surgeon in the surgical count" processes are currently being used as requirements for credentialing surgeons in Texas. The HRS Consulting team has experience in assessing over one million near-miss and "sentinel" events. Byrum is an expert in the evaluation of causal factors and the remediation of their impact.

Finally, several major insurers have recognized HRS Consulting tools for their ability to reduce losses; the use of these tools has led to medical malpractice premium reductions for physicians and facility premium reductions for individual hospitals and related healthcare entities.

Bahadir INOZU, PhD

Dr. Bahadir Inozu has worked with more than forty organizations to improve performance and reliability in the healthcare, aviation, defense, and maritime industries as well as in government. He is an internationally renowned expert in system reliability analysis and improvement as well as in the integration of best-of-breed methodologies for superior performance. He has conducted extensive research on best practices in several high-risk industries for safety and reliability improvements, including the shipping, nuclear power, and offshore industries in addition to the US Navy. He developed a reliability, availability, and maintainability data collection and analysis system and led its implementation at liquefied natural gas carriers. He also developed a failure reporting and corrective action system (FRACAS) for San Antonio–class amphibious transport dock (LPD) warships. He has provided process-improvement support for numerous hospitals both in the United States and abroad. He is the leading author of *Performance Improvement in Healthcare: Leading Change with Lean, Six Sigma, and Constraints Management* (McGraw-Hill, 2011).

Dr. Inozu has worked closely with the US Navy throughout his career. His hospital experience includes working with leaders of healthcare providers to customize and facilitate sustainable process improvements with system-level impact. He is the founder and CEO of SharpFocus, LLC, and cofounder and CEO of Sharp Focus, Inc. He is also the chief adviser and cofounder of NOVACES, LLC, and professor emeritus at the University of New Orleans.

He received a PhD in naval architecture and marine engineering from the University of Michigan (1990), an MSE in naval architecture and marine engineering (University of Michigan, 1986), and a BS in mechanical engineering (Technical University of Istanbul, 1982). His doctoral dissertation was a reliability and replacement analysis of Great Lakes marine diesels. His certifications include Lean Six Sigma Master Black Belt, Theory of Constraints (TOC) Jonah, and Enterprise AIRSpeed TOC supply chain technical expert (SCTE) and supply chain deployment expert (SCDE) from the Avraham Y. Goldratt Institute, LLP.

INDEX

Because of the variety of disciplines, words in the index may refer to discussions of the concept yet not use the indexed word.

Definitions or significant discussions are marked in bold.

Tables or figures are marked "t."

Made in the USA
Middletown, DE
04 June 2023

32023017R00318